WJ 151

Urinary Tract Infection in the Female

Publication has been supported by an educational grant from
Ocean Spray Cranberries, Inc.

Cover picture   Pseudopolyps on the bladder neck in a 23-year-old woman with recurrent
urinary tract infection

Urinary Tract Infection
in the Female

Edited by
Stuart L Stanton, FRCS, FRCOG
Professor of Pelvic Surgery and Urogynaecology
Urogynaecology Unit
St George's Hospital Medical School
London, UK
AND
Peter L Dwyer, FRCOG, FRACOG, CU
Director, Urogynaecology Department
Royal Women's Hospital and Mercy Hospital
for Women
Melbourne, Victoria, Australia

MARTIN DUNITZ

© Martin Dunitz Ltd 2000

First published in the United Kingdom in 2000
by Martin Dunitz Ltd, The Livery House, 7–9 Pratt Street, London NW1 0AE

Tel.:   +44-(0)20-74822202
Fax.:   +44-(0)20-72670159
E-mail: info@dunitz.co.uk
Website: http://www.dunitz.co.uk

Although every effort has been made to ensure that drug doses and other information are presented accurately in this publication, the ultimate responsibility rests with the prescribing physician. Neither the publishers nor the authors can be held responsible for errors or for any consequences arising from the use of information contained herein. For detailed prescribing information or instructions on the use of any product or procedure discussed herein, please consult the prescribing information or instructional material issued by the manufacturer.

A CIP record for this book is available from the British Library.

Distributed in the USA, Canada and Brazil by Blackwell Science Inc., Commerce Place, 350 Main Street, Malden, MA 02148–5018, USA.
Tel: 1-800-215-1000

ISBN 1 85317 689 3
Composition by Wearset, Boldon, Tyne and Wear
Printed and bound in Italy by Printer Trento

Contents

List of contributors

Edwin P Arnold
Department of Urology
Christchurch Hospital
Private Bag 4710
Christchurch 1, New Zealand

Jerry Avorn
Division of Pharmacoepidemiology and Pharmacoeconomics
The Brigham & Women's Hospital
221 Longwood Avenue, Room 341
Boston, MA 02115, USA

Kate Bourdeaux
Department of Nursing Studies
University of Wales College of Medicine
Heath Park
Cardiff CF4 4XN, UK

Charlotte Chaliha
Department of Obstetrics and Gynaecology
Kingston Hospital
Galsworthy Road
Kingston-upon-Thames, Surrey KT2 7QB, UK

Peter L Dwyer
Urogynaecology Department
Royal Women's Hospital and Mercy Hospital
for Women
132 Grattan Street
Carlton, Victoria 3052, Australia

Adrian GK Edwards
Department of General Practice
University of Wales College of Medicine
Health Centre
Maelfa, Llanedeyrn
Cardiff CF3 7PN

Suzanne M Garland
Departments of Microbiology and
Infectious Diseases
Royal Women's Hospital and Royal
Children's Hospital
132 Grattan Street
Carlton, Victoria 3052, Australia

Donna Gilmour
Department of Obstetrics and Gynaecology
1WK Grace Health Centre
5850/5980 University Avenue
Halifax, Nova Scotia B3J 3G9, Canada

Reuben Grüneberg
Department of Microbiology
University College Hospital
Grafton Way
London WC1E 8BD, UK

Phillip Hay
Department of Genito-Urinary Medicine
Courtyard Clinic
St George's Hospital
Blackshaw Road
London SW17 0QT, UK

Thomas M Hooton
Department of Medicine
University of Washington School of Medicine
Harborview Medical Center
Box 359930
325, 9th Avenue
Seattle, WA 98104, USA

Eric Knight
Internal Medicine
Dartmouth Medical School
Hanover, NH 03755, USA

Kelvin Lynn
Department of Nephrology
Christchurch Hospital
Private Bag 4710
Christchurch 1, New Zealand

Allan B MacLean
Department of Obstetrics and Gynaecology
Royal Free Hospital
Pond Street
London NW3 2QG, UK

Christopher Maher
Wesley Urogynaecological Unit
Wesley Hospital
Auchenflower, Queensland 4066
Australia

Kurt G Naber
Urology Clinic
St Elisabeth Hospital
St-Elisabeth-Str. 23
D-94315 Straubing, Germany

Lindsay E Nicolle
Department of Internal Medicine
University of Manitoba
GC430 Health Sciences Centre
820 Sherbrook Street
Winnepeg, Manitoba R3A 1R9, Canada

Mary O'Reilly
Department of Infectious Diseases
Box Hill Hospital
Melbourne, Victoria 3052, Australia

Allan Ronald
St Boniface General Hospital
Research, University of Manitoba Health
Sciences Centre
A-108 Chown Building
753 McDermot Avenue
Winnepeg, Manitoba R3E 0W3, Canada

Anna Rosamilia
Department of Urogynaecology
Royal Women's Hospital
132 Grattan Street
Carlton, Victoria 3052, Australia

Stuart L Stanton
Urogynaecology Unit
St George's Hospital Medical School
Cranmer Terrace
London SW17 0RE, UK

Kate Verrier Jones
KRUF Children's Kidney Centre for Wales
University of Wales College of Medicine
Heath Park
Cardiff CF4 4XN, UK

To my wife, Julia, a constant source of encouragement, and my children, Claire, Talia, Jo, Tamara and Noah

To my wife Pam, and children, Angela, Jeremy, Alastair, Holly, Patrick and Chloë, for their continuing support, love and tolerance

Preface

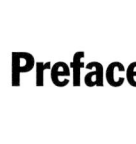

Urinary tract infection (UTI) is the most common infection
in women and is encountered on a daily basis by medical and
paramedical practitioners involved in their care. It is
estimated that 50 per cent of women will develop a UTI
during their lives, and up to 6 per cent of family practitioner
consultations concern UTIs. Non-infective sensory disorders
of the lower urinary tract also cause bladder pain and urinary
frequency; sometimes the cause is obvious, but in other
conditions (such as interstitial cystitis or the urethral
syndrome) the aetiology is poorly understood and the
treatment is often unsatisfactory.

Our aim in producing this book was to stimulate interest
in UTI and provide an extensive and up-to-date review
covering the spectrum of age from the neonate to the elderly
for all who see and treat this condition. Recent advances in
the epidemiology, prevention, diagnosis and treatment of
UTI in all ages have been reviewed by expert
multidisciplinary clinicians. The morbidity of UTI is
considered in the chapters on neonatal and childhood
infections (Chapter 6), recurrent infections (Chapter 13) and
kidney infections (Chapter 14) and underlines the seriousness
of this common condition. The risks and remedies of the

equally common procedure of catheterization are emphasized in Chapter 15. Alternative medicines, hardly written about in most textbooks of medicine, abound with simple and alternative remedies for UTI and are fully discussed in Chapter 16.

The decline in research activity into UTIs is outlined in Chapter 17 and may be a reflection of the medical community's apathy in the face of this common condition, although it may also reflect the fact that UTI is not the domain of any one group of medical practitioners and thus receives a low research priority from all. More research is needed into the pathogenesis of UTI, on better preventative strategies for recurrent UTI (other than antibiotics), and in the treatment of uncomplicated and complicated urinary infections by bacteria which are increasingly antibiotic-resistant. Allan Roland (Chapter 17) has challenged all involved in the care of women to look to multi-disciplinary cooperation for their research endeavours.

We wish to thank all our contributors for their patience and excellent work and for accepting the challenge we have set them. We would like to thank Martin Dunitz Publishers and their Commissioning Editor, Robert Peden, for help and advice. Finally, we thank our secretaries, Wendy Nash and Geraldine Rhoderick, who have been more than patient and good-humoured with their editors, and to whom we are most grateful.

Stuart L Stanton   *Peter L Dwyer*
London   *Melbourne*

Epidemiology

Thomas M Hooton

Contents

I Overview

Urinary tract infection (UTI) is one of the most common infections in girls and women and is associated with considerable morbidity. For example, Foxman and Frerichs (1985) found that on average each acute uncomplicated cystitis episode was associated with 6.1 days of symptoms, 2.4 days of restricted activity, 1.2 days in which they were not able to attend classes or work, and 0.4 bed days. The incidence of UTI increases in girls and women with age, especially with onset of sexual activity. UTIs in boys and young men, on the other hand, are very uncommon, although the rate approximates that of women among the elderly. Incidence data for healthy postmenopausal women are lacking, but the incidence of asymptomatic bacteriuria is high among the elderly, particularly those who are institutionalized. The epidemiology of UTI in women is reviewed in this chapter.

In any discussion of UTI, it is useful to distinguish between uncomplicated and complicated UTI since the approach to management is different with regard to pretreatment evaluation, choice of antibiotics, duration of therapy, and threshold for urologic evaluation. Basically, an uncomplicated UTI is one that occurs in a young, healthy non-pregnant woman who has no known functional or anatomic abnormality of the genitourinary tract. Such infections are usually successfully treated with a short-course regimen of an oral urinary tract antimicrobial without the need for pre- or post-treatment urine cultures. A complicated UTI, on the other hand, is associated with a condition that increases the risk of serious complications or treatment failure, and warrants pre- and post-treatment urine cultures, treatment with a broader spectrum antibiotic and for a longer duration, and a lower threshold for urologic evaluation. Patients with certain conditions such as those shown in *Table 1.1* are at greatly increased risk for serious complications of UTI and warrant special concern. On the other hand, many patients with 'complicated UTI' can be expected to respond to relatively short courses of oral antibiotics, especially a fluoroquinolone. Thus, while these definitions for uncomplicated and complicated infections are clearly oversimplified, they serve a useful purpose in the management of UTI.

II Pathogenesis

Most UTIs in healthy ambulatory women cannot be explained by underlying functional or anatomic abnormalities of the urinary tract. Vaginal colonization is a prerequisite to bladder infection, and factors which increase the risk of UTI generally do so at least in part by facilitating vaginal colonization. Vaginal colonization with uropathogens, however, does not inevitably lead to UTI. It is likely that other events, such as sexual intercourse,

Table 1.1
Conditions predisposing to complicated UTI*

Obstruction or other structural	*Urolithiasis*
	Malignancies
	Ureteric and urethral strictures
	Bladder diverticuli
	Renal cysts
	Fistulae
	Ileal conduits and other urinary diversions
Functional abnormality	*Neurogenic bladder*
	Vesicoureteric reflux
Foreign bodies	*Indwelling catheter*
	Ureteric stent
	Nephrostomy tube
Other conditions	*Diabetes mellitus*
	Pregnancy
	Renal failure
	Renal transplantation
	Immunosuppression
	Multidrug-resistant uropathogens
	Hospital-acquired infection

*Adapted from Ronald and Harding (1997) and Nicolle (1997b). Some factors complicate UTI through several mechanisms.

generally must occur to allow infection to occur. It remains to be determined, however, why vaginal colonization progresses to UTI in some women and not in others and why many women who have known risk factors for UTI never develop UTIs. The initial steps leading to uncomplicated UTI probably also occur in many persons who develop a complicated UTI, although the complicating conditions described below facilitate entry and persistence of uropathogens in the urinary tract.

III Diagnosis

The definitive diagnosis of UTI is made in the presence of typical UTI symptoms and significant bacteriuria, the definition of which remains somewhat controversial. The traditional standard for significant bacteriuria is $\geqslant 10^5$ uropathogens per ml of voided midstream urine, based on previous studies of women with acute pyelonephritis and asymptomatic bacteriuria (Norden and Kass, 1968). Several more recent studies have shown, however, that this is an insensitive standard when applied to acutely symptomatic women and that approximately one-third to one-half of cases of acute cystitis have $<10^5$ cfu per ml (Johnson and Stamm, 1987). Recent studies have shown that using a definition of $\geqslant 10^2$ uropathogens per ml for significant bacteriuria has the best combination of sensitivity (95%) and specificity (85%) for diagnosing acute cystitis in women (Stamm et al., 1982). In contrast to cystitis, 80–95% of episodes of pyelonephritis are associated with $>10^5$ cfu per ml of uropathogens (Kass, 1956). The Infectious Disease Society of America consensus definition of cystitis for use in antimicrobial treatment studies is $\geqslant 10^3$ cfu per ml and for pyelonephritis is $\geqslant 10^4$ cfu per ml (Rubin et al., 1992). Likewise, a colony count threshold of $\geqslant 10^3$ cfu per ml should be used to diagnose symptomatic complicated infection except when urine cultures are obtained through a catheter in which a level of $\geqslant 10^2$ cfu per ml is evidence of infection (Rubin et al., 1992). Asymptomatic bacteriuria is defined as the presence of two separate clean-voided urine specimens both with $\geqslant 10^5$ cfu per ml of the same

uropathogen in the absence of symptoms (Zhanel et al., 1990).

IV   Epidemiology

1.   Children

The overall incidence of neonatal bacteriuria has been reported to be 1.0 to 1.4% with the male-to-female ratio from 3:1 to 5:1 (Rushton, 1997). Population-based studies in Sweden in which suprapubic aspiration of urine was performed in children up to one year of age found screening bacteriuria in 2.5% of boys and 0.9% of girls. In addition, these studies have shown that approximately 1.1% of girls and 1.2% of boys up to age one have symptomatic UTI. During preschool and school age, the sex ratio for screening bacteriuria is reversed from that seen in infancy, ranging from 0.7% to 1.9% of girls and 0.02% to 0.04% of boys. These rates of asymptomatic bacteriuria are probably low estimates since the population-based Swedish studies have demonstrated that by the age of seven, almost 8% of girls and 2% of boys have had a culture-documented symptomatic UTI (Hansson et al., 1997), and asymptomatic bacteriuria occurs more often than symptomatic UTI. Of concern, approximately half of the children in the Swedish study experienced high fever with these infections suggesting that many of these episodes were pyelonephritis. Acute pyelonephritis in children, especially neonates and young infants, can cause irreversible renal scarring as documented by radionuclide scanning, even after a single severe episode. Furthermore, there is an association between the number of pyelonephritis attacks and the incidence of renal scarring. Vesicoureteric reflux, found in 25–50% of children with culture-documented UTI, 9% of children with asymptomatic bacteriuria, and < 2% of children without bacteriuria, is the most significant host risk factor in the aetiology of childhood pyelonephritis, and the risk for acute pyelonephritis and subsequent renal scarring is related to the severity of vesicoureteric reflux (Rushton, 1997). It appears that most of the renal damage from bacteriuria occurs during the first five years of life and that later progression is rare (Zhanel et al., 1990).

2. Uncomplicated UTI in adults

Urinary tract infection in adult women includes women with acute sporadic or recurrent uncomplicated cystitis, acute uncomplicated pyelonephritis, complicated urinary tract infection, and asymptomatic bacteriuria (Stamm and Hooton, 1993). Acute uncomplicated urinary tract infections are among the most common conditions causing individuals to seek outpatient medical care. In the United States, it is estimated from surveys of office practices, hospital-based clinics and emergency departments that there are over eight million episodes of urinary tract infection annually (personal communication, S.M. Schappert, National Ambulatory Medical Care Survey, 1996 Summary). Kunin has stated that about 40–50% of adult women report that they have had a UTI at some time in their life (Kunin, 1994). In a recent large prospective study of young sexually active women in a university student cohort and a large population-based health maintenance organization, the incidence of cystitis was approximately 0.5 per person-year (Hooton et al., 1996b). Given that in 1990, 53 million adolescent girls and women in the United States reported being sexually experienced, these incidence data suggest that many more millions of episodes of cystitis may occur annually among women in the United States than are reported on the basis of data obtained from office visits.

A recurrent UTI refers to a symptomatic UTI that follows clinical resolution of a previous UTI (generally after treatment, but not necessarily). Recurrent acute uncomplicated cystitis occurs in 12–27% of women after their first UTI and in 48% of women who have had a previous UTI (Foxman, 1990; Ikaheimo et al., 1996). A second recurrence occurred within six months in 2.7% of women following their first UTI (Foxman, 1990). In the Finnish study, the recurrence rate was 0.73 recurrences per patient-year (0.18 among those with first episode UTI and 0.89 among those with previous UTIs) (Ikaheimo et al., 1996). Among women at least 55 years of age, 53% had at least one recurrence whereas among those younger than 55, only 36% had a recurrence. The ratio of cystitis-to-pyelonephritis in studies of recurrent UTI has ranged from 18:1 (Stamm et al., 1991) to 28:1 (Ikaheimo et al., 1996). Overall, approximately 20–40% of women who experience an initial UTI develop recurrent UTIs (Mabeck, 1972), but it is not clear what proportion develop a pattern of high-frequency recurrences. Although epidemiologic data for older women are sparse, it is estimated that 10–15% of women over age 60 have frequent recurrences (Romano and Kaye, 1981).

Recurrent UTI may be due to relapse of the originally infecting uropathogen or to reinfection with the same or different strain as the originally infecting strain. It is generally not possible to distinguish between relapse and reinfection with the originally infecting strain (a negative urine culture between two UTIs suggests the recurrence is a reinfection) and, thus, relapse is often defined clinically as a recurrent UTI caused by the same species as that causing the original UTI within two weeks after treatment. A reinfection is a recurrent UTI caused by a different strain at any time or the originally infecting strain two or more weeks after therapy of the original UTI. Approximately 80–90% of recurrent UTIs are said to be reinfections, and in some studies one-third of recurrences have been found to be reinfections with the original strain (Brauner et al., 1992: Ikaheimo et al., 1996). Urovirulent strains may persist in the fecal flora and cause recurrent infection if they are not eradicated by antimicrobial therapy.

Although there are few data on the incidence of pyelonephritis, a recent population-based study in Canada showed that the overall rate of hospitalization for pyelonephritis in women was about 1 case per 1000 population (Nicolle et al., 1996). Pregnancy and diabetes contributed substantially to hospitalization rates, and Native American women were also overrepresented. This rate is almost certainly an underestimate since the study evaluated only patients with more severe disease who required hospitalization – in the United States, up to 75% of patients presenting to emergency departments with acute pyelonephritis do not require hospitalization (Safrin et al., 1988; Pinson et al., 1994). Data from the office practice survey of hospital-based clinics and emergency departments suggest that over 350 000 episodes of acute pyelonephritis occur annually in the United States (personal communication, S.M. Schappert, National Ambulatory Medical Care Survey, 1996 Summary).

3. Complicated UTI in adults

Complicated UTIs encompass an

extraordinarily broad range of infectious entities for which no population-based studies have been done and overall incidence data do not exist. A comprehensive discussion of complicated UTIs which are associated with conditions shown in *Table 1.1* is beyond the scope of this chapter. One of the most common types of complicated UTI, nosocomial UTI, occurs in approximately 5 per 100 admissions in a university tertiary-care hospital, with catheter-associated infections accounting for 88–95% of the infections (Bronsema et al., 1993; Richards et al., 1999). The incidence of bacteriuria associated with indwelling catheterization is 3–10% per day, and the duration of catheterization is the most important risk factor for the development of catheter-associated bacteriuria. Approximately 15–25% of patients in general hospitals have a catheter inserted at some time during their stay, and most are catheterized for only 2–4 days (Warren, 1997). Over 100 000 patients in nursing homes, on the other hand, are catheterized for months to years (Warren, 1997). Although fewer than 5% of catheter-associated bacteriuria episodes are complicated by bacteremia, catheter-associated bacteriuria is the most common source of Gram-negative bacteremia in hospitalized patients (Stamm and Hooton, 1993). Moreover, asymptomatic catheter-associated bacteriuria constitutes a huge reservoir of resistant bacteria in hospitals and nursing homes.

Persons with neurogenic bladder, such as those with spinal cord injury (SCI) and multiple sclerosis, are at very high risk for recurrent UTI. Eighty percent of persons with SCI have a UTI within 16 years of their injury (DeVivo et al., 1993). Spinal cord injury alters the dynamics of voiding, and the resulting use of catheters, elevated intravesical pressures, and increased postvoid residuals contribute to an increased risk and severity of urinary tract infections.

Urinary tract infection in pregnant women presents a special problem because of an increased risk of pregnancy and perinatal complications. Pregnant women appear to be at no greater risk of having asymptomatic bacteriuria than non-pregnant women (prevalence approximately 4–7%) (Patterson and Andriole, 1997a). Whether asymptomatic bacteriuria itself is associated with perinatal complications, such as premature delivery, remains controversial. However, pregnant women with asymptomatic bacteriuria, compared to those without bacteriuria, are at much greater risk of developing symptomatic UTI later in pregnancy (20–40% vs. 2%, respectively). Symptomatic UTI during pregnancy, especially pyelonephritis, is associated with an increased risk of premature delivery and possibly other maternal and fetal complications of pregnancy, and should be treated aggressively with regimens considered to be safe in pregnancy. Treatment of asymptomatic bacteriuria decreases the risk of subsequent UTI by up to 90% and, thus, the morbidity associated with symptomatic UTI.

4. Asymptomatic bacteriuria in adults

Asymptomatic bacteriuria is found in approximately 5% of young adult women but rarely in men less than age 50. In a recent study of young healthy women cultured monthly for six months, we found the incidence of episodes of $\geq 10^5$ uropathogens per ml to be 0.37 and 0.49 per person-year in a university student cohort and a population-based HMO cohort, respectively (Hooton et al., 1997). At least two consecutive episodes of asymptomatic bacteriuria with the same species (classic definition of asymptomatic bacteriuria) occurred in 5.2% of the university women and 4.5% of the HMO women. Persistent asymptomatic bacteriuria for several months was rare. In another recent population-based study of 1462 randomly selected women aged 38–60 in Sweden, bacteriuria was observed in 3–5% and increased with age (Bengtsson et al., 1998).

The prevalence of asymptomatic bacteriuria in women increases with age (Nicolle, 1997a). Thus, the prevalence in ambulatory non-catheterized women is reported to be approximately 6–10% among women over 60 years of age, 15–20% in women aged 65–90, and 22–43% in those age 90 or greater. The prevalence among institutionalized elderly women is even higher,

25–53%, varying with the underlying degree of disability (Nicolle, 1997a). Many episodes of asymptomatic bacteriuria in the elderly are transient (Abrutyn et al., 1991), although bacteriuria tends to be more persistent than in younger women. Asymptomatic bacteriuria is more likely to be persistent in those with chronic indwelling catheters.

Asymptomatic bacteriuria is generally assumed to be a benign condition in most clinical settings. No differences in mortality or incidence of severe kidney disease were found in the Swedish study during a 24-year follow-up between those with and those without bacteriuria at baseline (Bengtsson et al., 1998). Likewise, asymptomatic bacteriuria in the elderly does not appear to be associated with adverse long-term outcomes such as renal failure or genitourinary malignancy. Although early studies reported that asymptomatic bacteriuria in elderly men and women was associated with a higher mortality rate, this association has not been borne out in more recent studies in which underlying illness has been adjusted for. Asymptomatic bacteriuria, however, may lead to serious complications in some clinical conditions such as pregnancy, genitourinary manipulation and renal transplantation (Zhanel et al., 1990).

V   Aetiological agents

The spectrum of aetiological agents is similar in uncomplicated upper and lower urinary tract infection, with *E. coli* the causative pathogen in approximately 70–95% and *Staphylococcus saprophyticus* in 5% to more than 20% (Stamm and Hooton, 1993). Occasionally other Enterobacteriaceae such as *Proteus mirabilis* and *Klebsiella* sp. or enterococci are isolated from such patients. Group B streptococci also appear to cause occasional episodes and, rarely, *Pseudomonas aeruginosa*, *Citrobacter* sp., or other uropathogens cause uncomplicated UTI.

Unlike the narrow and predictable spectrum of causative agents in uncomplicated infection, a broad range of bacteria can cause complicated infections, and many are resistant to multiple antimicrobial agents. Although *E. coli* is the predominant uropathogen in complicated UTI, uropathogens other than *E. coli*, including *Citrobacter* sp., *Enterobacter* sp., *P. aeruginosa*, enterococci, and *S. aureus* account for a relatively higher proportion of cases compared with uncomplicated urinary tract infections (Nicolle, 1997b). *Candida* species are common in patients with indwelling urinary catheters, especially those who have had previous antibiotic therapy. *S. saprophyticus* is rarely isolated in the elderly. Patients with chronic conditions, such as spinal cord injury and neurogenic bladder, are relatively more likely to have polymicrobic and multidrug-resistant infections. The diversity and antimicrobial resistance of uropathogens reflect the fact that individuals with complicated UTIs tend to acquire their infections in the hospital setting and have frequent recurrences requiring multiple interventions (Nicolle, 1997b).

VI Risk factors for UTI in healthy premenopausal women

Most uncomplicated UTIs in women cannot be explained by underlying functional or anatomic abnormalities of the urinary tract. However, several host and uropathogen characteristics which appear to predispose women to uncomplicated UTI have been identified (Sobel, 1997). Not surprisingly, having a history of previous recurrent UTI is a strong risk factor for having a subsequent UTI (Hooton et al., 1996b). This could reflect a biological, behavioral or genetic predisposition of the host or a predisposition for persistent or recurrent colonization with a uropathogenic strain. Whether vaginal colonization and subsequent UTI occur is the result of a dynamic interaction between the host and uropathogen. The host risk factors discussed below appear to operate by facilitating this interaction.

1. Sexual intercourse and contraception

Sexual intercourse and spermicide use, especially in conjunction with diaphragm use, are factors most clearly demonstrated to predispose women to UTI (Hooton et al.,

1996b). Sexual intercourse, one of the strongest risk factors in almost all studies of UTI, appears to operate through a mechanical effect of introducing uropathogens into the bladder and possibly through a trauma effect (Foxman et al., 1997). Use of spermicides greatly increases the risk of vaginal colonization with uropathogens and UTI, independently of sexual intercourse. Even the relatively small amounts of spermicides coating condoms increase the risk of UTI (Fihn et al., 1996; Fihn et al., 1998). Based on clinical studies and in vitro data, it appears that the mechanism whereby spermicides predispose women who use these products to UTI is through an alteration of the vaginal ecosystem in favor of uropathogens (Hooton and Stamm, 1996a). Uropathogens from the fecal reservoir that come into contact with the vaginal introitus during insertion of a spermicide may be more likely to persist in the introitus because of a spermicide-associated reduction in colonization resistance attributable to a reduction in vaginal lactobacilli (especially H_2O_2-producing strains (Gupta et al., 1998)) and possibly an increased adherence to epithelial cells.

2. Antimicrobial use

Animal and human data suggest that use of certain antimicrobials may predispose women to UTI, apparently through their adverse effects on vaginal ecology (Herthelius et al.,

1988; Hooton and Stamm, 1996a). Data from studies in monkeys suggest that facilitation of vaginal *E. coli* colonization by beta-lactam antimicrobials may be due to alterations in the indigenous anaerobic flora of the vagina and, thus, altered colonization resistance. Trimethoprim and nitrofurantoin, which have much less effect on the periurethral anaerobic flora than does amoxicillin, did not result in enhanced vaginal colonization with *E. coli* in similar monkey experiments. In humans, studies demonstrate that administration of beta-lactam antibiotics induces marked changes in the indigenous genital flora of girls and a concomitant increase in genital uropathogen colonization. Administration of trimethoprim-sulfamethoxazole or fluoroquinolone, on the other hand, result in less vaginal colonization with uropathogens than beta-lactams. In a recent prospective study of premenopausal college women, we found that 326 women in a university cohort and 425 women in a health-maintenance organization cohort were at increased risk for UTI if antimicrobials had been taken during the previous 15–28 days but not during the previous 3, 7, or 14 days (when they may be protective) (Smith et al., 1997). The increased risks were noted both for women whose antimicrobial use was for treatment of previous UTI and for women who received antimicrobials for other illnesses.

3. Oestrogen

The role of oestrogens in predisposing premenopausal women to urinary tract infection is unclear (Hooton and Stamm, 1996a). In vitro studies have demonstrated that adherence of uropathogens to human vaginal or uroepithelial cells is facilitated by oestrogen. Moreover, several studies have shown that oestrogen treatment facilitates experimental urinary tract infection in animals. We have recently demonstrated a strong association between the time at which women present with acute cystitis and the time from the onset of their last menstrual period, but it is not clear whether this association was due to a hormonal mechanism or to changes in sexual behaviour in relation to the menstrual cycle (Hooton et al., 1996c). On the other hand, oestrogen deficiency in postmenopausal women appears to increase the risk of UTI, and the risk can be greatly diminished by topical application of oestrogen, apparently by normalizing vaginal flora (Raz and Stamm, 1993). It would appear therefore, that oestrogen is important in maintaining normal vaginal flora and, thus, reducing the risk of UTI, but that increased amounts may increase the risk of UTI, perhaps by facilitating adherence of uropathogens to uroepithelial cells.

VII Risk factors for recurrent UTI in healthy young women

Risk factors for recurrent UTI have received relatively little study. In a recent large case-control study of women with and without a history of recurrent UTI, the strongest risk factor for recurrent UTI in a multivariate analysis was the frequency of sexual intercourse (Scholes et al., 1997). Other risk factors were spermicide use during the past year, having a new sex partner during the past year, having a first UTI at or before 15 years of age, and having a mother with a history of UTIs. These latter two non-behavioural host factors were associated with two- to fourfold increases in risk and were the most strongly associated variables after sexual intercourse. These findings suggest the possibility that inherited factors may be important in some women with recurrent UTI, especially those with onset prior to sexual debut and spermicide exposure.

With regard to genetic factors, it has been shown that women with a history of recurrent UTIs are several times more likely to be non-secretors of histo-blood group antigens than are women without such a history (Kinane et al., 1982; Sheinfeld et al., 1989). Further, uropathogenic *E. coli* adhere better to uroepithelial cells from women who are non-secretors compared with cells from secretors (Lomberg et al., 1986). Recent data suggest that the biochemical explanation for the increased adherence of *E. coli* to non-secretors' uroepithelial cells and for the propensity of non-secretors to develop recurrent UTI is due to the presence of unique globoseries glycolipid receptors that bind uropathogenic *E. coli* (Stapleton et al., 1992). However, in our case-control study, no association was found between blood group phenotype or non-secretor phenotype and history of recurrent UTI. It is possible that non-secretor status may not figure prominently as a risk factor for recurrent infections in young women in whom sexual intercourse and spermicide exposures are more important (Scholes et al., 1997). In this regard, most studies showing an association between non-secretor phenotype and recurrent UTI have been performed in older women and in urology referral populations.

We also demonstrated no associations between history of recurrent UTI and pre- and post-coital voiding patterns, frequency of urination, delayed voiding habits, wiping patterns, douching, use of hot tubs, frequent use of pantyhose or tights, or body mass index (Scholes et al., 1997). In a subset of study participants evaluated for anatomical differences, the distance from the urethra to anus was found to be significantly shorter in cases than in controls, although the mean difference was only 2 mm (4.8 cm vs. 5.0 cm; $P = 0.03$) (Hooton et al., 1999). The difference was greater, however, among non-spermicide users, after controlling for sexual intercourse frequency. There were no differences between cases and controls in urethral length, postvoid urine residual, or urine voiding characteristics (e.g. peak flow rate, time to peak flow). These data suggest that a shorter distance between the urethra and anus may have a role in predisposing some young women to recurrent UTI, especially those who do not have exogenous risk factors for UTI.

VIII   Risk factors for recurrent UTI in healthy postmenopausal women

Stamm and Raz have described two groups of postmenopausal women with recurrent UTI: healthy postmenopausal women between the ages of approximately 50 and 70 years who are neither institutionalized nor catheterized; and elderly institutionalized women, who in many cases are catheterized (Stamm and Raz, 1999). In a recent case-control study of 149 postmenopausal women with a history of recurrent UTI and 53 controls without a history of UTI, several factors were identified as being associated with recurrent UTI. These factors were oestrogen deficiency, urogenital surgery, incontinence, presence of a cystocele, postvoid residual urine measured in a uroflow study, non-secretor status, and prior UTI (Stamm and Raz, 1999). In a multivariate analysis, urinary incontinence, history of UTIs before menopause, and non-secretor status were all strongly and independently associated with recurrent UTI in postmenopausal women.

IX Risk factors for complicated UTI

There are numerous factors that predispose individuals to complicated UTI (*Table 1.1*), but they all generally do so by one or more of the following mechanisms: causing obstruction and/or stasis of urine flow, facilitating entry of uropathogens into the urinary tract by bypassing normal host defence mechanisms, providing a nidus for infection that is not readily treatable with antimicrobials, or compromising the host immune system (Ronald and Harding, 1997; Nicolle, 1997b). Diabetes, in particular, is associated with several syndromes of complicated UTI, including intrarenal and perirenal abscess, emphysematous pyelonephritis and cystitis, and papillary necrosis (Patterson and Andriole, 1997b). Infection with multidrug-resistant uropathogens is more likely than with uncomplicated UTI, especially in those infections which develop in institutional settings and in patients exposed to frequent antimicrobial use.

X Risk factors for asymptomatic bacteriuria

Although little studied, risk factors for asymptomatic bacteriuria in young women appear to be the same as those for UTI, including diaphragm–spermicide or spermicide-alone use, recent sexual intercourse, and a history of recurrent UTI, although the associations are weaker (Hooton et al., 1997). The high prevalence of asymptomatic bacteriuria in elderly women is likely due to the high prevalence of conditions frequently seen in this age group, including obstructive uropathy, loss of oestrogen and resulting adverse effects on vaginal microflora, adverse effects on bladder emptying caused by uterine prolapse and cystocele, perineal soiling from fecal incontinence in demented individuals, and frequent instrumentation and bladder catheter use (Nicolle, 1997a). Risk factors shown to be important in nursing home residents include prior cerebrovascular accident, decreased functional status, decreased mental status, bladder catheterization, and prior antibiotic treatment (Wood and Abrutyn, 1998). The relative importance of these risk factors in the elderly is not known.

XI Uropathogen virulence determinants

Certain virulence determinants of uropathogens have been demonstrated to provide a selective advantage to those strains possessing them with regard to colonization and infections (Johnson, 1991; Svanborg and Godaly, 1997). These virulence determinants provide uropathogens with a survival advantage as they compete with other bacteria for a niche in the genitourinary flora. Virulence factors are much more important in the normal host than in the host who has a functional or anatomical abnormality of the genitourinary tract. Several bacterial properties (including P-fimbriae, type 1 fimbriae, hemolysin, aerobactin, serum resistance, and the K1 capsule) are fairly well established as virulence factors in acute symptomatic *E. coli* UTI (Johnson, 1991). It appears that, whereas P-fimbriae are important in development of pyelonephritis, type 1 fimbriae appear to be important in the development of cystitis. The pathogenesis of cystitis is less well understood compared with that of pyelonephritis, and there are no bacterial properties that identify 'cystitogenic' *E. coli* clones that clearly distinguish cystitis from pyelonephritis strains. The bacterial factors that result in asymptomatic bacteriuria remain unknown (Svanborg and Godaly, 1997).

XII   Conclusions

Uncomplicated UTI may involve the bladder (cystitis) or less commonly the kidney (pyelonephritis), are very common in girls and women, are associated with considerable morbidity, and frequently recur. *E. coli* and

S. saprophyticus cause most uncomplicated UTI whereas the microbiologic spectrum in complicated UTI is much more variable. Criteria for interpretation of midstream urine colony counts of uropathogens have been established for the diagnosis of uncomplicated cystitis and pyelonephritis, complicated UTI, and asymptomatic bacteriuria and those for symptomatic UTI are much more sensitive than traditional criteria. Most uncomplicated UTIs in women cannot be explained by underlying functional or anatomic abnormalities of the urinary tract. On the other hand, sexual intercourse, spermicidal product use, and a history of recurrent UTI are strongly associated with UTI. Recent antimicrobial therapy also appears to be a strong risk factor for UTI. Anatomic and functional factors, such as postvoid residual urine volume and urinary incontinence are more important risk factors for recurrent UTI in postmenopausal women. A genetic predisposition to recurrent UTI is suggested by the association of recurrent UTI in certain age groups with the blood group non-secretor phenotype, a maternal history of UTI, and early onset of UTI. Certain virulence determinants of uropathogens have been found to be associated with uropathogenic strains, particularly those causing pyelonephritis. These factors are much more important in the normal host than in the host who has a functional or anatomical abnormality of the genitourinary tract.

References

Abrutyn E, Mossey J, Levison M et al (1991) Epidemiology of asymptomatic bacteriuria in elderly women. *J Am Geriatr Soc* **39**: 388–93.

Bengtsson C, Bengtsson U, Bjorkelund C, Lincoln K, Sigurdsson JA (1998) Bacteriuria in a population sample of women: 24-year follow-up study: Results from the prospective population-based study of women in Gothenburg, Sweden. *Scand J Urol Nephrol* **32**: 284–9.

Brauner A, Jacobson SH, Kuhn I (1992) Urinary *Escherichia coli* causing recurrent infections – a prospective follow-up of biochemical phenotypes. *Clin Nephrol* **38**: 318–23.

Bronsema DA, Adams JR, Pallares R, Wenzel RP (1993) Secular trends in rates and etiology of nosocomial urinary tract infections at a university hospital. *J Urol* **150**: 414–16.

DeVivo MJ, Black KJ, Stover S (1993) Causes of death during the first 12 years after spinal cord injury. *Arch Phys Med Rehabil* **74**: 248–54.

Fihn SD, Boyko EJ, Normand EH et al (1996) Association between use of spermicide-coated condoms and *Escherichia coli* urinary tract infection in young women. *Am J Epidemiol* **144**: 512–20.

Fihn SD, Boyko EJ, Chen CL et al (1998) Use of spermicide-coated condoms and other risk factors for urinary tract infection caused by *Staphylococcus saprophyticus*. *Arch Intern Med* **158**: 281–7.

Foxman B (1990) Recurring urinary tract infection: incidence and risk factors. *Am J Public Health* **80**: 331–3.

Foxman B, Frerichs RR (1985) Epidemiology of urinary tract infection: I. Diaphragm use and sexual intercourse. *Am J Public Health* **75**: 1308–13.

Foxman B, Marsh J, Gillespie B et al (1997) Condom use and first-time urinary tract infection. *Epidemiology* 8: 637–41.

Gupta K, Stapleton AE, Hooton TM et al (1998) Inverse association of H_2O_2-producing lactobacilli and vaginal *Escherichia coli* colonization in women with recurrent urinary tract infections. *J Infect Dis* 178: 446–50.

Hansson S, Martinell J, Stokland E, Jodal U (1997) The natural history of bacteriuria in childhood. *Infect Dis Clin North Am* 11: 499–512.

Herthelius BM, Hedstrom KG, Mollby R et al (1988) Pathogenesis of urinary tract infections – amoxicillin induces genital *Escherichia coli* colonization. *Infection* 16: 263–6.

Hooton TM, Stamm WE (1996a) The vaginal flora and UTIs. In: Mobley HLT, Warren JW, eds. *UTIs: Molecular Pathogenesis and Clinical Management.* Washington DC: ASM Press, 67–94.

Hooton TM, Scholes D, Hughes JP et al (1996b) A prospective study of risk factors for symptomatic urinary tract infection in young women. *N Engl J Med* 335: 468–74.

Hooton TM, Winter C, Tiu F, Stamm WE (1996c) Association of acute cystitis with the state of the menstrual cycle in young women. *Clin Infect Dis* 23: 635–6.

Hooton TM, Scholes D, Stapleton AE et al (1997) A prospective study of asymptomatic bacteriuria in young sexually active women. Presented at the Infectious Diseases Society of America 35th Annual Meeting, 1997.

Hooton TM, Stapleton AE, Roberts PL et al (1999) Perineal anatomy and urine voiding characteristics of young women with and without recurrent urinary tract infections. *Clin Infect Dis* 29: 1600–1.

Ikaheimo R, Siitonen A, Heiskanen T et al (1996) Recurrence of urinary tract infection in a primary care setting: analysis of a 1-year follow-up of 179 women. *Clin Infect Dis* 22: 91–9.

Johnson JR (1991) Virulence factors in *Escherichia coli* urinary tract infection. *Clin Microbiol Rev* 4: 80–128.

Johnson JR, Stamm WE (1987) Diagnosis and treatment of acute urinary tract infections. *Infect Dis Clin North Am* 1: 773–91.

Kass EH (1956) Asymptomatic infections of the urinary tract. *Trans Assoc Am Phys* 69: 56.

Kinane DF, Blackwell CC, Brettle RP et al (1982) ABO blood group, secretor state, and susceptibility to recurrent urinary tract infection in women. *Br Med J* 285: 7–9.

Kunin CM (1994) Urinary tract infections in females. *Clin Infect Dis* 18: 1–12.

Lomberg H, Cedergren B, Leffler H et al (1986) Influence of blood group on the availability of receptors for attachment of uropathogenic *Escherichia coli*. *Infect Immun* 51: 919–26.

Mabeck CE (1972) Treatment of uncomplicated urinary tract infection in non-pregnant women. *Postgrad Med J* 48: 69–75.

Nicolle LE (1997a) Asymptomatic bacteriuria in elderly. *Infect Dis Clin North Am* 11: 647–62.

Nicolle LE (1997b) A practical guide to the management of complicated urinary tract infection. *Drugs* 53: 583–92.

Nicolle LE, Friesen D, Harding GKM, Roos LL (1996) Hospitalization for acute pyelonephritis in Manitoba, Canada, during the period from 1989 to 1992: impact of diabetes, pregnancy, and aboriginal origin. *Clin Infect Dis* 22: 1051–6.

Norden CW, Kass EH (1968) Bacteriuria of pregnancy – a critical appraisal. *Ann Rev Med* 19: 431–70.

Patterson TF, Andriole VT (1997a) Detection, significance, and therapy of bacteriuria in pregnancy. *Infect Dis Clin North Am* 11: 593–608.

Patterson JE, Andriole VT (1997b) Bacterial urinary tract infections in diabetes. *Infect Dis Clin North Am* 11: 735–50.

Pinson AG, Philbrick JT, Lindbeck GH, Schorling JB (1994) ED management of acute pyelonephritis in women: a cohort study. *Am J Emerg Med* 12: 271–8.

Raz R, Stamm WE (1993) A controlled trial of intravaginal estriol in postmenopausal women with recurrent urinary tract infections. *N Engl J Med* 329: 753–6.

Richards MJ, Edwards JR, Culver DH, Gaynes RP (1999) Nosocomial infections in medical intensive care units in the United States. National Nosocomial Infections Surveillance System. *Crit Care Med* 27: 887–92.

Romano JM, Kaye D (1981) UTI in the elderly: common yet atypical. *Geriatrics* 36: 113–15.

Ronald AR, Harding GKM (1997) Complicated urinary tract infections. *Infect Dis Clin North Am* 11: 583–92.

Rubin UH, Shapiro ED, Andriole VT, Davis RJ, Stamm WE (1992) Evaluation of new anti-infective drugs for the treatment of urinary tract infection. *Clin Infect Dis* 15: S216–27.

Rushton HG (1997) Urinary tract infections in children. *Pediatr Clin North Am* 44: 1133–69.

Safrin S, Siegel D, Black D (1988) Pyelonephritis in adult women: inpatient versus outpatient therapy. *Am J Med* 85: 793–8.

Scholes D, Hooton TM, Roberts PL et al (1997) Risk factors for recurrent UTI in young women (Abstract no. 459). *Clin Infect Dis* 25: 440.

Sheinfeld J, Schaeffer AJ, Cordon-Cardo C, Rogatko A, Fair WR (1989) Association of the Lewis blood-group phenotype with recurrent urinary tract infections in women. *N Engl J Med* **320**: 773–7.

Smith HS, Hughes JP, Hooton TM et al (1997) Antecedent antimicrobial use increases the risk of uncomplicated cystitis in young women. *Clin Infect Dis* **25**: 63–8.

Sobel JD (1997) Pathogenesis of urinary tract infection: role of host defenses. *Infect Dis Clin North Am* **11**: 531–49.

Stamm WE, Hooton TM (1993) Management of urinary tract infections in adults. *N Engl J Med* **329**: 1328–34.

Stamm WE, Raz R (1999) Factors contributing to susceptibility of postmenopausal women to recurrent urinary tract infections. *Clin Infect Dis* **28**: 723–5.

Stamm WE, Counts GW, Running KR et al (1982) Diagnosis of coliform infection in acutely dysuric women. *N Engl J Med* **307**: 463–8.

Stamm WE, McKevitt M, Roberts PL, White NJ (1991) Natural history of recurrent urinary tract infections in women. *Rev Infect Dis* **13**: 77–84.

Stapleton A, Nudelman E, Clausen H, Hakomori S, Stamm WE (1992) Binding of uropathogenic *Escherichia coli* R45 to glycolipids extracted from vaginal epithelial cells is dependent on histo-blood group secretor status. *J Clin Invest* **90**: 965–72.

Svanborg C, Godaly G (1997) Bacterial virulence in urinary tract infection. *Infect Dis Clin North Am* **11**: 513–29.

Warren JW (1997) Catheter-associated urinary tract infections. *Infect Dis Clin North Am* **11**: 609–22.

Wood CA, Abrutyn E (1998) Urinary tract infection in older adults. *Clin Geriatric Med* **14**: 267–83.

Zhanel GG, Harding GKM, Guay DRP (1990) Asymptomatic bacteriuria: which patients should be treated? *Arch Intern Med* **150**: 1389–96.

Pathogenesis and microbiology

Reuben Grüneberg

2

Contents

I Introduction

Urinary tract infection (UTI) is caused by aerobic Gram-negative rods and Gram-positive cocci derived from the bowel flora. The mix of species causing UTI differs (between UTI) in the community and in hospital practice and also varies through time. Such changes in species mix may change the pattern of antibiotic susceptibility of urinary pathogens overall, since some types of organisms have predictable sensitivities or resistance to particular antibiotics.

The antibiotic sensitivities of urinary pathogens are also different in community and hospital settings, and they too change with time. Some of these changes are owing to changes in species mix and some to changes within species.

The effects of antibiotics on the gut flora are central to understanding changes in the urinary flora. Since the overall picture is one of steadily progressive erosion of susceptibility to most, but not all antibiotics, action is needed. This chapter offers some suggestions for antibiotic prescribing in UTI which might delay the emergence of antibiotic resistance.

II General practice vs. hospital practice

Urinary tract infection (UTI) may affect either sex at any age. It is common, affecting perhaps 3% of humanity at any one time and perhaps 20–30% of all people during their lifetimes.

Because it is the only objectively defined bacterial infection which is common, it has been much studied. It is a major reason for consultation in primary care and a significant trigger for the prescription of antibiotics.

For the last three decades, the author has been studying (Grüneberg, 1976, 1980a, 1984, 1990, 1994) the pathogenic organisms isolated from infected urine samples handled by his laboratory. *Table 2.1* shows the organisms causing UTI in general practice and *Table 2.2*, those causing UTI in hospital practice.

In general practice (GP) (*Table 2.1*), *Escherichia coli* is responsible for about 75% of all UTI, a situation that has not changed in the years from 1971 to 1995. *Proteus mirabilis* which caused 9.2% of UTI in 1971 had fallen to 4.5% by 1995. *Klebsiella–Enterobacter* spp. represented 2.3% of UTI in 1971, rose to 5.9% by 1991 and had fallen to 4.7% by 1995. *Enterococcus* spp. have risen from about 2% to around 5% of GP UTI over the period. *Staphylococcus* spp. (mostly coagulase-negative species such as *S. epidermidis* and *S. saprophyticus*) rose from 5% to 12.8% by 1981, and declined to around 1% by 1995. Similar findings have been reported by others (de Mouy et al., 1988; Hannan et al., 1993; MacGowan et al., 1993; Barrett et al., 1997).

In hospital practice (*Table 2.2*), the situation is somewhat different. Again, *Escherichia coli* is numerically the most important urinary pathogen, representing 50–60% of isolates. The fall from prominence

Table 2.1
Organisms causing general practice UTI 1971–1995

Organism	1971		1981		1991		1995	
	n = 433	Percent	n = 829	Percent	n = 2165	Percent	n = 1920	Percent
Escherichia coli	340	78.5%	588	70.9%	1471	67.9%	1487	77.5%
Proteus mirabilis	40	9.2%	51	6.2%	95	4.4%	87	4.5%
Klebsiella–Enterobacter spp.	10	2.3%	41	4.9%	127	5.9%	90	4.7%
Enterococcus spp.	10	2.3%	14	1.7%	123	5.7%	95	4.9%
Staphylococcus spp.	22	5.1%	106	12.8%	99	4.6%	19	1.0%
Others	11	2.6%	29	3.5%	250	11.5%	142	7.4%

of *Proteus mirabilis* noted in the GP material has been seen in hospital isolates too, with a fall from 11% of isolates in 1971 to 4.5% in 1995. *Klebsiella–Enterobacter* spp. figure more prominently in the hospital material, representing 16.8% of isolates in 1971, falling to about 9% by 1981 and remaining at about that level since then. The rise of *Enterococcus* spp. as GP urinary pathogens is more strongly evident in hospital with 4% of isolates in 1971 and 9–11% in the 1990s. Staphylococci rose from 3% in 1971 to about 10% in 1991 and have fallen since to around 3%. *Pseudomonas aeruginosa* is represented in the hospital material by between 3 and 6% of isolates. Others have reported similar findings (de Mouy et al., 1988; Hannan et al., 1983; MacGowan et al., 1993).

A cursory inspection of the types of organisms shown as urinary pathogens in general practice and in hospital strongly suggests a faecal origin for this flora. The author's research conducted many years ago (Grüneberg et al., 1968) showed that in domiciliary practice, where cross-infection of the urinary tract is not likely, women acquired acute UTI with their prevalent faecal type of *Escherichia coli*. Moreover, the types of *E. coli* causing acute UTI reflect the prevalence of those types in the faecal flora of the community at the time (Grüneberg et al., 1968). As we shall see, this relationship between the urinary and faecal flora is central in the management of recurrent UTI and to

understanding the ecology of antibiotic resistance.

Inspection of *Tables 2.1* and *2.2* shows that, although there is quite a lot of stability in the types of organisms causing UTI in primary care and in hospital, there is also a change in the 'popularity' of some organisms with time. The reasons for this are not entirely clear but are presumably consequent upon changes in the bowel flora of the communities concerned over time. This has scarcely been studied at all. Apart from geographical differences (Grüneberg et al., 1968) there are likely to be dietary variations having an effect on faecal flora. Antibiotics will also have an effect, as will be seen.

III Antibiotic sensitivity

One effect of a change of species mix in the organisms causing UTI might be changes in antibiotic sensitivities. For example, *Klebsiella–Enterobacter* spp. are ampicillin/amoxycillin resistant so that a rise in the numbers of such organisms will lead to a reduction in β-lactam sensitivity. Similarly, staphylococci and enterococci are always resistant to nalidixic acid; staphylococci are generally β-lactamase producers and so resistant to ampicillin/amoxycillin; *Proteus mirabilis* is never fully sensitive to nitrofurantoin and is resistant to tetracycline, and so on.

Tables 2.3 and *2.4* show the sensitivities of all urinary pathogens isolated in the laboratory where the author worked from general

Table 2.2
Organisms causing hospital practice UTI 1971–1995

Organism	1971		1981		1991		1995	
	n = 552	Percent	n = 2194	Percent	n = 6898	Percent	n = 3146	Percent
Escherichia coli	306	55.4%	1235	56.3%	3329	48.3%	1975	62.9%
Proteus mirabilis	63	11.4%	169	7.7%	353	5.1%	143	4.5%
Klebsiella–Enterobacter spp.	93	16.8%	208	9.5%	594	8.6%	293	9.3%
Enterococcus spp.	22	4.0%	141	6.4%	780	11.3%	291	9.2%
Staphylococcus spp.	18	3.3%	181	8.2%	677	9.8%	86	2.7%
Pseudomonas aeruginosa	15	2.7%	135	6.2%	373	5.4%	118	3.8%
Others	35	4.4%	125	5.7%	792	11.5%	240	7.6%

practice and hospital practice, respectively, in the years 1971–1995. In general practice urinary pathogens (*Table 2.3*) some antibiotics still cover about as many organisms in 1995 as in 1971, e.g. nitrofurantoin. In other cases the situation shows marked deterioration. An example is ampicillin/amoxycillin, which in 1991 covered 88% of urinary pathogens, shrinking to 57% in 1995. Most other agents have suffered some loss of utility over the period, less marked than in the case of amoxycillin. *Table 2.4* shows the similar figures for the in vitro activity of antibiotics against hospital urinary pathogens, with nitrofurantoin at least maintaining its position, ampicillin/amoxycillin falling from 66% to 49% cover between 1971 and 1995 and most other drugs somewhere in between. If attention is paid not to the best case (nitrofurantoin) or the worst (amoxycillin) but to the average of all the drugs listed it can be seen that the utility of antibiotics in UTI overall is under severe threat, both in the community and in hospital. The rate of decay of usefulness of the average 'urinary' antibiotic is greater in primary care than in hospital.

Earlier it was suggested that one reason for changes in antibiotic sensitivities, whether beneficial or deleterious, might be a change in species mix of the organisms causing UTI. *Tables 2.5* and *2.6* present the changes in antibiotic sensitivities of urinary *E. coli* alone between 1971 and 1995 in community and hospital isolates, respectively. The tables show considerable reductions in the usefulness of many but not all drugs over the period, in both settings. That is to say, the changes in antibiotic sensitivity are a result of both a change in species mix and of changes within species.

IV   Repeated infections

A major problem in the management of UTI is the patient with repeated infection. Such repeated infection may be due to re-infection due to new pathogens or relapse of infection when the second episode is caused by the same organism as the first infection. When the organisms belong to different species, there is no problem about recognising that the patient has a re-infection. If the two pathogens from first and subsequent infection belong to the same species, e.g. *E. coli* it is necessary to apply differentiatory typing to establish whether the patient is suffering relapse or re-infection. This may be needed for clinical reasons because the treatment of the two conditions should be different, or in clinical trials to establish whether the initial organism has been eradicated or not.

A particular problem may be attempts to prevent repeated re-infections of the urinary tract. This may be important in adults to spare the patient recurrence of UTI symptoms. In children, there may be problems because recurrent infections of the urinary tract are nearly always due to

Table 2.3
Proportions of all urinary pathogens fully sensitive to various antimicrobials in general practice, 1971–1995

Drug	1971 n = 433	1981 n = 829	1991 n = 2165	1995 n = 1920
Ampicillin/amoxycillin	88.2%	66.2%	59.7%	56.9%
Cephaloridine	87.5%	85.1%	87.5%	86.9%
Ciprofloxacin	–	–	91.5%	90.3%
Co-trimoxazole	96.6%	95.7%	80.3%	86.8%
Nalidixic acid	90.7%	81.8%	79.2%	85.7%
Nitrofurantoin	85.6%	84.1%	88.4%	88.4%
Sulphonamide	76.4%	74.2%	65.6%	64.5%
Tetracycline	72.5%	72.3%	65.7%	65.0%
Trimethoprim	94.0%	91.1%	78.1%	74.0%

Table 2.4
Proportions of all urinary pathogens fully sensitive to various antimicrobials in hospital practice, 1971–1995

Drug	1971 n = 552	1981 n = 2194	1991 n = 6898	1995 n = 3146
Ampicillin/amoxycillin	66.1%	53.7%	51.0%	48.8%
Cephaloridine	69.9%	71.6%	76.5%	73.1%
Ciprofloxacin	–	–	85.9%	83.3%
Co-trimoxazole	83.9%	81.4%	75.2%	74.1%
Nalidixic acid	84.8%	74.3%	64.6%	73.5%
Nitrofurantoin	70.3%	71.3%	79.3%	79.3%
Sulphonamide	61.9%	59.7%	57.0%	55.5%
Tetracycline	55.8%	58.3%	56.9%	57.9%
Trimethoprim	79.9%	74.4%	68.7%	64.9%

Table 2.5
The percentage of urinary E. coli from general practice, 1971–1995 fully sensitive to various antimicrobials

Year	Strains (n)	Ampicillin/ amoxycillin	Cephaloridine	Ciprofloxacin	Co-trimoxazole	Nalidixic acid	Nitrofurantoin	Sulphonamide	Tetracycline	Trimethoprim
1971	340	91.4%	91.2%	–	99.2%	99.1%	97.6%	77.3%	81.2%	98.5%
1981	558	75.6%	86.6%	–	98.4%	99.5%	95.3%	71.5%	79.4%	95.7%
1991	1471	64.7%	92.9%	99.8%	81.8%	98.7%	97.0%	65.3%	73.8%	80.1%
1995	1487	58.4%	90.8%	99.1%	86.8%	96.8%	95.0%	64.5%	68.3%	74.1%

Table 2.6

The percentage of urinary E. coli from hospital practice, 1971–1995 fully sensitive to various antimicrobials

Year	Strains (n)	Ampicillin/ amoxycillin	Cephaloridine	Ciprofloxacin	Co-trimoxazole	Nalidixic acid	Nitrofurantoin	Sulphonamide	Tetracycline	Trimethoprim
1971	306	84.4%	86.6%	–	97.0%	98.1%	95.7%	75.3%	75.8%	96.8%
1981	1235	64.3%	78.0%	–	90.9%	97.7%	89.4%	62.6%	71.7%	86.2%
1991	3329	57.4%	88.7%	99.7%	76.7%	97.4%	94.2%	62.1%	68.6%	75.1%
1995	1975	52.2%	86.7%	97.2%	77.3%	93.8%	92.6%	57.9%	66.7%	68.1%

re-infection, sometimes asymptomatic, and are capable of causing renal scarring or increasing the extent of pre-existing renal scars, particularly in the presence of vesico-ureteric reflux. One strategy which is widely applied is to give the re-infection-prone child a long-term low-dose prophylactic antimicrobial agent in an attempt to prevent further episodes. *Table 2.7* presents data on the effectiveness of such prophylaxis with various antibiotics in a high-risk group of children studied for many years by my colleague Dr Jean Smellie. The right-hand column of *Table 2.7* shows the mean re-infection interval in child-months, with various antibiotics – the higher the figure in that column, the more effective the antibiotic is as a preventative of re-infection of the urinary tract. Co-trimoxazole (and trimethoprim, probably) and nitrofurantoin are shown to be very good at preventing re-infection, ampicillin and tetracycline are very poor at prevention, and sulphonamides are in an intermediate position.

V   Differences in prophylaxis

Why should there be such differences in prophylactic effectiveness? An ideal prophylactic agent would be administrable by mouth, absorbed from the gut, excreted in high concentration in the urine and active against urinary pathogens (as well, of course, as being acceptable to patients so ensuring

compliance, producing few and trivial adverse events, and costing little). All the antimicrobial agents listed in *Table 2.7* broadly fit the description. A further requirement is that the antibiotic should select little or no resistance to itself in the aerobes of the intestinal flora, the reservoir from which new infecting urinary pathogens will be derived. A good prophylactic agent, such as nitrofurantoin or co-trimoxazole, will select little resistance to itself in the gut flora so that a gut-derived organism gaining access to the urinary tract will be eliminated by the urine which contains high concentrations of the antibiotic to which it is still sensitive. A poor prophylactic agent such as ampicillin/amoxycillin will produce a gut flora which is resistant to the drug. Organisms from the gut flora will then be able to establish themselves easily in the urinary tract because they are resistant to the drug in the urine.

VI   Conclusions

To draw the central conclusion from all this: If our medical practices lead to the aerobic bacterial flora becoming antibiotic resistant, urinary tract pathogens will go on becoming more resistant and effective treatment of UTI will become ever more difficult. Of course, the intestinal flora will be affected by antibiotics prescribed for indications other than UTI. In relation to antibiotic prescribing for UTI, however, some prescribing policies can be

Table 2.7
The effectiveness of various antibiotics in long-term low-dosage prophylaxis of urinary tract re-infection in children

Drug	Child months of treatment (A)	Breakthrough infections (B)	Mean re-infection interval (A/B) in child-months
Co-trimoxazole[1-3]	2637	6	439
Nitrofurantoin[4]	1117	4	279
Sulphonamide[4]	4962	34	145
Ampicillin[4]	208	9	23
Tetracycline[4]	13	2	6
Trimethoprim[5]	92	0	> 92

1, Grüneberg et al. (1975); 2, Smellie et al. (1976); 3, Grüneberg et al. (1979); 4, Grüneberg et al. (1973); 5, Grüneberg (1980b).

suggested which might help to minimize the problem without jeopardizing patient welfare:

- Always send urine for culture before starting antibiotic treatment.
- If the urine yields no bacterial growth, stop the antibiotic treatment (50% of patients with frequency-dysuria syndrome do not have UTI).
- If the organism grown is resistant to the prescribed antibiotic stop the treatment, re-culture and re-treat with laboratory guidance, if necessary.
- Use minimum effective therapy – single-dose treatment with many antibiotics is little or no worse than extended courses.
- Asymptomatic bacteriuria should only be treated in children, pregnant women, or those whose urinary tract is about to be catheterized or operated upon.
- Antibiotics should not be given to patients with UTI associated with urethral catheters unless they are very ill with it.
- 'Green' antibiotics, i.e. those which will not select much resistance to themselves in the aerobes of the gut flora, should be preferred to drugs which select a great deal of resistance.

References

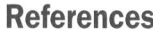

Barrett SP, Andrews N, Joshi A, Nathwani A, Shrimpton SB (1997) Reported antimicrobial sensitivities of urinary pathogens to orally administrable agents in Britain in 1995. *Br J Clin Res* **8**: 47–55.

de Mouy D, Auriol JC, de Clercq G et al (1988) Fréquence d'isolement de germes d'infection urinaire en practique de ville et leur sensibilité aux différents antibiotiques. *Pathol Biol* **36**: 1011–15.

Grüneberg RN (1976) Susceptibility of urinary pathogens to various antimicrobial substances: a four year study. *J Clin Pathol* **29**: 292–5.

Grüneberg RN (1980a) Antibiotic sensitivities of urinary pathogens 1971–8. *J Clin Pathol* **33**: 853–8.

Grüneberg RN (1980b) Recurrent urinary tract infection. *Tijdschr Geneesk* **36**: 1207–11.

Grüneberg RN (1984) Antibiotic sensitivities of urinary pathogens, 1971–82. *J Antimicrob Chemother* **14**: 17–23.

Grüneberg RN (1990) Changes in the antibiotic sensitivities of urinary pathogens, 1971–1989. *J Antimicrob Chemother* **26**(Suppl F): 3–11.

Grüneberg RN (1994) Changes in urinary pathogens and their antibiotic sensitivities, 1971–1992. *J Antimicrob Chemother* **33**(Suppl A): 1–8.

Grüneberg RN, Leigh DA, Brumfitt W (1968) *Escherichia coli* serotypes in urinary tract infection: studies in domiciliary, antenatal and hospital practice. In: O'Grady F, Brumfitt W, eds, *Urinary Tract Infection.* Oxford: Oxford University Press, 68–79.

Grüneberg RN, Smellie JM, Leakey A (1973) Changes in the antibiotic sensitivities of faecal organisms in response to treatment in children with urinary tract infection. In: Brumfitt W, Asscher AW, eds, *Urinary Tract Infection*. London: Oxford University Press, 131–6.

Grüneberg RN, Leakey A, Bendall MJ, Smellie JM (1975) Bowel flora in urinary tract infection: effect of chemotherapy with special reference to co-trimoxazole. *Kidney Internat* **8:** S122–9.

Grüneberg RN, Smellie JM, Leakey A, Atkin WS (1979) Trimethoprim-sulfamethoxazole for treatment of urinary tract infections: some bacteriologic considerations. In: Kass EH, Brumfitt W, eds, *Infections of the Urinary Tract*. Chicago and London: University of Chicago Press, 74–7.

Hannan M, Cormican M, Flynn J (1993) Comparison of antimicrobial sensitivities of urinary pathogens for the years 1980 and 1990. *Irish J Med Sci* **162:** 499–501.

MacGowan AP, Brown NM, Holt HA et al (1993) An eight-year survey of the antimicrobial susceptibility patterns of 85,971 bacteria isolated from patients in a district general hospital and the local community. *J Antimicrob Chemother* **31:** 543–57.

Smellie JM, Grüneberg RN, Leakey A, Atkin WS (1976) Long term low dose co-trimoxazole in prophylaxis of childhood urinary tract infection: clinical aspects. *Br Med J* **ii:** 203–6.

Investigations

Edwin P Arnold

3

Contents

I Introduction

The point of investigating any clinical problem is not only to select appropriate treatment, but also to determine if there is an underlying cause which, if corrected, would prevent recurrence of that clinical problem or its sequelae.

Investigations should always begin with a careful history and clinical examination. Symptoms of burning, frequency, nocturia, urgency and strangury sometimes associated with haematuria are typical of a urinary tract infection proven on microbiological assessment (Gallagher et al., 1965; MRC Bacteriuria Committee, 1979). However, the classic symptoms of frequency, burning and suprapubic discomfort are not universally present in women with a proven lower urinary tract infection. Burning may be less of a feature, particularly in elderly women.

Young children often do not or cannot complain of the burning, but because of the pain, they may stop the flow by reflexly shutting the voluntary external urethral sphincter and then restarting the flow, and this intermittency is repeated throughout the cycle of voiding. This is called sphincter-active voiding. This pattern may persist into older childhood after treatment of the infection (van Gool and Tanagho, 1977). They may become febrile and ill. The onset of secondary enuresis or daytime incontinence, having previously gained control, should lead to the search for a urinary tract infection.

In the frail and elderly, loss of bladder control or sensory urge incontinence may develop, because it is too painful to hold on or because they lack the mobility to get to a toilet in time. For others, poor mentation makes them unaware of bladder urgency and leakage follows.

Symptoms of urgency and burning seem to rely on the combination of an inflamed urethra/trigone/bladder with an acid urine. Alkalinization of the urine provides rapid relief of symptoms well before any resolution of cystitis could occur. Conversely, renal TB is classically accompanied by a 'sterile' acid pyuria, but does not produce burning unless there is bladder involvement as well.

The presence of loin pain and tenderness, fever and malaise raises the possibility of acute pyelonephritis.

A previous history of past infections, previous surgery, diabetes, immunodeficiency states and drug treatment or radiotherapy are clearly important.

Factors associated with developing recurrent urinary infections should be sought and might include relationship to sexual intercourse, menstrual cycle or postmenopausal status.

The presence of hesitancy, poor stream, the need to strain to void and any feeling of incomplete emptying should be noted. It is clearly important to know whether a catheter is used, either indwelling or intermittently passed.

Abdominal examination may reveal suprapubic and pelvic tenderness due to infection or chronic retention of urine or may reveal another predisposing cause like salpingitis, a tubo-ovarian abscess or a pelvic mass. The external genitalia should be carefully examined. Congenital hypospadias or an intravaginal urethral meatus might predispose to urinary tract infections after intercourse. Evidence of vulvovaginitis, trauma, urethral diverticulum and the presence of incontinence should be sought. Pelvic examination should be included to detect pelvic masses, tenderness or constipation. The tone of the pelvic musculature should also be noted as changes might indicate a neuropathic cause.

II Factors predisposing to urinary tract infection

Possible predisposing causes of urinary tract infection are listed in *Tables 3.1* and *3.2*. Investigations need to be tailored to the individual according to clinical presentation, so any cause can be found and treated appropriately.

III Investigations

1. Urinalysis

The bacteriological definition of infection and its diagnosis has been addressed in detail in Chapter 1.

(i) Collection of urine specimens

The aim is to obtain a specimen of bladder urine free of contamination from urethral/vulval secretions or organisms. The technique should be as patient friendly as possible commensurate with an accurate diagnosis.

(a) Bag urine specimen
Adhesive plastic bags can be used to collect urine specimens from babies, infants and

Table 3.1
Factors predisposing to urinary tract infection: congenital abnormalities

Urethra/bladder	Exstrophy, hypospadias, epispadias
Ureter	Vesicoureteric reflux
	Ectopic ureters
	Primary obstructive megaureter
Pelvis	Pelvic–ureteric junction obstruction
Nervous system	Meningomyelocoele
	Tethered cord syndrome

Table 3.2
Factors predisposing to urinary tract infection: acquired causes

Traumatic	Operations including intestinal segments, substitutions
	Sexual intercourse, or abuse
	Foreign bodies, catheters, stents, etc.
Inflammatory	Immunodeficiency states
	Vulvo urethritis:
	Sexually transmitted disease
	Sexual abuse
	Urinary incontinence
	Chronic inflammations:
	TB
	Syphilis
	Schistosomiasis
	Interstitial cystitis
	Cystitis cystica
	Radiotherapy
	Fistula between bowel/bladder
Metabolic	Stones in kidneys, ureters or bladder
	Diabetes
	Drugs, e.g. cyclophosphamide and tioprofenic acid
Functional	Residual urine
	Postobstruction, e.g. urethral diverticulum, cystocele
	Impaired contractility with ageing
	Sphincter-active voiding
	Immobility, bedridden status and constipation
	'Cameloid' bladder, indicating the infrequent voiding syndrome
Malignant	Bladder tumours, especially carcinoma in situ (C_{is})
	Adjacent cancer invading the bladder

young children. The perineum needs to be adequately washed and cleaned and there is clearly a significant risk of contamination if the bag is left on for any length of time. The bag should be frequently inspected and removed as soon as the child has voided. The urine is transferred into a sterile container and sent to the laboratory as soon as possible.

(b)   Midstream urine (MSU)

The midstream urine (MSU) technique was developed to avoid contaminating the bladder urine with urethral or vulval organisms, particularly in the obese. In the usual method, the patient passes some urine and then stops. She then restarts with the container ready to collect the sample. She then stops again and empties her bladder to completion in the toilet. Urine reports often indicate epithelial cells which imply that such contamination has occurred.

The clean-catch modification of the MSU means asking the patient to clean the vulva, separate the labia with one hand and pass urine with an uninterrupted flow, in the middle of which the sterile container is placed under the flowing stream to collect the midstream sample.

If results remain unclear or contamination persists, then it should be repeated. In cases of doubt a bladder puncture urine is the best way to resolve the issue.

(c)   Suprapubic bladder puncture

This is most often used in children where the diagnosis of infection from bag urine is inconclusive or in a sick child where accurate, rapid diagnosis is needed prior to antibiotics being given. In infants and young children under two years of age, the bladder is an abdominal organ and the puncture is done 1–2 cm above the symphysis in the midline with a 22 gauge 38 mm needle directed at right angles to the skin. It is done 15 minutes after a feed so that there is some urine in the bladder.

The bladder puncture urine should be sterile and any white cells or organisms found in it can be considered abnormal, unless the adjacent bowel has been inadvertently punctured during the aspiration attempt, which is a rare event.

In adults bladder puncture is often used in spinal cord injury patients where voluntary voiding is not possible. A 20 gauge spinal needle 90 mm long is inserted 2 cm above the symphysis. In non-neuropathic patients, because the bladder is in the pelvis, the needle needs to be directed slightly caudally at about 20°. If lumbar lordosis is present secondary to spinal cord injury, the needle should be inserted at right angles to the skin.

(d)   Early morning urine specimens (EMUs)

The concentrated first specimen in the morning is used to culture for mycobacterium tuberculosis. Specimens are collected daily for 3–6 days.

(e)   Catheter specimens

An in-and-out catheter is occasionally needed to obtain a specimen. There is a small risk of introducing organisms and obtaining a false-positive result.

Patients with permanent indwelling catheters often have commensal organisms which cause no symptoms and are best not treated, treatment being reserved for those with symptoms. In closed systems of drainage the tubing can be clamped, and swabbed after a quarter of an hour, and a specimen is aspirated from the tubing with a needle and syringe. Some systems have a sampling port.

In patients with an ileal conduit some have advocated using a two-catheter technique, one inside the other larger diameter 'sump' with side holes, to allow collection of specimen via the smaller tube close to the ureterointestinal anastomosis.

Specimens can also be obtained for microbiology from any urine-draining catheter, e.g. nephrostomy tube or suprapubic catheter.

(f)   Localizing the site of a urinary infection
The site of infection is usually clear from the clinical history of pain or X-ray changes like a staghorn calculus. Needle puncture of the renal pelvis is rarely indicated and is not entirely risk free. Collection of ureteric catheter specimens for microbiology testing is sometimes useful (Stamey et al., 1965). Alternatively, Fairley et al. (1967) advocated bladder washouts with antibiotics followed by copious saline washouts to clear the antibiotics and then collection of a catheter specimen of urine, but this is seldom used in practice.

(ii)   Microscopy and culture

The microbiology and definition of infection have been discussed fully in Chapter 2. There is an important group of patients who have symptoms suggesting infection but in whom no organisms can be found. This group of patients needs careful further investigation. A search for schistosomiasis ova should be requested from those at risk. Lowenstein-Jensen cultures of early morning urines should be performed if TB needs consideration. Faecal debris may be seen in fistula cases.

(iii)   Dipstick tests

This non-culture method tests bacterial conversion of nitrates to nitrites and, in some, the consumption of the minimal urinary glucose concentration. There is an unacceptably high false-negative rate of 40–80% (Stevens, 1989), but the test can be useful evidence of urinary tract infection in certain circumstances and for checking that a course of antibiotics completed more than two days earlier has actually cleared the infection.

(iv)   Exfoliative cytology

A smear is made from the centrifuged deposit of a freshly voided urine sample and stained by the Papanicolau technique. It will show any abnormal cells shed from the surface of a bladder cancer, especially if poorly differentiated or carcinoma in situ. The recently developed urine assay for nuclear matrix protein 22 (NMP22) has been shown to have a greater sensitivity and specificity than cytology (Landman et al., 1998).

(v) Other tests

Urinary glucose and protein should be tested to screen for diabetes/renal failure as possible predisposing causes, especially where infections are recurrent.

2. Blood tests

Patients admitted with acute and severe symptoms suggesting pyelonephritis should have blood drawn for a complete blood count, creatinine and electrolytes together with blood cultures before administration of appropriate antibiotics. Although there is little evidence to show that acute pyelonephritis causes measurable long-term renal damage in an otherwise normal adult kidney, the extent of segmental or global pyelonephritis, as seen by defects on a DMSA scan, correlates with the magnitude of elevation of C-reactive protein (CRP) in the serum. CRP was elevated in 57 of 66 women with acute pyelonephritis (86%). It was significantly higher in those with defects seen on subsequent DMSA scans (Bailey et al., 1996). This may have some practical value in research, and in spinal cord-injured patients unable to localize the site of pain and who have acute fever and a proven urinary bacterial infection. It may also help to distinguish lower urinary tract infection from an acute pyelonephritis.

3. Voiding function

Tests of voiding function are required only occasionally. Some children develop sphincter-active voiding after a urinary tract infection and this can predispose to further attacks.

(i) Voiding flow rate

The patient is asked to attend with a full bladder (more than 150 ml) and to void in privacy on a commode chair, under which is a beaker seated on a load cell transducer. The rate of change of weight provides a flow rate pattern and curve. This is the most widely used type of flow meter although there are other types.

Sphincter-active voiding indicates that the sphincter is contracting instead of relaxing throughout the voiding cycle (van Gool and Tanagho, 1977). It is common in neuropaths and spinal cord injury patients but also occurs in some children and adults who have had a urinary infection. As micturiction is painful, they stop and start several times during voiding. This pattern can become imprinted, persisting after the urinary infection has been cleared.

If this diagnosis is suspected a flow rate might help by showing an interrupted or staccato pattern to the voiding. Such a pattern in an older woman might suggest she is using abdominal straining to empty her bladder

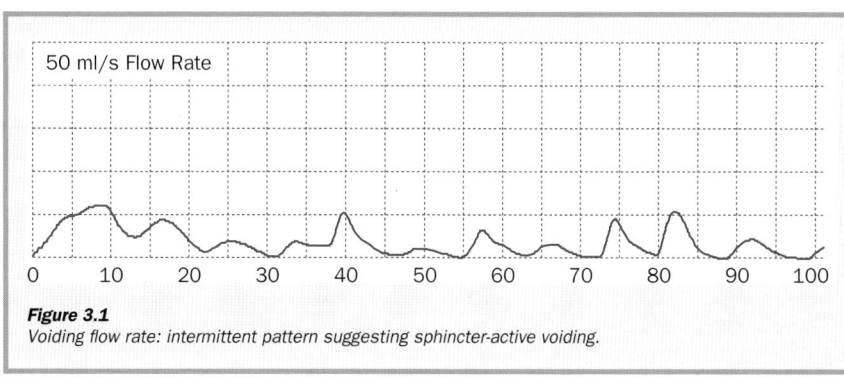

Figure 3.1
Voiding flow rate: intermittent pattern suggesting sphincter-active voiding.

rather than a detrusor contraction (*Figure 3.1*) A prolonged slow flow might suggest obstruction or reduced contractility, either of which can cause a postvoid residual urine and predilection to urinary infection.

(ii)   Postvoid residual urine

This can be readily measured by ultrasound. However, there is considerable intraindividual variability, so repeat testing is advisable. The presence of a residual urine does predispose to urinary infection in some women and regular emptying and flushing out is one of the bladder defences in preventing multiplication of organisms and the establishment of infection. Residual urine has been identified as a predisposing factor in developing urinary infections in patients with a neuropathic

bladder or diabetes. Regular emptying of the bladder using intermittent self-catheterization may suffice to stop the urinary infection. The relation of residual urine to infection has been questioned by Hampson et al. (1992), in the non-neuropathic state.

(iii)   Cystography

This requires catheterization so the bladder can be filled with X-ray contrast to look for vesicoureteric reflux and diverticula of the bladder and urethra and to delineate any cystocoele (*Figure 3.2*). In many centres, it is combined with pressure studies which help in the assessment of the neuropathic bladder or the presence of obstruction.

The video cystourethrogram will detect vesicoureteric reflux if present, although

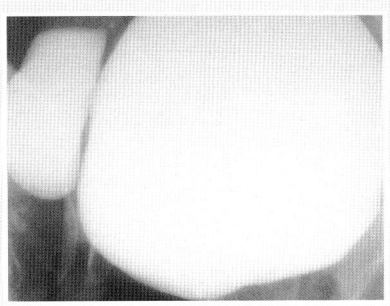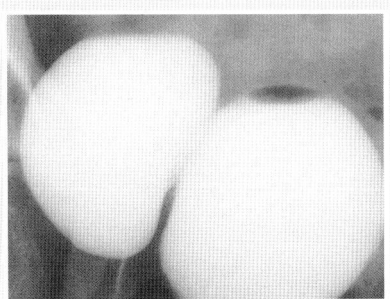

Figure 3.2
Bladder diverticulum: (left) at the end of filling; (right) during micturition (the diverticulum is larger because some urine passes into it with the rise in bladder pressure)

sometimes reflux is intermittent. It can show urethral diverticula if present (*Figure 3.3*) and also demonstrate widening of the proximal urethra in patients with an overactive bladder. It is believed this proximal urethral dilatation occurs when the bladder contracts and the patient tries to stop leakage by voluntarily holding on with the external sphincter. This leads to what is termed a 'spinning top' deformity.

Voiding studies will demonstrate the activation of the detrusor reflex and whether emptying is achieved by urethral relaxation or by abdominal straining. The configuration of the urethra during voiding can be documented and the presence of any

diverticula of the urethra can be noted. If sphincter-active voiding is present, this too can be readily seen.

Finally, the efficiency of bladder emptying can be assessed by measuring the postvoid residual urine. The test should be deferred until after any acute infection has settled, as it might cause anomalies unrelated to any predisposing causes for the infection.

In the elderly, there is not infrequently a combination of detrusor hyperactivity (DH) with uninhibited detrusor contractions in the filling phase and impaired contractility (IC) leaving a postvoid residual. The combination of DHIC was highlighted by Resnick and Yalla (1987).

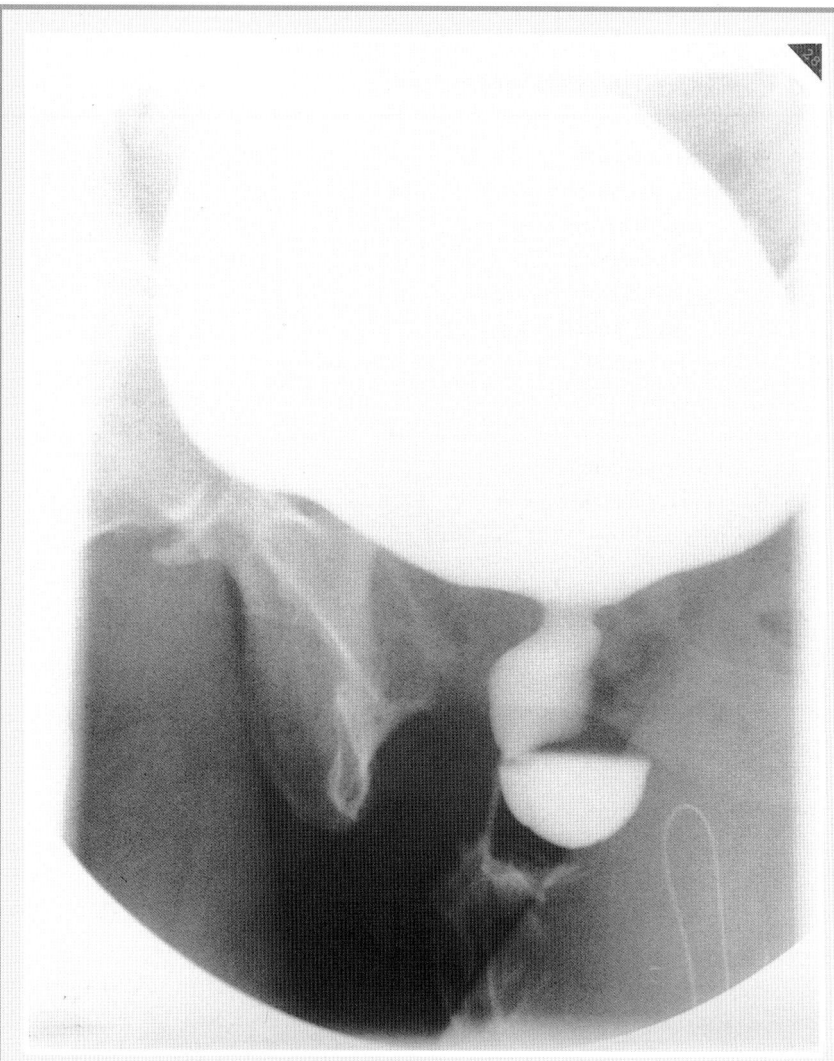

Figure 3.3
Micturating cystogram in the standing position showing a fluid level in a urethral diverticulum and distal urethral stenosis.

Incontinence can lead to vulvovaginitis and this can predispose to ascending urinary tract infections. Sphincter competence can be evaluated clinically by observation during cough/strain at stages through filling. The influence of coughing and passive posture change can be recorded. The degree of prolapse can be assessed radiologically and its mobility during cough/strain evaluated. The rationale of these pressure recordings is to evaluate the storage function of the bladder and to determine whether urethral sphincter incompetence is the cause of any leakage or whether it is due to detrusor instability where bladder contractions occur at times when the bladder should be relaxed.

4. Plain abdominal X-ray (KUB)

If stones are present in the kidney, ureters or bladder, 90% will show on plain abdominal X-ray because they contain calcium or cystine which, although radio-opaque, is less dense than are stones containing calcium. Tomography can clarify the detail of any renal calculi if needed. Uric acid stones are radiolucent. Other causes of opacities include calcified mesenteric lymph nodes, phleboliths, calcified uterine fibroids and calcium in ovarian cysts (eg teratoma). These different calcifications can usually be distinguished from the urological causes. Calcification in renal tumours occasionally occurs, particularly in the cystic type.

Multiple caliceal stones can develop due to papillary necrosis (*Figure 3.4*).

Calcification along the line of the psoas muscle often indicates a previous ileopsoas abscess arising from a tuberculous spine and may be a marker to TB of the kidney. Tuberculous pyonephrosis often progresses to non-function and thence to dystrophic calcification of the kidney, the so-called autonephrectomy.

In patients with emphysematous pyelonephritis, the plain X-ray may show a mottled appearance due to gas in the collecting tubules, pelvis and calyces. The infecting organism is usually a gas-forming *Escherichia coli*. Diabetics are more prone to this condition. In some, gas is apparent in the bladder on plain X-ray.

In the rare but serious condition of xanthogranulomatous pyelonephritis, the kidney is usually enlarged, stones are present and sometimes also gas. The kidney is non-functioning. It is most often seen in elderly women and usually requires a nephrectomy.

Schistosomiasis and the associated chronic inflammation often lead to calcification of the bladder or ureteric walls.

A stone in the lower third of the ureter can produce symptoms indistinguishable from a urinary tract infection. Frequency and hypersensitivity at the urethral meatus worsening during voiding can result because both the lower ureter and the urethral meatus

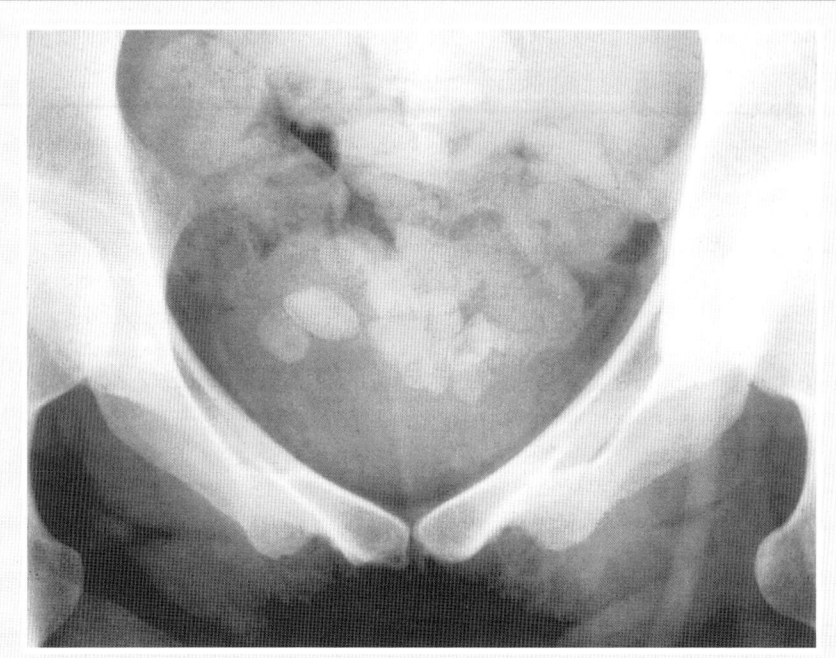

Figure 3.4
Plain X-ray showing multiple bladder stones.

are supplied by the same nerve distribution (S2 and S3). The pain from a stone in the lower third of the ureter can therefore be referred to the external meatus.

5.   Ultrasound of kidneys and bladder

This is usually the first imaging test done in combination with the plain X-ray, for women with recurrent urinary infection. This will show dilatation of the renal pelvic calyces but only in the ureter if gross. If a stone is present in the kidney or bladder this will produce a focus of bright echoes with associated acoustic shadowing.

Ultrasound is a useful non-invasive method of assessing postvoid residual urine (PVR) and the efficiency of voiding. However, PVR can have significant intraindividual variations.

Bladder wall thickness can be assessed by ultrasound and recent work suggests it correlates with bladder outlet obstruction and detrusor instability (Kaefer et al., 1997; Khullar et al., 1996). More validation of this non-invasive method is needed before general acceptance.

Urinary infection can occur as a complication of a tumour. Ultrasound is a good test for renal parenchymal tumours but less good at detecting urothelial tumours of the renal pelvis or ureter. A bladder tumour can often be seen if large enough to produce a filling defect on ultrasound. However, it has low specificity.

Dilatation of the lower ureters or the presence of a ureterocele can be demonstrated on bladder ultrasound.

6. Intravenous urogram (IVU)

The indications for IVU have diminished to a degree since the advent of cheaper, less invasive and good-quality ultrasound which in many cases is now more accurate than the IVU.

Intravenous non-ionic iodine-containing contrast is filtered by the glomerulus and concentrated by the tubules and then outlines the calyces, pelvis, ureters and bladder. In acute pyelonephritis, the kidney is enlarged and function may be delayed or reduced globally or segmentally depending on the distribution of the inflammatory change. If obstruction is present due to calculus, the nephrogram is delayed in appearance, denser than the unobstructed side and is present for longer than the unobstructed side. There is a delay in appearance of the contrast in the renal pelvis.

Clubbing of calyces and caliceal stones can indicate papillary necrosis, secondary to infection and local ischaemia. It is a common feature of diabetes and analgesic nephropathy.

Currently, an IVU is still used as the main imaging modality for patients with haematuria which persists after cure of the urinary tract infection or which has occurred spontaneously. When some abnormality is shown on ultrasound, the IVU may be needed to further evaluate it. For example, if a hydronephrosis is seen, an IVU is useful to document the site of obstruction.

It is used in most centres to evaluate ureteric stones and in patients with acute ureteric colic. Many centres now use spiral computerized tomography for this purpose.

Where infection complicates an

obstruction, urgent proximal drainage is required by a nephrostomy.

If percutaneous nephrolithotomy (PCN) is planned an IVU is helpful in delineating calyces and planning the radiological approach for developing the track into the calyx.

7. Nuclear medicine scans

A nuclear medicine scan can be used to detect or confirm obstructed drainage from the upper urinary tract, suspected on ultrasound. Secondly, it can determine differential function between the various areas of interest, either the right compared to the left kidney or upper versus lower poles. Finally, it can demonstrate renal scars if present. Dimercaptosuccinic acid (DMSA) scans are not indicated in adult women with acute pyelonephritis where there is a rapid response to appropriate antibiotics but should be considered where the illness is severe or protracted (Bailey et al., 1996).

In a patient with recent acute pyelonephritis, the reduced perfusion of the whole kidney or of the segment affected can be seen. When DSMA scans were done in 81 adult women with acute pyelonephritis, 37 had abnormalities. A single segment of reduced perfusion was seen in 19 and multiple areas were seen in 12. There were five with pre-existing scars of reflux nephropathy and one shrunken kidney (Bailey et al., 1996). In children such areas of reduced perfusion resolved in 34–60% of cases. In the

majority of the adults, however, they had returned to normal within three months (Baily et al., 1996; Rushton et al., 1992).

A patient who has had a bout of pyelonephritis and in whom a renal ultrasound shows some dilatation may need to undergo a nuclear medicine scan to document if obstruction is present. This can be documented from the delayed washout of the isotope from the renal pelvis using radioactive technetium-labelled diethyltriaminepentaacetic acid (DTPA) or, more recently, with mercaptoacetyl triglycine (MAG3). If equivocal, the injection of a diuretic (frusemide) may clarify ambiguous findings.

MAG3 and DMSA scans are the most useful for showing areas of reduced uptake and renal scars. Computer enhancement and manipulation allows comparison of areas of interest and comparison of function in each kidney.

8. Computed tomography (CT) scans

CT scans are useful occasionally in urinary infections to delineate the extent of changes seen in acute pyelonephritis and to determine if they are bilateral changes, focal or diffuse and the extent of any renal enlargement (Talner et al., 1994). If a spiral CT is used, it can also show any predisposing cause like ureteric stones causing obstruction or a pelvic–ureteric junction obstruction, as well

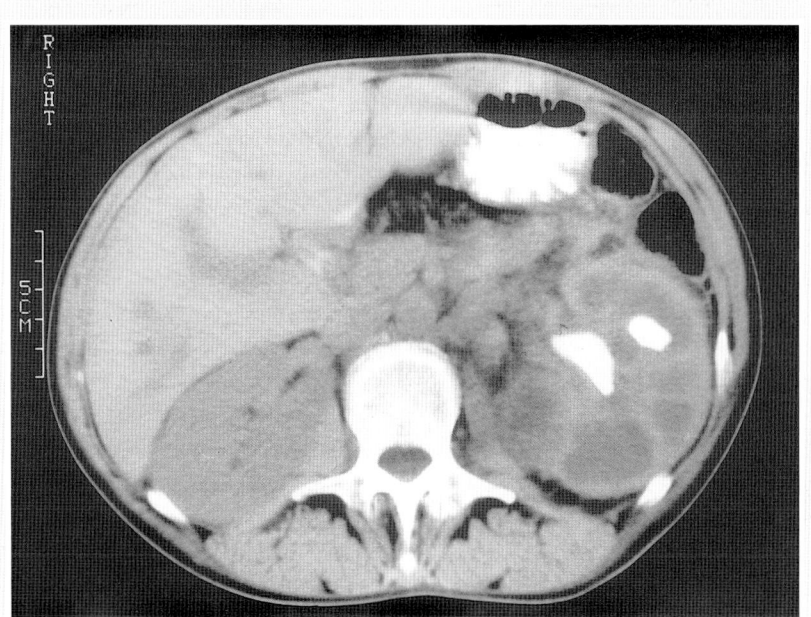

Figure 3.5
CT showing two large left renal stones, a renal carbuncle and perinephric abscess formation.
Histology after nephrectomy showed xanthogranulomatous pyelonephritis.

as the associated renal changes. It will also define whether a renal or perinephric abscess is present and any gas formation (*Figure 3.5*).

While the diagnosis is usually clear, sometimes infection can occur in a renal cancer and cause some difficulty in diagnosis of the malignancy.

9. Cystoscopy

Cystoscopy is rarely helpful in diagnosis or treatment of women with uncomplicated urinary tract infections but is indicated in cases where symptoms persist or recur frequently or in the absence of proven urinary tract infections or if microscopic haematuria persists after satisfactory treatment of the urinary tract infection.

Facilities for cystoscopy under local anaesthesia using a flexible (or rigid) cystoscope are readily available in most centres and will allow exclusion of any sinister pathology and even allow small biopsies to be performed. This can also be undertaken more adequately under a general anaesthetic with a rigid cystoscope.

IV Who needs investigating and how?

1. Proven bacterial infections

In general, the following patients should be fully investigated.

- All children with urinary infections and males of any age.
- Women of reproductive age, if recurrent urinary infections are not responding to adequate courses of antibiotics (and/or antibiotic prophylaxis) or if a proteus is the recurring uropathogen, as this may be associated with stones.
- Any woman who has persistent haematuria, macroscopic or microscopic, after clearance of a urinary infection. Patients with proteinuria require nephrological review.

(i) Neonates and young children less than two years of age

After appropriate treatment for the infection, investigation should be pursued because infection in a young child should be considered a marker for possible underlying structural or functional abnormalities in the urinary tract, the detection of which may alter management. In young children with bacteriuria or urinary infections, the incidence of radiological abnormalities, including reflux, is around 40–60% and is a little lower in children over the age of six (Whitaker and Sherwood, 1984).

In neonates and children up to the age of two, appropriate investigation includes renal ultrasound and a micturating cystourethrogram (MCU) to seek for possible reflux. The bladder is filled with iodine-containing contrast fluid via a urethral catheter or sometimes a suprapubic puncture. It is reasonably well established that a combination of urinary tract infection with vesicoureteric reflux and intrarenal reflux is associated with the development of reflux nephropathy. Such renal damage is most likely to occur in children under the age of five and probably under the age of two. Reflux in older children, whilst sometimes accompanied by infection, only occasionally results in new scars or progression of older ones. The reason for this might well relate to the higher voiding pressures observed in younger children, particularly if associated with sphincter-active voiding. There is some evidence that vesicoureteric reflux might result from transient fetal urethral obstruction (Avni and Schulmann, 1996). Reflux nephropathy is sometimes associated with renal failure and hypertension.

If renal ultrasound is abnormal, then a DMSA scan or IVU may be indicated. If dilatation of the renal pelvis is noted, then an IVU is indicated to detect the site of any obstruction, e.g. congenital hydronephrosis due to pelvic–ureteric junction obstruction or a ureterocoele.

Reflux might predispose to urinary tract infection because of a residual urine and the system not emptying completely, with the ureter acting like a diverticulum into which urine passes during voiding and from which it empties back into the bladder after voiding.

Not all patients with reflux will have a urinary tract infection and the incidence of reflux lessens as the child grows. The older patient with endstage renal failure due to reflux nephropathy often has no clear history of urinary infection in childhood.

Family members of those found to reflux should be assessed initially by an ultrasound and other studies if this is abnormal. Reflux appears to be genetically determined with an autosomal mode of inheritance. The incidence in families varies between 15% and 30%.

(ii) Girls aged 2–5 years

In children older than two, most units limit investigations to a plain X-ray, renal ultrasound and a DMSA scan. Detection of any abnormality might lead on to an IVU or other appropriate tests as indicated.

Micturating cystourethrograms are indicated if urinary tract infections are recurrent but it appears that reflux is rarely associated with development of new scars of reflux nephropathy after the age of two and a rather uncomfortable X-ray can be avoided safely in most cases (***Figure 3.6***).

(iii) Girls over the age of five

In the absence of obstruction, urinary tract infection over the age of five will rarely cause renal damage but can be associated with significant morbidity. Predisposing factors need to be sought, in particular vulvitis, possible sexual abuse, thread worms, diabetes and foreign bodies. Investigations should include vulval swabs and anal skin test for worm ova if appropriate.

A plain abdominal X-ray (kidneys, ureters, bladder or KUB) is undertaken to seek for stone or foreign body. A renal ultrasound is used to detect any dilatation of the upper tracts and any significant PVR. This can be combined with a flow rate. If the pattern of voiding flow is intermittent this would suggest sphincter-active voiding. Detection of a

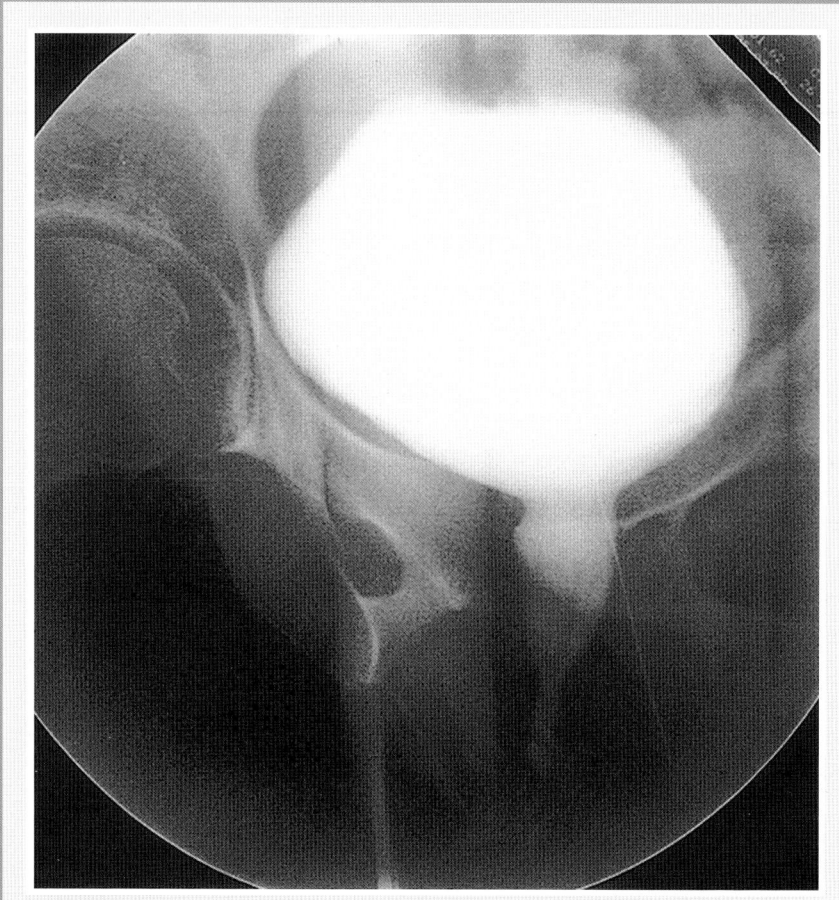

Figure 3.6
Voiding cystourethrogram showing sphincter-active voiding.

dilated upper urinary tract would lead to an IVU and a possible MCU and DMSA scan.

If sphincter-active voiding is suspected on history or flow rate, an MCU, preferably with pressure measurements, should be performed (Allen, 1977; van Gool and Tanagho, 1977). Some have used electromyography (EMG) of the sphincter with needle or skin disc electrodes but these investigations can be uncomfortable and produce artefacts by their very presence. They add little to what can be discovered by routine video urodynamic studies. Sphincter-active voiding is best managed by patient education and retraining, sometimes with biofeedback. Children and adults can simply listen to the sound of the urine stream on the potty or toilet and concentrate on relaxing the pelvic floor and making a continuous sound. This type of biofeedback can be performed using more complicated apparatus of flow meters and pressures in tertiary referral centres. Neuromodulation has been used in refractory cases and in adults (Schmidt and Tanagho, 1981).

Secondary enuresis can be cause by urinary tract infections but can also occur as a result of disorganized voiding due to neurological causes like tethered cord syndrome. Urodynamic studies should be performed if a neurological disorder is suspected.

Urinary incontinence both day and night might lead to excoriation and vulvitis and predispose to urinary tract infection. An ectopic ureter should be suspected and an IVU arranged. A duplex system with a dilated upper segment may be the clue to an ectopic ureter opening below the sphincter mechanism.

Over half the children with proven urinary infections have no anatomic abnormality. Some of these will have functional sphincter-active voiding. Some will need suppressive antibiotics for 6–12 months.

(iv) Women in the reproductive years

Where urinary tract infection is proven in a woman with fever and loin pain and a clinical diagnosis of acute pyelonephritis is made, appropriate antibiotics should be administered. If the infection is an uncomplicated one and resolves promptly, no further investigations are warranted. However, if prompt resolution does not occur or in recurrent cases, an urgent plain film to exclude stones and an ultrasound to exclude obstruction should be performed. A DMSA scan might then be useful in selected cases in detecting areas of reduced perfusion and areas of scarring. Abnormal scans need to be repeated approximately three months after acute pyelonephritis. Serum C-reactive protein (CRP) is often elevated in acute pyelonephritis.

Recurrent infections with proteus often indicate a urinary stone. Vulvovaginal examination can sometimes reveal local anomalies like a minor degree of hypospadias where the meatus opens more proximally along the vaginal wall.

Associated vulvovaginitis and urethritis

should lead to tests to exclude sexually transmitted infections and diabetes. If there is also urinary incontinence this can cause excoriation and the patient should undergo investigations of the problem, including urodynamic studies.

Prolapse of the bladder base (cystocele) can lead to PVR and predispose to urinary tract infections, as can chronic constipation.

A urethral diverticulum can present as a painful swelling in the anterior vaginal wall if it gets infected. If more chronic, it can present with a urinary flow which is slow and often slows down towards the end of micturition as the diveticulum fills and presses on the urethra, causing obstruction. After voiding, a urethral discharge of the urine in the diverticulum can occur, leading to what is thought initially to be a vaginal discharge. If suspected, these can be difficult to image radiologically but a micturating cystourethrogram using undiluted contrast often outlines them (see *Figure 3.3*). A catheter with two balloons, one for the bladder neck and one at the meatus with an opening of the catheter between the two for injecting contrast, has been advocated by some to produce a positive pressure urethrogram.

Where urinary tract infections become recurrent, a flexible cystoscopy should be suggested to exclude infections secondary to stones or growths. Infection can occur on the encrusted surface of a tumour.

(v)   Postmenopausal women

Women confined to bed for medical reasons and who have to perch on a bedpan rarely empty their bladders completely; as a result of the persistent PVR, urinary tract infections in hospital medical wards are very common.

Recurrent urinary infections or symptoms suggesting it in the absence of a proven infection can sometimes be alleviated by hormone replacement therapy (HRT), either orally or by vaginal cream/pessaries. If vulvovaginitis is present, vaginal swabs to exclude candida, etc. should be undertaken, diabetes should be excluded and, if associated with incontinence, urodynamic investigations should be undertaken.

If haematuria has occurred, then urinary cytology, an IVU and cystoscopy should be undertaken to exclude tumour or stone.

(vi)   Patients at any age with neurological symptoms or signs

Neurological problems can predispose to a urinary tract infection causing incomplete bladder emptying or relative mucosal ischaemia from prolonged periods of high bladder pressure, which reduces the natural bladder defences against bacterial infection.

These patients should have an independent flow rate, plain X-ray and ultrasound and a urodynamic study looking for dyssynergia of the external sphincter, impaired bladder emptying, and to exclude stone or reflux. Therapeutic measures may be required to lower high bladder pressure by anticholinergics with or without intermittent self-catheterization to improve bladder emptying.

(vii)   Communication between bowel and bladder or incorporation of intestinal segments in the urinary tract

(a)   Fistula between bowel and bladder

Colonic diverticulitis, Crohn's disease or bowel cancer can cause pericolic abscess which then ruptures into the bladder. Fistulae may also be a complication of pelvic irradiation. The diagnosis can be made by history and presence of associated pneumaturia. A barium enema or colonoscopy is needed to define the cause of the bowel lesion. A cystoscopy and biopsy of the edge of a fistula can be useful in differentiating benign from malignant causes in these cases.

(b)   Enterocystoplasty

Operations to replace the excised bladder completely or to augment its capacity use a defunctional segment of small and/or large bowel taken out of circuitry and incorporated into the neobladder. About 30% of such patients develop persistent or recurrent urinary tract infections. There is also an increased risk of tumour development in the

new bladder, so many authors suggest a cystoscopy be undertaken every two years after the first five years from the operation.

(c)   Intestinal conduit urinary diversion

Urine in an ileal conduit often has a resident flora. Most ureterointestinal anastomoses allow free reflux to the kidneys and thus episodes of urinary tract infection are not uncommon. Infection in combination with mucus can predispose to developing infective renal stones.

(d)   Ureterosigmoidostomy

This is an operation not often performed now because of the complicating problems with ascending infection, ureterosigmoidostomy obstruction and stone disease and sometimes renal failure. Again, some of these patients develop tumours at the site of the ureterosigmoidostomy anastomosis. Regular sigmoidoscopy is advocated.

2.   Fungal infections in the urinary tract

These are common after antibiotic treatment of bacterial infections where the absence of normal flora allows candida to grow. Diabetic women and women with long-term catheters or stents, and the immunocompromised are at special risk. The organism once cleared from the urinary tract can recolonize from the bowel or vagina so that if bladder washouts are done for the candida cystitis, oral and vaginal antifungals like mycostatin should also be given.

3. Symptoms but sterile urine

Non-infective causes, such as urethral syndrome, interstitial cystitis, bladder and ureteric stones, tumours and foreign bodies, together with drug-induced cystitis, will be addressed in Chapter 9.

(i)   Tuberculosis

Unfortunately tuberculosis is increasing worldwide again. Some symptomatic patients in whom infection is not confirmed on routine testing but who do have persistent pyuria will have TB. Unless specifically sought by several (3–6) early morning urine samples and appropriate Lowenstein-Jensen (LJ) culture, it may remain undetected. An IVU and a cystoscopy should be performed. The IVU may show strictures at the caliceal neck, pelvic–ureteric junction, along the ureter at the pelvic brim or at the ureterovesical junction. They are often multiple. There may be associated pyocalyx, pyonephrosis or non-function. If biopsied, a tuberculous bladder ulcer will show changes typical of TB and allow more prompt therapy than is possible if one needs to await the urinary TB cultures which cannot be considered negative until up to eight weeks later.

(ii)   Viral

Herpes zoster viral infections of the sacral dorsal nerve roots can lead to typical skin rashes (shingles) on sacral segments but can also be associated with similar vesicles on the trigone with intense frequency and urgency. The disorder can also render the bladder areflexic.

(iii)   Schistosomiasis

This parasite is spreading worldwide and all travellers should be warned against the risks of swimming in fresh water in Africa and Asia. Equally, urologists should be aware of the condition and test urine specifically looking for ova in any person at risk after an overseas trip. Such patients should have upper tract imaging, usually an IVU as haematuria is common and may be caused by ureteric strictures predisposing to stones as well as the chronic inflammation caused by the ova. Cystoscopy and biopsy of any suspicious areas of 'sandy patch' change or ulceration may need to be done in order to make the diagnosis and to exclude any sinister causes.

V   Conclusion

Any urinary tract infection in infants and young children might prove to be a marker of underlying congenital or acquired pathology and should always be fully investigated.

In older women, lower urinary tract symptoms are usually due to ascending infection. UTIs are the cause of a great deal of discomfort and morbidity but usually respond well to antibiotics unless complicated by anatomical abnormalities. If they become recurrent, they need to be investigated to detect any predisposing cause.

References

Allen TD (1977) The non-neurogenic bladder. *J Urol* 117: 232–8.

Avni EF, Shulmann CC (1996) The origin of vesico-ureteric reflux in male newborns: further evidence in favour of a transient fetal urethral obstruction. *Br J Urol* 78: 454–9.

Bailey RR, Lynn KL, Robson RA, Smith AH, Maling TMJ, Turner JG (1996) DMSA renal scans in adults with acute pyelonephritis. *Clin Nephrol* 46: 99–104.

Fairley KF, Bond AG, Brown RB, Haber S, Berger P (1967) Simple test to determine site of urinary tract infection. *Lancet* ii: 427.

Gallagher DJA, Montgomery SZ, North JDK (1965) Acute infections in the urinary tract and the urethral syndrome in general practice. *BMJ* 1: 622–6.

Gillenwater JY, Wein AJ (1988) Summary of the National Institute of Arthritis, Diabetes, Digestive and Kidney Diseases Workshop on interstitial cystitis. *J Urol* 140: 203–6.

Hampson SJ, Noble JG, Rickards D, Milroy EJG (1992) Does residual urine predispose to urinary tract infection? *Br J Urol* 70: 506–8.

Kaefer M, Barnewolt C, Retik AB, Peters CA (1997) The sonographic diagnosis of intravesical obstruction in children: evaluation of bladder wall thickness indexed to bladder filling. *J Urol* 157: 989–91.

Kullar V, Cardozo LD, Salvatore S, Hill S (1996) Ultrasound: a non-invasive screening test for detrusor instability. *Br J Obstet Gynaecol* 103: 904–8.

Landman J, Kavaler E, Chang Y, Droller MJ, Liu BC-S (1998) Sensitivity and specificity of NMP-22, telomerase, and BTA in the detection of human bladder cancer. *J Urol* 159(5) (suppl): 245.

Resnick NM, Yalla SV (1987) Detrusor hyperactivity with impaired contractile function: an unrecognised but common cause of incontinence in elderly patients. *JAMA* **257**: 3076–81.

Rushton HG, Majd M, Jantausch B, Weidermann BL, Belman AB (1992), Renal scarring following reflux and non-reflux pyelonephritis in children with a ^{99m}technetium-dimercapto succinic acid scintigraphy. *J Urol* **147**: 1327.

Schmidt RA, Tanagho EA (1981) Urethral syndrome or urinary tract infection? *Urology* **18**: 424–7.

Stamey TA, Govan DE, Palmer JM (1965) The localisation and treatment of urinary tract infections: the role of bactericidal urine levels as opposed to serum levels. *Medicine* **44**: 1.

Stevens M (1989) Screening urines for bacteriuria. *Med Lab Sci* **46**: 194–206.

Talner CB, Davidson AJ, Lebowitz RL, Dalla-Palma L, Goldman SM (1994) Acute pyelonephritis: can we agree on terminology? *Radiology* **192**: 297–305.

van Gool J, Tanagho EA (1977) External sphincter activity and recurrent urinary tract infection in girls. *Urology* **10**: 348.

Whitaker RH, Sherwood T (1984) Another look at diagnostic pathways in children with urinary tract infections. *BMJ* **288**: 839.

Antibacterial therapy of uncomplicated acute cystitis

Kurt G Naber

4

Contents

I Introduction

Acute lower uncomplicated urinary tract infection, i.e. acute uncomplicated cystitis, is one of the most common bacterial infections in women. It was estimated that 20 to 30% of adult women experience one or more episodes of dysuria yearly and most of these episodes represent acute uncomplicated cystitis (Sandford, 1975). Since Grüneberg and Brumfitt conducted the first single-dose clinical trial in 1967 (Grüneberg and Brumfitt, 1967), a large number of studies have assessed the efficacy of single-dose antibacterial treatment of acute cystitis in women (Bailey, 1990). In recent years, a 3-day therapy was recommended for some antibacterial agents because in comparative clinical studies better results were achieved by 3-day regimens than with single dose. Single-dose or short-term (3-day) therapeutic regimens are attractive as they insure compliance, reduce costs, have less impact on the normal fecal and vaginal flora and possibly decrease the emergence of resistant organisms.

Before a specific antibacterial agent can be recommended for a single-dose or short-term therapeutic regimen, the cure rate should be equivalent to those of conventional 5- or 7-day treatments and confirmed by well designed studies of adequate sample size. Unfortunately only a few studies satisfy these requirements (Fihn and Stamm, 1985). To minimize the type II or β-error the results of comparable studies are usually cumulated for meta-analysis, yet this is a compromise. Having this in mind, this review tries to find out which oral antibacterial agents should be recommended for a single-dose or a short-term regimen for the treatment of acute uncomplicated cystitis in women.

II Amoxicillin, classical oral cephalosporins, co-trimoxazole, nitrofurantoin

Amoxicillin and co-trimoxazole have widely been used as oral agents for single-dose, short-term and conventional regimens. Reviewing several studies, Philbrick and Bracikowski (Philbrick and Bracikowski, 1985) concluded that single-dose amoxicillin is less effective than conventional therapy, but single-dose co-trimoxazole is as effective as a multiple dose. In a meta-analysis, Leibovici and Wysenbeek (Leibovici and Wysenbeek, 1991) analysed the data of 25 controlled studies in order to compare the efficacy of a single-dose regimen versus longer treatment courses, e.g. a 3-day course or conventional course (≥5 days) of therapy. A considerable difference between a single dose and a 3-day course or conventional course of therapy was found in the two subgroup analyses performed with amoxicillin and trimethoprim-sulfamethoxazole (co-trimoxazole).

Similar findings were made by Norrby

Table 4.1
Eradication of bacteriuria in patients treated with trimethoprim (TMP) alone or in combination with a sulfonamide, such as sulfamethoxazole

TMP-sulfa time	Follow-up			
	< 2 weeks		≥ 2 weeks	
Single dose	267/300	(89.0%)	114/176	(81.8%)
3-day course	139/147	(94.6%)	117/138	(84.8%)
≥ 5-day course	294/308	(95.5%}	170/187	(90.9%)
From Norrby (1990).				

(Norrby, 1990) who reviewed 28 trials in which trimethoprim, usually in combination with sufonamides, and beta-lactam antibiotics were used and various treatment durations were compared. When analysing the results with all antibacterial agents, he postulated that a single dose was less effective than a 3-day course of therapy. This was less pronounced for co-trimoxazole than for beta-lactams. With co-trimoxazole the early eradication of bacteriuria (< 2 weeks) after a single dose was 89%, compared to 94.6% for a 3-day course and 95.5% for conventional treatment (≥ 5 days) (*Table 4.1*). It was concluded that co-trimoxazole treatment should not be continued for longer than 3 days because of comparable cure rates but with lower risk of adverse reactions. The statistical difference between a single dose and a 3-day course was significant ($P < 0.05$) with 95% confidence

interval points of 0.5% and 10.5%. However, the clinical relevance of this finding can be questioned, especially when considering the shortcomings mentioned above. For example, in one of the studies (Fihn et al., 1988) a single dose of co-trimoxazole was compared with a 10-day course in a randomized double-blind manner. The patients were followed on days 3, 13 and 42. There was no statistically significant difference in symptoms cured or improved at any time. Only at day 13 was there a statistically ($P < 0.01$) higher risk of failure/recurrence in the group treated with a single dose. However, at this time in the group treated with single dose, the antibacterial treatment had already been discontinued for 12 days, whereas in the group treated for 10 days the treatment had only been discontinued for 3 days. Therefore, the results have to be interpreted with caution.

Table 4.2
Eradication of bacteriuria in patients treated with an oral β-lactam antibiotic, such as amoxicillin, or with one of the first generation oral cephalosporins

β-lactams time	Follow-up			
	< 2 weeks		≥ 2 weeks	
Single dose	53/80	(66.3%)	126/175	(72.0%)
3-day course	282/343	(82.2%)	117/156	(75.0%)
≥ 5-day course	370/423	(87.5%)	175/226	(77.4%)

From Norrby (1990).

In the meantime, there is enough evidence to suggest that trimethoprim combined with or without sulfonamides should best be administered for 3 days.

When aminopenicillins and classical oral first-generation cephalosporins were used as a single dose, the cure rates were unacceptably low (*Table 4.2*). As a compromise Norrby (Norrby, 1990) recommended a 3-day therapy which, although less effective, caused fewer adverse effects than a conventional (≥5 days) therapy. As few studies have been conducted to evaluate the newer cephalosporins no conclusion can be drawn at this moment.

Only a few studies evaluating short-term nitrofurantoin therapy have been performed. One study (Gossius, 1984) compared nitrofurantoin single dose to a 10-day regimen. There was no statistical difference in eradication rates, but the study was of insufficient power. There was, however, a significantly higher rate of adverse events with the longer term therapy, 4/104 (4%) versus 15/114 (13%). A randomized trial of 3-day regimens comparing trimethoprim/sulfamethoxazole (160/320 mg twice daily), macrocrystalline nitrofurantoin (100 mg four times daily), cefadroxil (500 mg twice daily), or amoxicillin (500 mg three times daily) was performed by Hooton and colleagues (Hooton et al., 1995). They found that a 3-day regimen of trimethoprim/sulfamethoxazole was more effective and less expensive than 3-day regimens of nitrofurantoin, cefadroxil, or amoxicillin.

III   Fluoroquinolones

The fluoroquinolones are rapidly absorbed from the gastrointestinal tract, penetrate well into body fluids, are widely distributed and

Table 4.3
Antibacterial activity as minimal inhibitory concentration (MIC) of norfloxacin at different pH values in various media against 22 clinical isolates

pH	MIC (mg/litre) geometric mean	
	Mueller–Hinton	Urine
8.4	0.17	0.33
7.4	0.20	0.34
6.5	0.39	4.11
5.8	2.00	10.27
5.2	6.00	23.30

From Machka and Braveny (1984).

Table 4.4
Median urinary concentrations (mg/litre) of fluoroquinolones*

Time (h)	Norfloxacin (800 mg)	Ciprofloxacin (500 mg)	Enoxacin (400 mg)	Fleroxacin (400 mg)	Ofloxacin (200 mg)
0–4	422	150	423	210	458
4–8	147	108	278	186	215
8–12	58	51	109	99	93
12–24	22	10	43	116	76
24–48	nd	2.6	4.6	40	nd
48–72	nd	nd	nd	11	nd

* In volunteers (11,12) after oral dose. nd = not done.
From Naber (1989).

attain high urinary concentrations that exceed several times the minimal inhibitory concentrations (MIC) for the commonly encountered urinary tract pathogens. However, the antibacterial activity of the fluoroquinolones is generally much lower in urine than in nutrient broth, and in acid rather than in alkaline milieu (Machka and Braveny, 1984). This results in an up to 100-fold increase of MIC in the clinical situation (*Table 4.3*). The currently available fluoroquinolones have different urinary concentrations (*Table 4.4*) (Sörgel et al., 1989; Naber, 1989). In general, however, they are suitable antibacterial agents for short-term therapy of uncomplicated acute cystitis in women (Andriole, 1991; Bailey, 1992).

Norfloxacin was mainly studied (Reeves et al., 1984; Ganguli et al., 1985; Rugendorff and Schneider, 1985; Bischoff, 1985; Stein et al., 1987; Inter-Nordic Urinary Tract Infection Study Group, 1988; Pippo et al., 1990; Miano et al., 1990; Reynaert et al., 1990; Saginur and Nicolle, 1992; Del Rio et al., 1996) in a 3-day course (*Table 4.5*) with an overall bacteriological eradication rate at early follow-up ($\leqslant 2$ weeks) of 95% and cumulatively at late follow-up (> 2 weeks) of 87%. In two studies, a single-dose regimen (800 mg) was used (Rugendorff and Schneider, 1985; Saginur and Nicolle, 1992); the results were inferior to the 3-day course. Only one of four studies comparing a 3-day course with conventional therapy (7–14 days) showed, at late follow-up, significantly better results in the conventional arm; otherwise, the 3-day course was comparable to conventional therapy. However, in two studies the eradication rates of *Staphylococcus saprophyticus* were inferior in the 3-day arm (Inter-Nordic Urinary Tract Infection Study Group, 1988; Pippo et al, 1990).

For enoxacin, a twice-daily regimen over 3 days, when compared with single-dose enoxacin therapy, may be preferable in cases of *S. saprophyticus* infection, although clinical and bacteriologic responses were not significantly different (Backhouse and Matthews, 1989).

Ciprofloxacin was studied with single-dose regimens ranging from 100 to 750 mg. Most of the early studies (*Table 4.6*), however, had only small sample sizes (Garlando et al., 1987; Martin et al., 1987; Gellermann et al., 1988; Raz et al., 1989; Dedinsky and Bittner, 1989) resulting in an overall eradication rate of 83% at early follow up (< 2 weeks). From three recent studies (Iravani et al., 1995a) with larger sample sizes using single-dose (500 mg), 3-day courses (100–250 mg twice daily and 500 mg once daily), a 5-day (500 mg once daily) and a 7-day course (250 mg twice daily) the authors concluded that for ciprofloxacin, a 3-day course with either 250 mg or 100 mg (minimum effective dose) twice daily is an appropriate dosage regimen (*Table 4.7*). There was no evidence that a 3-day regimen of ciprofloxacin 100 mg twice daily would be any less efficacious in treating *S. saprophyticus* than in treating *E. coli* infections. The risk factors that might predict bacteriologic failure included initial colony counts ($\geqslant 10^5$ cfu/ml), UTI within the previous 6 weeks, frequency of intercourse, the use of a diaphragm and in one study age over 40 years. In two further studies (Iravani et al., 1995b) the 3-day regimen of ciprofloxacin, 100 mg twice daily, was compared in one study with 7-day courses of trimethoprim/sulfamethoxazole, 160/800 mg twice daily, and nitrofurantoin, 100 mg twice daily, and in the other study with 3-day courses of trimethoprim/ sulfamethoxazole, 160/800 mg twice daily,

Table 4.5
Norfloxacin: eradication of bacteriuria by short-term therapy in uncomplicated lower UTI

Drug	Dose (mg)/ course duration	≤2 weeks	> 2 weeks*	Year	Reference
Nor	400 bd/3 days	53/55 (96%)	40/45 (89%)	1984	Reeves et al.
Nal	660 q8 h/3 days	45/55 (82%)	29/43 (67%)		
Nor	400 bd/3 days	48/50 (96%)	48/50 (96%)	1985	Ganguli et al.
Nor	800 sd	23/27 (85%)	21/24 (88%)	1985	Rugendorff et al.
Nor	400 bd/3 days	30/32 (94%)	28/30 (93%)		
Nor	400 bd/3 days	45/50 (84%)	–	1985	Bischoff
Nor	400 bd/3 days	71/74 (96%)	67/74 (91%)	1987	Stein et al.
T/S	960 bd/10 days	81/81 (100%)	78/81 (96%)		
Nor	400 bd/3 days	181/193 (94%)	157/193 (81%)	1988	Inter-Nordic UTI Study Group
Nor	400 bd/7 days	169/180 (97%)	165/180 (92%)		
Nor	400 bd/3 days	159/163 (98%)	143/164 (87%)	1990	Piippo et al.
Nor	400 bd/7 days	158/162 (98%)	149/163 (91%)		
Nor	400 bd/3 days	93/94 (99%)	60/65 (92%)	1990	Miano et al.
Nor	400 bd/2 weeks	72/72 (100%)	52/56 (93%)		
Nor	400 bd/3 days	14/16 (87%)	9/16 (56%)	1990	Reynaert et al.
Fos	3000 sd	14/16 (87%)	13/16 (81%)		
Nor	800 sd	59/73 (81%)	53/73 (78%)	1992	Saginur and Nicolle
Nor	400 bd/3 days	78/83 (94%)	73/83 (88%)		
Nor	400 bd/3 days	73/74 (99%)	52/55 (95%)	1996	Del Rio et al.
Ruf	400 sd	77/82 (94%)	61/69 (88%)		
Total					
Nor	400 bd/3 days	842/884 (95%)	677/775 (87%)		
Nor	800 sd	80/100 (80%)	74/97 (76%)		

* Cumulative results (treatment failures were forwarded; non-compliant patients were not included in the baseline).
sd = single dose; bd = twice daily.
Nor = norfloxacin; Nal = nalidixic acid; T/S = trimethoprim/sulfamethoxazole (co-trimoxazole); Fos = fosfomycin trometamol; Ruf = rufloxacin.

Table 4.6
Ciprofloxacin: eradication of bacteriuria (< 2 weeks) by short-term therapy in uncomplicated lower UTI

Drug	Dose (mg)	Single dose	3 days	≥5 days	Year	Reference
Cip	100 sd	16/19 (84%)			1987	Garlando et al.
Cip	250 sd	17/19 (89%)				
Cip	500 sd	21/23 (91%)			1987	Martin et al.
Cip	100 bd			20/20 (100%)		
Cip	125 sd	20/32 (64%)			1988	Gellermann et al.*
Cip	250 sd	37/42 (88%)				
Cip	250 bd		26/30 (85%)			
Cip	250 sd	43/53 (81%)			1989	Raz et al.**
Cip	750 sd	38/46 (85%)				
Cip	500 sd	6/6 (100%)			1989	Dedinsky et al.
T/S	960 sd	5/6 (83%)				
Cip	Total	198/240 (83%)				

Cip = ciprofloxacin; T/S = trimethoprim/sulfamethoxazole (co-trimoxazole).
sd = single dose; bd = twice daily.
* Including elderly.
** Including recurrent UTI.

and of ofloxacin, 200 mg twice daily. The 3-day courses of ciprofloxacin were as effective as that of the other 3-day and 7-day regimens. The overall results for patients treated with ciprofloxacin, 100 mg twice daily, for 3 days were 92% at early and 83% at late follow-up.

Ofloxacin (*Table 4.8*) showed comparable overall eradication rates at early follow-up (< 2 weeks) with single dose (88%) and 3-day courses (89%). (Black et al., 1987; Ludwig and Panthner, 1987; Naber, 1987; Ode, 1987; Teare and Tettmar, 1989; Moorehouse et al., 1989; Naber, 1990; Hooton et al., 1991; Asbach, 1991; Naber and Koch, 1993; Raz et al., 1994). In one study, however, ofloxacin 100 mg single dose was significantly inferior to a conventional course of cotrimoxazole (Ode, 1987). In the study (Hooton et al., 1991) comparing 400 mg single dose with 200 mg twice daily for

Table 4.7
Ciprofloxacin: eradication of bacteriuria by short-term therapy in uncomplicated lower UTI

Drug	Dose (mg)/ course duration	5–9 days	4–6 weeks*	Year	Reference
Cip	500 qd/3 days	137/149 (92%)	107/133 (80%)	1995	Iravani et al.
Cip	500 qd/5 days	134/149 (90%)	91/129 (71%)		
Nor	400 bd/7 days	133/141 (94%)	99/118 (84%)		
Cip	500 sd	95/107 (89%)	80/99 (81%)	1995	Iravani et al.
Cip	250 bd/7 days	101/103 (98%)	89/96 (92%)		
Cip	100 bd/3 days	98/105 (93%)	73/84 (87%)	1995	Iravani et al.
Cip	250 bd/3 days	95/105 (90%)	69/91 (76%)		
Cip	250 bd/7 days	98/106 (93%)	77/91 (85%)		
Cip	100 bd/3 days	148/168 (88%)	118/150 (79%)	1995	Iravani et al.
T/S	960 bd/7 days	161/174 (93%)	113/157 (72%)		
Ntf	100 bd/7 days	153/177 (86%)	115/165 (70%)		
Cip	100 bd/3 days	215/228 (94%)	173/207 (84%)	1995	Iravani et al.
T/S	480 bd/3 days	224/230 (97%)	175/207 (85%)		
Ofx	200 bd/3 days	211/228 (93%)	155/201 (77%)		
Total Cip	100 bd/3 days	461/501 (92%)	364/441 (83%)		

* Cumulative results (treatment failures were forwarded; non-compliant patients were not included in the baseline).
Cip = ciprofloxacin; T/S = trimethoprim/sulfamethoxazole (co-trimoxazole); Nor = norfloxacin; Ntf = nitrofurantoin;
Ofx = ofloxacin.
sd = single dose; bd = twice daily; qd = once daily.

3 days, the early eradication rates were comparable. At 5 weeks post-treatment, 81% treated with single dose and in 89% treated with 3 days of ofloxacin, and 98% treated with co-trimoxazole for 7 days were cured ($P = 0.03$, single-dose ofloxacin group versus co-trimoxazole group). Thus, 100 mg or 200 mg twice daily for 3 days can be considered the appropriate dose for ofloxacin.

Lomefloxacin was used as a 3-day regimen in two studies (Neringer et al., 1992; Nicolle et al, 1993). A 3-day course was bacteriologically less effective than a 7-day course, 180/196 (92%) versus 190/194 (98%); $P = 0.006$, but showed a lower rate of adverse events (25% versus 31%, statistically not significantly different) (Neringer et al., 1992). If the 3- and 7-day courses of

Table 4.8
Ofloxacin: bacteriological eradication (< 2 weeks) by short-term therapy in uncomplicated lower UTI

Drug	Dose (mg)/ course duration	Single dose	3 days	≥5 days	Year	Reference
Ofx	100 bd		89/97 (92%)		1987	Block et al.
T/S	960 bd		81/92 (88%)			
Ofx	100 bd		34/42 (81%)		1987	Ludwig and Pauthner
Ntf	100 td			21/32 (66%)		
Ofx	100 sd	25/29 (86%)			1987	Ludwig et al.
Ofx	100 bd		27/30 (90%)			
Ofx	100 sd	26/28 (93%)			1987	Naber
T/S	1000 sd	33/36 (92%)				
Ofx	100 sd	44/60 (73%)			1987	Ode et al.
T/S	960 bd			55/59 (93%)		
Ofx	200 bd		18/20 (90%)		1989	Teare and Tettmar
Tmp	200 bd		24/27 (89%)			
Ofx	200 sd	9/9 (100%)			1989	Moorhouse et al.
Amx	3000 sd	6/8 (75%)				
Ofx	200 sd	98/107 (92%)			1990	Naber and Thyroff-Friesinger
T/S	960 sd	93/105 (89%)				
Fos	3000 sd	182/213 (85%)				
Ofx	400 sd	42/45 (93%)			1991	Hooton et al.
Ofx	200 bd		44/48 (92%)			
T/S	960 bd			42/44 (95%)		
Ofx	200 sd	17/19 (89%)			1991	Asbach
T/S	960 sd	16/19 (84%)				
Cfm	400 sd	17/19 (89%)				
Plo	– sd	5/19 (26%)				
Ofx	100 bd/3 days		57/64 (89%)		1992	Naber and Koch
Cfx	125 bd/3 days		53/66 (80%)			
Ofx	200 bd		43/50 (86%)		1994	Raz et al.
Cfm	400 qd		41/49 (83%)			
Total Ofx			261/297 (88%)	312/351 (89%)		

sd = single dose; bd = twice daily; qd = once daily; Tmp = trimethoprim; T/S = trimethoprim/sulfamethoxazole in combination with a sulfonamide (sulfamethoxazole or sulfadiazine); Ntf = nitrofurantoin; Amx = amoxicillin; Fos = fosfomycin trometamol; Cfm = cefixime; Cfx = cefuroxime axetil; Ofx = ofloxacin; Plo = placebo.

lomefloxacin were pooled (Neringer et al., 1992; Nicolle et al., 1993), then there was no difference between lomefloxacin and norfloxacin (98% versus 97%), but norfloxacin showed lesser adverse events than lomefloxacin (24% versus 35%); $P \leqslant 0.001$.

Pefloxacin is almost completely absorbed after oral administration. Plasma elimination half-life ranges between 7.2 and 12 h after a single oral dose. Pefloxacin is excreted and concentrated in urine at about 14% as parent drug and about 20% as the major metabolite N-demethylpefloxacin (norfloxacin) (Lode et al., 1990; Hofbauer et al., 1997). Urinary bactericidal activity is maintained for 5 to 7 days after administration of a single oral 800 mg dose (Guibert et al., 1989; Hofbauer et al., 1997). A meta-analysis (Naber et al., 1994) comprising seven clinical trials (five controlled and two non-comparative multicentre clinical trials) with a total of 1578 women enrolled, revealed a pooled rate of bacteriological eradication of 77% as compared to 74% using co-trimoxazole for 3–7 days at 4–6 weeks follow-up. In one study, pefloxacin single dose (800 mg) was compared with norfloxacin 400 mg twice daily over 5 days (Van Balen et al., 1990). Bacteriological eradication at 4–6 weeks follow-up was achieved in 54% and 58% in pefloxacin and norfloxacin patients, respectively. It should be noted that in this meta-analysis patients not compliant were rated as failures.

In another study (Jardin and Cesana, 1995) pefloxacin (800 mg single dose) was compared with rufloxacin (400 mg single dose). Of 178 patients in the intention-to-treat group and treated with pefloxacin, 136 (84%) and 165 patients treated with rufloxacin 127 (88%) showed bacteriological eradication at 7 to 10 days after treatment. At 4 weeks post-treatment, the bacteriological success was reduced to 78% and 80%, respectively, if patients with reinfections were considered treatment failures. The study confirmed also a good cure for *S. saprophyticus* and *P. mirabilis* infections. This was explained by the particularly high and prolonged concentrations of both fluoroquinolones in urine.

Fleroxacin is almost totally absorbed after oral administration with about the same half-life (8–12 h) as pefloxacin, but in contrast to pefloxacin almost completely excreted in the urine as the parent drug by glomerular filtration (Sörgel et al., 1989). In a total of eight studies (*Table 4.9*), fleroxacin was tested in single doses of 200–600 mg, usually 400 mg, with an overall eradication rate of 92% at early and 86% at late follow-up (Weissenbacher et al., 1987; Kosmidis et al., 1988; Moller et al., 1988; Walstad et al., 1989; Whitby, 1989; Bailey et al., 1989; Kajanoja et al., 1990; Iravani, 1993). In one study (Iravani, 1993) the results obtained by single dose were inferior to those of conventional therapy. This, however, was not true for the late follow-up investigation.

Table 4.9
Fleroxacin: bacteriological eradication by single-dose therapy in uncomplicated lower UTI

Drug	Dose (mg)/ course duration	≤2 weeks	> 2 weeks*	Year	Reference
Flx	2000 sd	17/20 (85%)	–	1987	Weissenbacher et al.
Flx	400 sd	10/10 (100%)	–	1989	Kosmodis et al.
Flx	600 sd	10/10 (100%)	–		
Amx	3000 sd	10/10 (100%)	–		
Flx	200 sd	4/4 (100%)	–	1988	Moller et al.
Flx	400 sd	13/15 (87%)	–		
Flx	200 sd	24/24 (100%)	20/24 (83%)	1989	Walstad et al.
Flx	400 sd	33/37 (89%)	29/37 (78%)		
Flx	400 sd	32/33 (97%)[a]	20/22 (91%)	1989	Whitby
Amx	3000 sd	22/39 (56%)	8/26 (31%)		
Flx	400 sd	16/17 (94%)	–	1989	Bailey et al.
Tmp	600 sd	16/18 (89%)	–		
Flx	200 sd	52/54 (96%)	–	1990	Kajanoja et al.
Flx	400 sd	63/66 (95%)	–		
Flx	400 sd	151/172 (88%)[b]	40/44 (91%)	1993	Iravani
Flx	200 qd/7 days	173/180 (96%)	56/63 (89%)		
Cip	500 qd/7 days	196/204 (96%)	56/60 (93%)		
Total					
Flx	200 sd	97/102 (95%)	20/24 (83%)		
Flx	400 sd	318/350 (91%)	89/103 (86%)		
Flx	total	425/462 (92%)	109/127 (86%)		

* Cumulative results (treatment failures were forwarded; non-compliant patients were not included in the baseline).
[a] P > 0.001; [b] P > 0.05.
Flx = fleroxacin; Amx = amoxicillin; Tmp = trimethoprim; Cip = ciprofloxacin.
sd = single dose; qd = once daily.

Rufloxacin, a fluoroquinolone with an even longer half-life (about 28 h) (Wise et al., 1991), was used as single dose of 400 mg and compared in one study with a 3-day course of norfloxacin (400 mg twice daily) (Del Rio et al., 1996) and in another study with pefloxacin

Table 4.10
Eradication rates of fosfomycin trometamol (single dose). 3 g as fosfomycin, in adult females with acute lower UTI

	3–10 days	3–6 weeks
Eradication rate	87%	79%
Range	75–100%	62–93%
Patients (eradication/total)	475/544	461/583
Number of trials	12	12

From Naber (1992).

(800 mg single dose) (Jardin and Cesana, 1995). In both studies, the clinical and bacteriological results were comparable (no statistically significant difference). In the group treated with rufloxacin, however, a higher rate (20.4%) of patients reported adverse events compared with those (12%) treated with norfloxacin. A statistically significant difference ($P = 0.001$) was found when comparing patients reporting adverse reactions related to the central nervous system between the group treated with rufloxacin (11.7%) and that treated with norfloxacin (0%).

IV Fosfomycin trometamol

Fosfomycin trometamol is an orally absorbable derivate of the drug fosfomycin, a broad-spectrum antibiotic, with a bioavailability of about 50% and with high and long-lasting urine concentrations,

resulting in bactericidal activity in urine without regrowth within 24 h (bladder model) (Greenwood, 1990). A review of 12 comparative studies (eight open and four double blind) with a total of 1733 adult females enrolled, revealed comparable eradication rates for a single dose (3 g) of fosfomycin trometamol as compared to the reference drugs (Naber, 1992). The bacteriological eradication rates at about 1 week (3–10 days) of follow-up with fosfomycin trometamol ranged from 75 to 100% and at 4 weeks of follow-up from 62 to 93% (*Table 4.10*). It should be noted that in not all studies were the patients investigated at early as well as at late follow-up.

Stein (Stein, 1998) analysed three randomized, double-blind, placebo-controlled trials of single-dose (3 g) fosfomycin trometamol which have been conducted in the USA, but none of these studies has been published. Fosfomycin trometamol was

Table 4.11
Clinical success and bacteriological eradication rates one week post-treatment of fosfomycin trometamol (single dose), 3 g as fosfomycin, in women with uncomplicated urinary tract infection as compared to nitrofurantoin (7 days); ciprofloxacin (7 days) and trimethoprim/sulfamethoxazole (10 days)

Drug	Duration	Patients	Clinical success (per cent)	Bacteriological eradication (per cent)
Fos	sd	260	69%	83%
Ntf	7 days	237	70%	76%
Fos	sd	268	76%	83%
Cip	7 days	245	82%	97%
Fos	sd	273	73%	86%
T/S	10 days	239	75%	93%

Fos = fosfomycin trometamol; Ntf = nitrofurantoin; Cip = ciprofloxacin; T/S = trimethoprim/sulfamethoxazole. sd = single dose. From Stein (1998).

compared with nitrofurantoin (7 days), ciprofloxacin (7 days), and trimethoprim-sulfamethoxazole (10 days) in women who had uncomplicated UTIs with symptoms of less than 4 days' duration (*Table 4.11*). These studies found that clinical cures were similar for fosfomycin trometamol and the comparative agents. Microbiological eradication was superior for ciprofloxacin and trimethoprim-sulfamethoxazole compared with fosfomycin trometamol.

V   Discussion

Acute uncomplicated cystitis usually is a self-limiting infection with a high spontaneous cure rate. In only a few studies compared with unspecific, nonantibacterial therapy (Rugendorff et al., 1983; Naber et al., 1985; Asbach, 1991) could it, however, be demonstrated that antibacterial agents are superior in achieving earlier relief of symptoms and bacterial eradication. Nevertheless, it can be assumed that within one week of onset about 20–50% of the patients become asymptomatic without antibacterial therapy. Therefore, only highly effective and well-tolerated antibacterial regimens should be recommended for treatment of acute uncomplicated cystitis, because the main aim of the treatment of acute uncomplicated cystitis is prompt release of symptoms and reduction of morbidity.

Numerous antibacterial agents have been

used in the past for this indication, but not all substances are equally suitable for single-dose or short-term therapy. This may be owing to their pharmacokinetic properties and mode of antibacterial activity in urine. According to his clinical results, Kumamoto (Kumamoto, 1992) postulated that antibiotics which produce long-lasting effective urinary concentrations are preferable. The possible higher initial urinary concentrations of antibacterial agents with shorter half-lives and more rapid renal excretion obviously cannot compensate for that. This may explain why the beta-lactams such as amoxicillin and the classical oral cephalosporins are not the ideal agents for single-dose or short-term therapy.

Although trimethoprim has a long half-life, its mode of antibacterial activity in urine is only bacteriostatic and the elimination of bacteria from urine is achieved relatively late (Helm et al., 1979). Nevertheless, it could be demonstrated that therapy no longer than 3 days is necessary when trimethoprim is combined with sulfamethoxazole (Norrby, 1990). On the other hand, studies with substances such as fosfomycin trometamol and some of the fluoroquinolones, especially when using substances with prolonged half-lives such as pefloxacin, fleroxacin and rufloxacin, have demonstrated that single-dose therapy is as effective as other standard regimens. Fluoroquinolones with shorter half-lives, such as norfloxacin, ciprofloxacin, ofloxacin, and lomefloxacin, are better administered in a 3-day regimen.

A relative comparison between different substances concerning their antibacterial urinary activity in vivo can be achieved by determining urinary bacterial titres over time after drug administration. Comparing norfloxacin and pefloxacin in this manner we could demonstrate (Hofbauer et al., 1997) that pefloxacin exhibits much longer antibacterial activity in urine (up to 5 days (median) against a susceptible *E. coli* and up to 2 days against *S. saprophyticus*) than norfloxacin. The time in which norfloxacin is bactericidal may be already too short for a less-susceptible *S. saprophyticus* strain which seems to be reflected in inferior clinical results compared to UTI caused by *E. coli*. These results may explain why a 1-day regimen with pefloxacin might be equally effective as a 3-day regimen with norfloxacin. A comparison of pefloxacin and fleroxacin in this manner could show that half the dose of fleroxacin exhibits about the same urinary bacterial titres over time as does a full dose of pefloxacin (Naber et al., 1998).

Whether a single-dose or 3-day is chosen, it should be explained to the patient that the inflammatory process might last longer than the time of bacterial eradication and that the symptoms may disappear only in about 80% of cases within 2 days and that they may last somewhat longer in the remaining ones (Brumpt et al., 1988). A review of the literature on uncomplicated urinary tract infections revealed no cases of resistance development in association with single-dose or short-term therapy with fluoroquinolones in contrast to those with amoxicillin (Hooton et al., 1995).

Postmenopausal women, in contrast to younger women, have relatively high rates of failure or reinfection, and therefore some authors consider UTIs in such patients as complicated cystitis (Raz and Rozenfeld, 1996). Raz and Rozenfeld enrolled 250 postmenopausal women in a clinical study. Most of the women (87%) had recurrent cystitis. Women were excluded from the study if they had renal insufficiency, neurogenic bladder, nephrolithiasis, a permanently indwelling catheter, diabetes or any other immunosuppressive disease, cystoceles grades II–III, or the presence of urinary pathogens resistant to one of the agents used in the study. They compared a 3-day course of 200 mg of ofloxacin once daily with a 7-day course of 500 mg of cefalexin four times a day. The bacterial spectrum consisted of 190/223 *E. coli*, 19/223 *K. pneumoniae*, 9/223 *P. mirabilis* and 5/223 *M. morganii*. Of the 223 women evaluable for treatment outcome at 3–5 days after therapy, 77% showed bacterial eradication with ofloxacin and 64% with cefalexin. The authors concluded that treatment with ofloxacin was more effective and cheaper than that with cefalexin. The authors compared their results with those found by Iravani et al. (1995) who

used two different fluoroquinolones in women ⩾40 years old. The eradication rates with ciprofloxacin (0.5 g once a day) administered for 3 and 5 days were 75% and 63%, respectively. A 7-day course of 400 mg of norfloxacin twice a day was more effective, leading to a 93% eradication rate.

It has been shown that oestrogen (e.g. as an intravaginal cream) can reduce recurrences. Where treatment of premenopausal and postmenopausal patients are compared in clinical studies, it is important to separate these two groups. Whether postmenopausal women with an episode of cystitis without underlying nephropathy or uropathy should be defined as having complicated UTI remains questionable as a conventional treatment course with a suitable antibacterial agent gives better short- and long-term results than can be achieved in patients with complicated UTI owing to urological abnormalities (Frankenschmidt et al., 1997).

Since acute uncomplicated cystitis in women is a very common infection, any improved management is favourable both for the individual patient but also for the health care system. Only a few studies have addressed these aspects. Hooton et al. (1995) performed a randomized computer trial with cost analysis of 3-day antimicrobial regimens with co-trimoxazole (160 mg/800 mg twice daily), cefadroxil (500 mg twice daily), or amoxicillin (500 mg three times daily). Six weeks after treatment 32 (82%) women treated with co-trimoxazole were cured compared with 22 (61%) treated with nitrofurantoin ($P = 0.04$ vs. co-trimoxazole), 21 (66%) treated with cefadroxil ($P = 0.11$ vs. co-trimoxazole), and 28 (67%) treated with amoxicillin ($P = 0.11$ vs. co-trimoxazole). Persistence of significant bacteriuria was less common with co-trimoxazole (3%) and cefadroxil (0%) as compared with nitrofurantoin (16%; $P = 0.05$ vs. co-trimoxazole) and amoxicillin (14%; $P = 0.11$ vs. co-trimoxazole). Persistence of bacteriuria was associated with amoxicillin-resistant strains in the amoxicillin group, but with nitrofurantoin-susceptible strains in the nitrofurantoin group. Co-trimoxazole was more successful in eradicating *E. coli* from rectal cultures soon after therapy and from urethral and vaginal cultures at all follow-up visits compared with the other treatment regimens. Adverse effects were reported by 16 (35%) patients receiving co-trimoxazole, 18 (43%) receiving nitrofurantoin, 12 (30%) receiving cefadroxil and 13 (25%) receiving amoxicillin. The mean costs per patient were less with co-trimoxazole ($114) and amoxicillin ($131) compared with nitrofurantoin ($155) and cefadroxil ($155). The authors concluded that a 3-day regimen of co-trimoxazole is more effective and less expensive than 3-day regimens of nitrofurantoin, cefadroxil, or amoxicillin for treatment of acute uncomplicated cystitis in women. The increased efficacy of co-trimoxazole was believed to be related to its antimicrobial effects against *E. coli* in the rectum, urethra and vagina.

Rosenberg and Waugh (1996) performed a cost-benefit and cost-effectiveness analysis comparing a 3-day course of ofloxacin with 7-day courses of co-trimoxazole, ampicillin and nitrofurantoin. They found that ofloxacin was the most cost-effective antibiotic for empirical treatment of uncomplicated UTIs. In their analysis costs of patients' evaluation, treatment, and outcomes were taken from published literature. Antibiotic susceptibilities were determined from 1000 samples from four areas in the USA. The results were robust over a broad range of values; the main findings that might have altered these conclusions were the antimicrobial sensitivity of *E. coli* strains susceptible to co-trimoxazole over ofloxacin and co-trimoxazole. A rate of more than 92% of *E. coli* strains susceptible to co-trimoxazole would have favoured co-trimoxazole over ofloxacin. Therefore, the authors recommended that antimicrobial sensitivities which might vary should be determined as a first step.

Only in a few less studies were the MICs determined for the uropathogens correlated with the clinical outcome. However, it is not clear a priori whether the breakpoints used in any system, e.g. NCCLS, DIN, etc. are relevant also for the treatment of acute uncomplicated cystitis. Such data are usually not available because of several reasons.

- In only a few laboratories, uropathogens cultured from women with acute uncomplicated cystitis were determined and analysed separately.
- Since the treatment of acute uncomplicated cystitis is empirical, in most cases no urine cultures are taken either at all, or only in cases with treatment failures.
- The susceptibility data are extrapolated from other urine cultures obtained from outpatients or inpatients, which might be misleading.

In one multicentre study (Naber and Thyroff-Friesinger, 1992) we determined the MICs of various antibiotics for 249 uropathogens cultured from women with acute uncomplicated cystitis. In this study, for the total bacterial spectrum the resistance rate of ofloxacin was 0% and that of co-trimoxazole 4%. A few years later a similar study (Naber and Koch, 1993) showed a resistance rate for co-trimoxazole of 12% and that for ofloxacin of 3.4%.

VI Conclusion

Acute uncomplicated cystitis in premenopausal women can be treated effectively by short-term therapy if suitable antibacterial agents and dosage regimens are used. Short-term therapy has clearly advantages over conventional treatment, mainly by reduction of adverse events. Therefore, short-term therapy should be considered the treatment of choice for this kind of infection. From the results of all these studies, a 3-day regimen can be recommended for trimethoprim alone or in combination with a sulfonamide, such as sulfamethoxazole, and for fluoroquinolones with moderately long half-lives, such as ciprofloxacin, enoxacin, lomefloxacin, norfloxacin and ofloxacin. A single dose may be recommended for those fluoroquinolones with longer half-lives, such as pefloxacin, fleroxacin and rufloxacin. Fosfomycin trometamol may also be an alternative for a single-dose therapy.

As long as the resistance rate for *E. coli* against trimethoprim is low (< 10%), trimethoprim alone or in combination with a sulfonamide may be considered the first-line drug. Otherwise, one of the fluoroquinolones or fosfomycin trometamol should be considered as alternatives according to the tolerability of each drug and its cost. Agents which have not been shown to be effective in any of these short-term regimens should no longer be propagated for the treatment of acute uncomplicated cystitis. Consequently, no further studies using conventional therapy of acute uncomplicated cystitis are necessary in the future.

References

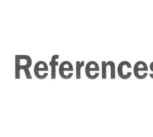

Andriole VT (1991) Use of quinolones in treatment of prostatitis and lower urinary tract infections. *Eur J Clin Microbiol Infect Dis* April: 342–50.

Asbach HW (1991) Single dose oral administration of cefixime 400 mg in the treatment of acute uncomplicated cystitis and gonorrhoea. *Drugs* 42(Suppl 4): 10–13.

Backhouse EI, Matthews JA (1989) Single-dose enoxacin compared with 3-day treatment of urinary tract infection. *Antimicrob Agents Chemother* 33: 877–80.

Bailey RR (1990) Review of published studies on single dose therapy of urinary tract infections. *Infection* 18(suppl 2): 53–6.

Bailey RR (1992) Quinolones in the treatment of uncomplicated urinary tract infections. *Int J Antimicrob Agents* 2: 19–28.

Bailey RR, Peddie BA, Davies PR (1989) Randomized trial comparing single dose fleroxacin (Quinodis) and trimethoprim (Triprim) for treatment of bacterial cystitis. *Clin Trials* 26: 411–16.

Bischoff W (1985) Norfloxacin-Behandlung der akuten Zystitis der Frau und der bakteriellen Prostatitis. *Fortschr Med* 103: 225–8.

Block, Walstad RA, Bjertnaes A, Hafstad PE, Holte M, Ottemo I, Svarva PL, Rolstad T, Peterson LE (1987) Ofloxacin vs. trimethoprim-sulphamethoxazole in acute cystitis. *Drugs* 34(Suppl 1): 100–6.

Brumpt I, Guibert J, Delleur G (1988) Etude clinique de la péfloxacine en prise unique de 800 mg dans le traitement de la cystite bactérienne de la femme. *Temps Méd* 320: 74–80.

Dedinsky B, Bittner MJ (1989) One-dose ciprofloxacin or trimethoprim-sulfamethoxazole therapy of urinary tract infections with analysis of drug resistance and urinalysis findings in the rural Dominican Republic. *Clin Res* **27**: 973A.

Del Rio G, Dalet F, Aguilar L, Caffaratti J, Dal-Re R (1996) Single dose rufloxacin versus 3-day norfloxacin treatment of uncomplicated cystitis: clinical evaluation and pharmacodynamic considerations. *Antimicrob Agents Chemother* **40**: 408–12.

Fihn SD, Stamm WE (1985) Interpretation and comparison of treatment studies for uncomplicated urinary tract infections in women. *Rev Infect Dis* **7**: 468–78.

Fihn SD, Johnson C, Roberts PL, Running K, Stamm WE (1988) Trimethoprim-sulfamethoxazole for acute dysuria in women: a single-dose or 10-day course. A double-blind, randomized trial. *Ann Intern Med* **108**: 350–7.

Frankenschmidt A, Naber KG, Bischoff W, Kullmann K (1997) Once-daily fleroxacin versus twice daily ciprofloxacin in the treatment of complicated urinary tract infections. *J Urol* **158**: 1494–9.

Ganguli LA, Keaney MGL, Gould LJ (1985) Norfloxacin: a three-day course for the treatment of urinary tract infection. *Drugs Exp Clin Res* **9**: 177–9.

Garlando F, Rietiker S, Täuber MG, Flepp M, Meier B, Lüthy R (1987) Single-dose ciprofloxacin at 100 vs. 250 mg for treatment of uncomplicated urinary tract infection in women. *Antimicrob Agents Chemother* **31**: 354–6.

Gellermann HJ, Grote J, Peters-Haertel W, Verbeek H (1988) Kurzzeit-Therapie von unkomplizierten Harnwegsinfektionen der Frau mit Ciprofloxacin. *Med Welt* **39**: 1586–91.

Gossius G (1984) Single-dose nitrofurantoin therapy for urinary tract infections in women. *Curr Therapeut Res* **35**: 925–31.

Greenwood D (1990) Fosfomycin trometamol: activity in vitro against urinary tract pathogens. *Infection* **18**(Suppl 2): S60–S65.

Grüneberg RN, Brumfitt W (1967) Single dose treatment of acute urinary tract infection. *Br Med J* **3**: 649–51.

Guibert J, Kitzis MD, Brumpt I, Cara JF (1989) Activité antibactérienne de la péfloxacine dans l'urine durant sept jours aprés prise orale unique de 800 mg. *Path Biol* **37**: 406–10.

Helm EB, Munk I, Shah PM, Stille W (1979) Elimination of bacteria during antibacterial chemotherapy, a neglected parameter of chemotherapy. *Infection* (Suppl 5): 492–4.

Hofbauer H, Naber KG, Kinzig-Schippers M, Sörgel F, Rustige-Wiedemann C, Wiedemann B, Reiz A, Kresken M (1997)

Urine bactericidal activity of pefloxacin versus norfloxacin in healthy female volunteers after a single 800-mg oral dose. *Infection* **25**: 121–6.

Hooton TM, Johnson C, Winter C, Kuwamura L, Rogers ME, Roberts PL, Stamm WE (1991) Single-dose and three-day regimens of ofloxacin vs. trimethoprim-sulfamethoxazole for acute cystitis in women. *Antimicrob Agents Chemother* **35**: 1479–83.

Hooton TM, Winter C, Tiu F, Stamm WE (1995) Randomized comparative trial and cost analysis of 3-day antimicrobial regimens for treatment of acute cystitis in women. *JAMA* **273**: 41–5.

The Inter-Nordic Urinary Tract Infection Study Group (1988) Double-blind comparison of 3-day versus 7-day treatment with norfloxacin in symptomatic urinary tract infections. *Scand J Infect Dis* **20**: 619–24.

Iravani A. (1993) Multicenter study of single-dose and multiple-dose fleroxacin vs. ciprofloxacin in the treatment of uncomplicated urinary tract infections. *Am Med* **94**(Suppl 3A): 89–96.

Iravani A, Tice AD, McCarty J, Sikes DH, Nolen T, Gallis HA, Whalen EP, Tosiello RL, Heyd A, Kowalsky SF, Echols RM (1995a) Short-course ciprofloxacin treatment of acute uncomplicated urinary tract infection in women. The minimum effective dose. *Arch Intern Med* **155**: 485–94.

Iravani A, Heyd A, Tosiello RL, Block AL, Echols RM (1995b) Low-dose, short-course ciprofloxacin treatment of acute urinary tract infection in women. Poster. Presented at the 19th International Congress of Chemotherapy, Montreal, Canada.

Jardin A, Cesana M (1995) Randomized, double-blind comparison of single-dose regimens of rufloxacin and pefloxacin for acute uncomplicated cystitis in women. French Multicenter Urinary Tract Infection-Rufloxacin Group. *Antimicrob Agents Chemother* **39**: 215–20.

Kajanoja P, Kivinen S, Ranta T, Hulkko S, Walstag RE, Stramboulian D, Valdes EF, Moeller BR (1990) Treatment of uncomplicated urinary tract infections of females by a single oral dose of fleroxacin; comparison of two doses, 200 mg and 400 mg. Abstract no. 231. Presented at the 3rd International Symposium on New Quinolones, Vancouver, Canada, 12–14 July 1990.

Kosmidis J, Gargalianos P, Adamis G, Petropoulou D, Makris D (1988) Fleroxacin in single dose oral therapy of uncomplicated lower urinary tract infection. *J Antimicrob Chemother* **22**(Suppl D): 219–21.

Kumamoto Y (1992) Single-dose treatment of female acute uncomplicated cystitis. *Infection* **20**(Suppl 3): 173–4.

Leibovici L, Wysenbeek AJ (1991) Single-dose antibiotic treatment for symptomatic urinary tract infections in women: a meta-analysis of randomized trials. *Q J Med New Series* **78**: 43–57.

Lode H, Höffken G, Boeck M, Deppermann N, Koeppe P (1990) Quinolone pharmacokinetics and metabolism. *J Antimicrob Chemother* **26**(Suppl B): 41–9.

Ludwig G, Pauthner H (1987) Clinical experience with ofloxacin in upper and lower urinary tract infections. A comparison with co-trimoxazole and nitrofurantoin. *Drugs* **34**(Suppl 1): 95–9.

Machka K, Braveny I (1984) Inhibitorische Wirkung verschiedener Faktoren auf die Aktivität von Norfloxacin. In: Stille W, Adam D, Eickenberg HU, Knothe H, Ruckdeschl G, Simon C, Gyrase-Hemmer I, eds. *Fortschritte der Antimikrobiellen und Antineoplastischen Chemotherapie*, FAC 3-5. Munich: Futuramed, 557–62.

Martín G, Kobelt R, Carmona O (1987) Ciprofloxacin con dosis unica y convencional en el tratamiento de infeccion urinaria aguda. Sensibilidad comparativa de uropatogenos hospitalarios. *Acta Physiol Pharmacol Latinoam* **37**: 67.

Miano L, Goldoni S, Tubaro A, Paradiso Galatioto G, Gandolfi P (1990) Review of norfloxacin in lower urinary tract infections. *Eur Urol* **17**(Suppl 1): 13–18.

Moller BR, Kaspersen P, Mamsen A, Korsager B, Quitzau K (1988) Fleroxacin in the treatment of uncomplicated acute cystitis in women. *J Antimicrob Chemother* **22**(Suppl D): 215–18.

Moorhouse EC, McNamara C, Clarke PC (1989) A comparison of the efficacy of single dose treatment of ofloxacin with amoxycillin in the treatment of acute lower urinary tract infection. Abstract no. 188. Presented at the 16th International Congress of Chemotherapy, Jerusalem, Israel, June.

Naber KG, Asbach HW, Burchhardt P, Schneider H-J, Weidner W, Weißbach L (1985) Single dose therapy and reinfection prophylaxis of acute bacterial cystitis in females. In: *Proceedings of the 36th Congress of the German Society for Urology, Bremen, 3–6 October 1984*, Berlin: Springer, 363–71.

Naber KG (1987) Single dose therapy with ofloxacin vs. cotrimazine in the treatment of acute cystitis in female. Proceedings of the 15th International Congress of Chemotherapy, Istanbul, Turkey, 19–24 July 1987. *Progress in Chemotherapy*. Antimicrobial Section 1, Landsberg, Germany: Ecomed, 1282–4.

Naber KG (1989) Use of quinolones in urinary tract infections and prostatitis. *Rev Infect Dis* **11**(Suppl 5): 1321–37.

Naber KG, Thyroff-Friesinger U (1990) Fosfomycin trometamol vs. ofloxacin/co-trimoxazole as single dose therapy of acute uncomplicated urinary tract infection in females: a multicenter study. *Infection* **18**(Suppl 2): 70–6.

Naber KG (1992) Fosfomycin trometamol in treatment of uncomplicated lower urinary tract infections in adult women – an overview. *Infection* (Suppl 4): 310–12.

Naber KG, Koch EMW (1993) Cefuroxime axetil versus ofloxacin for short-term therapy of acute uncomplicated lower urinary tract infections in women. *Infection* **21**: 34–9.

Naber KG, Thynroff-Friesinger U (1992) Spectrum and susceptibility of pathogens causing acute uncomplicated lower UTI in females and its correlation to bacteriologic outcome after single dose therapy with fosfomycin trometamol versus ofloxacin/co-trimoxazole. *Infection* **20**(Suppl 4): S297–S301.

Naber KG, Theuretzbacher U, Kinzig M, Savoy O, Sörgel F (1998) Urinary excretion and bactericidal activity of a single oral dose of 400 milligrams of fleroxacin versus a single oral dose of 800 milligrams of pefloxacin in healthy volunteers. *Antimicrob Agent Chemother* **42**: 1659–65.

Naber KG, Baurecht W, Fischer M, Kresken M (1994) Pefloxacin single-dose in the treatment of acute uncomplicated lower urinary tract infections in women: a meta-analysis of seven clinical trials. *Int J Antimicrob Agents* **4**: 197–202.

Neringer R, Forsgen A, Hanson C, Ode B, The South Swedish Lolex Study Group (1992) Lomefloxacin versus norfloxacin in the treatment of uncomplicated urinary tract infections: three-day versus seven-day treatment. *Scand J Infect Dis* **24**: 773–80.

Nicolle LE, Dubois J, Martel AY, Harding GKM, Shafran SD, Conly JM (1993) Treatment of uncomplicated urinary tract infections with 3 days of lomefloxacin compared with treatment with 3 days of norfloxacin. *Antimicrob Agents Chemother* **37**: 574–9.

Norrby SR (1990) Short-term treatment of uncomplicated lower urinary tract infections in women. *Rev Infect Dis* **12**: 458–67.

Ode B, Walder M, Forsgren A (1987) Failure of a single dose of 100 mg ofloxacin in lower urinary tract infections in females. *Scand J Infect Dis* **19**: 677–9.

Philbrick J, Bracikowski JP (1985) Single dose antibiotic treatment for uncomplicated urinary tract infections. Less for less? *Arch Intern Med* **145**: 1672–8.

Piipo T, Pitkäjärvi T, Salo SA (1990) Three-day versus seven-day treatment with norfloxacin in acute cystitis. *Curr Therapeut Res* **47**: 644–53.

Raz R, Rozenfeld S (1996) 3-day course of ofloxacin versus cefalexin in the treatment of urinary tract infections in postmenopausal women. *Antimicrob Agents Chemother* 40: 2200–1.

Raz R, Stamm WE (1993) A controlled trial of intravaginal estriol in postmenopausal women with recurrent urinary tract infections. *N Engl J Med* 329: 753–6.

Raz R, Rottenstreich F, Hefter H, Knees Y, Potasman I (1989) Single-dose ciprofloxacin in the treatment of uncomplicated urinary tract infection in women. *Eur J Clin Microbiol Infect Dis* 8: 1040–2.

Raz R, Rottensterich E, Leshem Y, Tabenkin H (1994) Double-blind study comparing 3-day regimens of cefixime and ofloxacin in treatment of uncomplicated urinary tract infections in women. *Antimicrob Agent Chemother* 38: 1176–7.

Reeves DS, Lacey RW, Mummery RV, Mahendra M, Bint AJ, Newson SWB (1984) Treatment of acute urinary infection by norfloxacin or nalidixic acid/citrate: a multi-centre comparative study. *J Antimicrob Chemother* 13(Suppl B): 99–105.

Reynaert J, van Eyck D, Vandepitte J (1990) Single dose fosfomycin trometamol vs. multiple dose norfloxacin over three days for uncomplicated UTI in general practice. *Infection* 18(Suppl 2): 77–9.

Rosenberg M, Waugh MS (1996) Antibiotic choice in empiric treatment of urinary tract infections: a cost-benefit and cost-effectiveness analysis. Poster. Presented at the Interscience Conference on Antimicrobial Agents and Chemotherapy (ICAAC), New Orleans, Louisiana, USA, September 15–18, 1996.

Rugendorff EW, Schneider HJ (1985) Randomized comparison of single-dose versus short-term norfloxacin therapy in acute urinary tract infections. Presented at the 14th International Congress of Chemotherapy, Kyoto 23–28 June.

Rugendorff EW, Naber KG, Späth A, Stürmer K, Ahrens T, Dietlein G (1983) Antibakterielle Behandlung von unkomplizierten Harnwegsinfektionen mit einem neuen Cephalosporin: Cefroxadin (CGP 9000). In: Stille W, ed. *Kurzzeittherapie von Harnwegsinfektionen*. Munich: Zuckschwerdt, 112–21.

Saginur R, Nicolle LE (1992) Single-dose compared with 3-day norfloxacin treatment of uncomplicated urinary tract infection in women. *Arch Intern Med* 152: 1233–7.

Sandford JP (1975) Urinary tract symptoms and infections. *Annu Rev Med* 26: 485–98.

Sörgel F, Faehde K, Naber KG, Stephan U (1989) Pharmacokinetic disposition of quinolones in human body fluids and tissues. *Clin Pharmacokin* **16**(Suppl 1): 5–24.

Stein GE (1998) Single-dose treatment of acute cystitis with fosfomycin tromethamine. *Ann Pharmacother* **32**: 215–19.

Stein GE, Mummaw N, Goldstein EJC, Boyko EJ, Reller LB, Kurtz TO, Miller K, Cox CE (1987) A multicenter comparative trial of three-day norfloxacin vs. ten-day sulfamethoxazole and trimethoprim for the treatment of uncomplicated urinary tract infections. *Arch Intern Med* **147**: 1760–2.

Teare EL, Tettmar R (1989) A comparison of the efficacy and safety of ofloxacin or trimethoprim in treatment of uncomplicated lower urinary tract infection. Abstract no. 183. Presented at the 16th International Congress of Chemotherapy, Jerusalem, Israel, June.

Van Balen FAM, Touw-Otten FWMM, de Melker RA (1990) Single-dose pefloxacin vs. 5-days treatment with norfloxacin in uncomplicated cystitis in women. *J Antimicrob Chemother* **26**(Suppl B): 153–60.

Walstad RA, Bjertnaes A, Block JM, Hofstad PE, Julsrud E, Ottemo I (1989) Single dose therapy with fleroxacin (RO 23-6240) in patients suffering from community acquired acute, uncomplicated urinary tract infection. A double-blind dose range finding study. In: Rubinstein E et al., eds. *Recent Advances in Chemotherapy Antimicrobial*, Section 1. Presented at the 16th International Congress on Chemotherapy, Jerusalem, Israel, 1989. Tel-Aviv, Israel: E. Lewin-Epstein, 1989, 288.1–288.3.

Weissenbacher ER, Gutschow K, Wachter I, Schneider A, Gotz A, Tsutsulopulos C (1987) Single application of RO 23-6240 (200 mg) in acute lower urinary tract infections (UTI). In: Berkada P et al., eds. *Progress in Antimicrobial and Anticancer Chemotherapy*, Vol. 2. Proceedings of the 15th International Congress on Chemotherapy, Istanbul, Turkey, 19–24 July 1987. Landsberg, Germany: Ecomed: 1987: 1094–5.

Whitby M (1989) Fleroxacin vs. amoxicillin in single dose therapy of uncomplicated urinary tract infection. In: Rubinstein E et al., eds. *Recent Advances in Chemotherapy*, Jerusalem, Israel, 1989, 290.1–290.3.

Wise R, Johnson J, O'Sullivan N, Andrews JM, Imbimbo BP (1991) Pharmacokinetics and tissue penetration of rufloxacin, a long acting quinolone antimicrobial agent. *J Antimicrob Chemother* **28**: 905–9.

Prevention

Lindsay E Nicolle

5

Contents

I Introduction

Urinary infection is a common bacterial infection, which may be associated with substantial morbidity and, occasionally, mortality. The prevention of urinary infection and its complications is beneficial to both the individual and society but it is a realistic goal for only selected clinical groups with frequent episodes. In some situations efforts to prevent infection have not been shown to be beneficial.

This chapter summarizes current knowledge and practice relevant to prevention of urinary infection in women. Specific clinical presentations discussed include recurrent acute uncomplicated urinary infection (acute cystitis), acute pyelonephritis in pregnancy and some aspects of complicated urinary tract infection.

II Prevention of acute uncomplicated urinary infection

1. General considerations

Women who experience recurrent acute, uncomplicated urinary infection repeatedly have usually been advised to modify selected behaviours to prevent infection (*Table 5.1*). These behavioural interventions have frequently been reinforced by the medical establishment, as well as the popular media. Proposed

interventions have included drinking large quantities of fluids, voiding frequently, diet, type of underwear, avoiding baths, wiping from front to back after toileting, and use of specific soaps. The evidence, however, does not support a benefit of these interventions in decreasing the frequency of urinary infection (Foxman and Frerichs, 1985b; Remis et al., 1987). These case control studies of premenopausal women with and without recurrent urinary infection found no significant difference between groups in behaviours including beverage use, tampon or soap use, type of underwear or frequency of urination. Thus, these modifications should not be promoted as a means to prevent symptomatic recurrence and women should be reassured that these personal practices are not a cause of infections.

Certain other activities, however, are associated with an increased frequency of urinary infection. A strong association between sexual intercourse and urinary infection, with increasing frequency of both symptomatic and asymptomatic episodes of infection with increasing frequency of infection, has been repeatedly reported (Foxman and Frerichs, 1985a; Hooton et al., 1996; Leibovici et al., 1987; Nicolle et al., 1982). Thus, abstaining from sexual intercourse is one possible 'preventive measure' but is not a realistic intervention for the majority of women. While early studies suggested that immediate postintercourse voiding may decrease the frequency of urinary infection in women with

Table 5.1
Prevention of recurrent acute, uncomplicated urinary infection

Effective	Not effective
Avoid spermicide or diaphragm	Frequency of voiding
Prophylactic antimicrobials:	Increasing fluids
long term	Avoiding baths
postintercourse	Menstrual hygiene
	Perineal hygiene
	Clothing
	Postcoital voiding

frequent, recurrent infections (Strom et al., 1987), this has not been confirmed in subsequent studies (Hooton et al., 1996). The use of spermicides as foam, gel or with a diaphragm is associated with an increased frequency of urinary infection (Foxman and Frerichs, 1985a; Hooton et al., 1991, 1996) and the use of a diaphragm by itself may be associated with some increased risk (Foxman and Frerichs, 1985a; Hooton et al., 1991, 1996; Remis et al., 1987). Other methods for birth control, including a condom without spermicide, the birth control pill (Hooton et al., 1991; Leibovici et al., 1987; Remis et al., 1987) and the cervical cap (Hooton et al., 1996), are not associated with an increased frequency of infection. Thus, avoiding spermicide-based birth control measures is a reasonable intervention to prevent urinary infections in some women.

2.   Antimicrobial therapy for prevention

Clinical trials have consistently documented that continuous low-dose prophylactic antimicrobials will prevent about 95% of symptomatic episodes of cystitis in women with frequent, recurrent episodes (Brumfitt and Hamilton-Miller, 1995; Nicolle, 1992; Nicolle and Ronald, 1987; Raz and Boger, 1991). Antimocrobial prophylaxis to prevent infection is usually considered if there have been at least two episodes in the past six months or three in the past 12 months. Prophylactic regimens with efficacy documented in clinical trials are listed in *Table 5.2*. Trimethoprim/sulfamethoxazole, trimethoprim, and nitrofurantoin are considered first-line therapy. The daily medication is usually taken at bedtime. Duration of prophylaxis is variable but

Table 5.2
Antimicrobial regimens effective for prevention of recurrent acute uncomplicated urinary infection.

Agent	Dose
Long-term low dose	
Trimethoprim/sulfamethoxazole	$^1/_2$ (80/400 mg) daily or 3 × weekly
Trimethoprim	100 mg daily
Nitrofurantoin	50 mg daily
Nitrofurantoin macrocrystals	100 mg daily
Cephalexin	125–250 mg daily
Norfloxacin	200 mg 3 × weekly
Ciprofloxacin	250 mg 3 × weekly
Postintercourse	
Trimethoprim/sulfamethoxazole	$^1/_2$ regular strength (80/400 mg) tablet
Trimethorpim	100 mg
Cephalexin	250 mg
Ciprofloxacin	250 mg
Ofloxacin	200 mg
Norfloxacin	200 mg

initially six months or one year is recommended.

Prophylactic antimicrobial therapy appears to be effective through at least two mechanisms. The source of organisms causing uncomplicated urinary infection, usually *Escherichia coli*, is the gut. Women with infection are frequently colonized in the vagina and periurethral area with *E. coli* or other potential uropathogens. Antimicrobials such as TMP/SMX (Stamey et al., 1977) and the quinolones (Nicolle et al., 1989) decrease colonization of aerobic Gram-negative flora of the bowel and vagina. Thus, these agents are

effective through eradication of potential uropathogens from the reservoir. Nitrofurantoin has no impact on colonization but in clinical trials is as effective as other agents in prevention of infection (Stamm et al., 1980). Thus, it appears to be effective through intermittent sterilization of the urine.

Long-term low-dose prophylactic antimicrobial therapy remains effective while the woman continues to take the medication but the prophylactic course does not alter the subsequent frequency of recurrent infection once the antimicrobial is discontinued. Approximately 50% of women will have a symptomatic episode of infection within three months following discontinuation of prophylactic therapy (Stamm et al., 1980). This incidence is similar to that prior to initiation of prophylactic therapy. Thus prophylaxis does not alter the natural history of recurrent acute uncomplicated urinary infection in the individual woman. When early recurrence occurs following discontinuation of prophylaxis, the antimicrobial therapy may be reinstituted. Prophylaxis may be continued for as long as two (Harding et al., 1982) or five (Nicolle et al., 1988) years with efficacy maintained and without an increased occurrence of colonization with resistant organisms or adverse effects.

Prophylactic antimicrobial therapy is also effective when given as a single postintercourse dose (see *Table 5.2*) (Pfau and Sacks, 1991; Stapleton et al., 1990; Vosti, 1975). Long-term low-dose antimicrobials and postintercourse prophylaxis have not been evaluated directly in comparative trials but non-comparative reports suggest the approaches are equally effective. For women with frequent recurrent infection the choice of preventive strategy, either long-term low-dose prophylaxis or postintercourse prophylaxis, is an individual one. Different women will have different needs and preferences based on lifestyle and other factors.

While low-dose prophylactic antimicrobial therapy is very effective in decreasing the frequency of symptomatic infection, occasional infections will occur in women receiving prophylaxis. The rate of infection is usually reported as 0.1–0.2 infections per patient-year (Nicolle and Ronald, 1987). When a woman receiving low-dose atimicrobial prophylaxis experiences symptomatic infection, the infecting organism will frequently be resistant to the prophylactic antimicrobial. If empiric treatment for the symptomatic episode is given, it should be with a different class of antimicrobial. Following therapy for the symptomatic episode, prophylactic therapy is reinstituted.

3. Other approaches

Topical antimicrobials applied to the periurethral area have been proposed as an approach for prevention of recurrent urinary infection, as periurethral colonization usually precedes urinary infection (Meyhoff et al., 1981). A comparative clinical study with periurethral application of povidone-iodine compared to oral trimethoprim prophylaxis has been reported (Nicolle and Ronald, 1987). While this study suggested the two regimens were equivalent, the infection frequency for either regimen was substantially higher than reported in other studies of prophylaxis. In addition, there is a risk of hypersensitivity reactions of the genital mucosa with topically applied agents. Thus, topical approaches are not currently recommended.

Recurrent acute uncomplicated urinary infection in premenopausal women is frequently associated with an abnormal vaginal flora. Lactobacilli spp., the normal predominant flora of the vagina which maintains the acidic environment, are replaced by *E. coli* and other organisms associated with the syndrome of bacterial vaginosis (Hooton et al., 1994). Thus, it has been proposed that reconstitution of the normal lactobacilli vaginal flora may prevent recurrent urinary infection. This approach has found its way into folk remedies which suggest that yogurt intake or intravaginal lactobacilli suppositories may prevent infection. Studies are currently exploring characteristics of lactobacilli such as hydrogen peroxide production and adhesiveness to understand how these organisms colonize and maintain residence in the normal premenopausal vaginal environment. Clinical studies, however, have not yet confirmed the feasibility or effectiveness of 'vaginal flora reconstitution' and these strategies are not yet a therapeutic option.

The multiple strains of *E. coli* isolated from acute urinary infection have complicated efforts to develop antibacterial vaccines as an approach to the prevention of acute cystitis. Investigators, have, however, been addressing this problem through development of systemic (Schluman et al., 1993) and intravaginal (Uechlin et al., 1994) vaccines derived from multiple strains. Clinical trials have not yet reported the efficacy of such vaccines. Any vaccine would have to be highly effective for a prolonged period of time to match the efficacy of antimicrobial prophylaxis. Thus, vaccination is not currently a realistic preventive approach.

III Prevention of pyelonephritis in pregnancy

1. Background

Normal physiologic changes in the genitourinary tract in pregnancy result in decreased smooth muscle tone with stasis in the genitourinary tract and, occasionally, ureteric reflux of urine. Pressure of the gravid uterus may also produce ureteric obstruction at the pelvic brim, usually on the right side. These changes are greatest at the end of the second trimester and early in the third trimester (Patterson and Andriole, 1997) and increase the likelihood of acute pyelonephritis at this time in gestation. The presence of asymptomatic bacteriuria early in pregnancy substantially increases this risk for pyelonephritis. Acute pyelonephritis, as with any other acute febrile infection later in pregnancy, may precipitate premature labour and delivery. Urinary tract infection in pregnancy has also been associated with intrauterine growth retardation and perinatal wastage (Patterson and Andriole, 1997). Screening for and treatment of asymptomatic bacteriuria in early pregnancy is effective in decreasing the incidence of pyelonephritis later in pregnancy (Nicolle, 1994). Thus strategies to prevent pyelonephritis are a goal of prenatal care.

2.   Screening for bacteriuria

The prevalence of asymptomatic bacteriuria in pregnant women in the first trimester varies from 2% to 11% (Patterson and Andriole, 1997). Women with a past history of recurrent urinary infection or from lower socioeconomic groups have a higher prevalence. If asymptomatic bacteriuria early in pregnancy is untreated, about one-third of these women will develop pyelonephritis.

Pregnant women should have a urine specimen for culture obtained at 12–14 weeks gestation, to identify the presence of asymptomatic bacteriuria. If $\geq 10^5$ cfu/ml of organisms are isolated, a second urine culture to confirm the presence of asymptomatic bacteriuria should be obtained (*Figure 5.1*). Women who have experienced an episode of asymptomatic bacteriuria should have urine cultures obtained post-treatment at least monthly throughout the duration of the pregnancy. Women with symptomatic infection early in pregnancy are also at increased risk of recurrent infection after treatment and warrant continued screening throughout the pregnancy.

3.   Treatment of asymptomatic bacteriuria

Identification and treatment of asymptomatic bacteriuria early in pregnancy, with continued post-treatment monitoring for recurrent infection, decreases the incidence of acute pyelonephritis later in pregnancy by about 67% (Nicolle, 1994). Suggested treatment regimens for asymptomatic bacteriuria are provided in *Table 5.3*. Beta-lactam antibiotics and nitrofurantoin are considered safe in pregnancy. Nitrofurantoin, if used for prophylaxis, should be discontinued close to term because of the possibility of haemolytic anaemia due to glutathione instability with immature erythrocyte enzyme systems. While trimethoprim and trimethoprim/sulfamethoxazole have been considered contraindicated in pregnancy, they have been widely used and no adverse fetal outcomes have been observed. Quinolone antimicrobials are contraindicated in pregnancy. Women with recurrent infection after treatment should be retreated and then placed on prophylactic therapy for the duration of the pregnancy.

IV   Prevention of complicated urinary infection

1.   General

Intermittent complete voiding is the major mechanism by which a sterile urinary tract is maintained. Any genitourinary abnormality which impairs complete voiding increases the risk of urinary infection. Complicated urinary infection is urinary infection which occurs in the presence of functional or structural abnormalities of the urinary tract (Rubin et al., 1992). The most important principle of prevention of complicated urinary infection is identification and correction of the underlying genitourinary abnormality which promotes infection. In some cases, such as removal of an indwelling catheter or obstructing stone, correction is straightforward. In other cases, such as an individual with an ileal conduit or with a neurogenic bladder with voiding maintained by intermittent catheterization, removal of complicating factors may not be a realistic goal. Long-term antimicrobial therapy is not generally recommended for the prevention of complicated urinary infection as the risk of recurrent urinary infection remains

as long as the abnormality persists. If long-term antimicrobials are given, infections which occur will be with organisms of increasing resistance. There is, however, evidence to support interventions to prevent infection in some selected clinical situations.

2. Postoperative urosepsis

Mucosal trauma in the presence of urinary infection carries a high risk of bacteremia, occasionally complicated by sepsis and septic shock. Thus, instrumentation of the genitourinary tract in someone with urinary infection has a high risk of serious complications. Antimicrobial therapy initiated immediately prior to the interventional procedure will prevent bacteremia and its complications (Cafferkey et al., 1982). While this is primarily a concern for men undergoing urologic procedures, the

Table 5.3
Antimicrobial treatment for prevention of pyelonephritis in pregnancy

Treatment of asymptomatic bacteriuria
Amoxycillin 500 mg tid 3–7 days
Nitrofurantoin 100 mg qid 3–7 days
Cephalexin 250–500 mg qid 3–7 days
Amoxycillin/clavulanic acid* 250/125 mg tid 3–7 days

Prophylaxis for recurrent infection
Nitrofurantoin 50–100 mg
Cephalexin 125 mg

* Limited experience in pregnancy but likely safe.

principles of management are similar for women. The use of preprocedure antimicrobial prophylaxis will decrease the occurrence of symptomatic invasive infection from 5–10% to less than 1%. A single dose given shortly before the intervention is optimal and prolonged postprocedure therapy does not provide additional benefit. If therapy is started too early before the interventional procedure, infection with a resistant organism may develop. Thus, it is recommended that the antimicrobial be given only one hour prior to the procedure. The antimicrobial agent selected for preprocedure prophylaxis is determined by the susceptibilities of the infecting organism, as a urine culture should be obtained as part of the preoperative assessment. Alternatively, empirical therapy with a single dose of gentamicin or another aminoglycoside may be considered,

3. Catheter-acquired urinary infection

Intermittent catheterization of the genitourinary tract carries a high risk of acquisition of urinary infection, with infection rates of 4.1/100 patient-days (Mohler et al., 1987) or 17.2/patient-year (Waites et al., 1993). Most episodes of infection are asymptomatic. In randomized clinical trials, prophylactic antimicrobial therapy in the early spinal cord injury period decreased the frequency of symptomatic infection but was

associated with an increased frequency of emergence of resistant organisms (Gribble and Puterman, 1993). Thus, routine antimicrobial prophylaxis is not recommended for individuals undergoing intermittent catheterization for bladder emptying. Treatment of asymptomatic bacteriuria in subjects maintained on intermittent catheterization as 'prophylaxis' for symptomatic infection or other morbidity is also not recommended (Cardenas and Hooton, 1995). A study in a nursing home population addressed the question of whether sterile technique for intermittent catheterization was associated with fewer infections than clean technique (Duffy et al., 1995). Intermittent catheterization with clean or sterile technique was associated with a similar occurrence of urinary tract infection, while the clean method was less costly. Thus sterile technique for intermittent catheterization in nursing home subjects is not recommended as a means of preventing infection.

The risk of acquisition of bacteriuria with an indwelling urethral catheter is higher for women than for men, approximating 5% per day (Warren, 1997). For short-term indwelling urethral catheters, infection is decreased in frequency by maintaining a closed drainage system and is less frequent in the first four days of catheterization in individuals who receive systemic antimicrobials. More prolonged use of antimicrobials, however, is not associated with a decreased frequency of catheter-acquired infection and is associated with isolation of more resistant organisms. Thus, prophylactic antimicrobial therapy is not recommended to decrease the occurrence of urinary infection in catheterized subjects. The use of antimicrobial substances such as antibiotic-impregnated catheters and silver-impregnated catheters or local perineal antibacterial care does not decrease the occurrence of infection. The most effective way of preventing urinary tract infections associated with a chronic indwelling catheter is to limit the duration of catheter use to as short a time as possible.

4. Elderly women

Well, elderly women living in the community have a prevalence of asymptomatic bacteriuria approaching 10%. The prevalence of bacteriuria in women resident in nursing homes is approximately 50%. There are no studies which suggest that this high prevalence of infection in the general population can be decreased. In addition, asymptomatic bacteriuria does not appear to be associated with substantial morbidity and thus there is no evidence for benefits from 'prophylactic' treatment of asymptomatic infection to prevent adverse outcomes (Nicolle, 1997). In the nursing home, treatment of asymptomatic bacteriuria does not prevent symptomatic episodes but does lead to infection with

organisms of increased antimicrobial resistance and increased adverse drug effects. Thus, treatment of asymptomatic bacteriuria to prevent morbidity or mortality of urinary infection is not indicated.

There has been interest in the use of 'natural antiseptics', such as cranberry juice, for the prevention of urinary infection. One prospective, randomized study compared the effectiveness of cranberry juice with placebo in preventing infection in elderly women in a nursing home (Avorn et al., 1994). While the prevalence of pyuria associated with bacteriuria was decreased, the prevalence of bacteriuria was not decreased and there was no decrease in symptomatic episodes.

In selected elderly women with a high frequency of recurrent urinary infection, the use of topical estrogen therapy decreases the frequency of both symptomatic and asymptomatic infections (Raz and Stamm, 1993). It is not clear how generally applicable this strategy is to the wider postmenopausal population. There are no comparative studies of the relative efficacy of topical estrogen with long-term low-dose antimicrobial prophylaxis. Elderly women who have recurrent episodes of acute cystitis may benefit from long-term prophylactic antimicrobial therapy similar to younger women with acute uncomplicated urinary infection (Nicolle, 1992).

V   Conclusion

The goal for the prevention of urinary tract
infection is to decrease morbidity and,
potentially, mortality associated with urinary
tract infection. Antimicrobial therapy has
been shown to be effective in prevention of
urinary infection for women with acute
uncomplicated urinary infection.
Asymptomatic bacteriuria is very common but
has only been shown to place individuals at
risk if they are pregnant women or if they are
undergoing genitourinary procedures with
mucosal trauma. In these two situations,
asymptomatic bacteriuria should be treated as
a strategy to prevent complications of urinary
infection. In other situations, asymptomatic
bacteriuria has not been shown to be
associated with poorer outcomes. For
indwelling urethral catheters, limitation in
catheter use and maintenance of a closed
drainage system are the most effective
strategies for prevention of infection.

References

Avorn J, Monane M, Gurwitz JH et al. (1994) Reduction of bacteriuria and pyuria after ingestion of cranberry juice. *JAMA* **271**: 751–5.

Brumfitt W, Hamilton-Miller JMT (1995) A comparative trial of low-dose cefaclor and macrocrystalline nitrofurantoin in the prevention of recurrent urinary tract. *Infection* **23**: 99–102.

Cafferkey MT, Falkiner FR, Gillespie WA, Murphy PM (1982) Antibiotics for the prevention of septicaemia in urology. *Antimicrob Chemother* **9**: 471–7.

Cardenas DD, Hooton TM (1995) Urinary tract infection in persons with spinal cord injury. *Arch Phys Med Rehab* **76**: 272–80.

Duffy LM, Cleary J, Ahern S et al. (1995) Clean intermittent catheterization: safe, cost-effective bladder management for male residents of VA nursing homes. *J Am Geriatr Soc* **43**: 865–70.

Foxman B, Frerichs RR (1985a) Epidemiology of urinary tract infection. I. Diaphragm use and sexual intercourse. *Am J Public Health* **75**: 1306–13.

Foxman B, Frerichs RR (1985b) Epidemiology of urinary tract infections. II. Diet, clothing and urinary habits. *Am J Public Health* **75**: 1314–17.

Gribble M, Puterman M (1993) Prophylaxis of urinary tract infection in persons with recent spinal cord injury: a prospective, randomized, double-blind, placebo-controlled study of trimethoprim–sulfamethoxazole. *Am J Med* **95**: 141–52.

Harding GKM, Ronald AR, Nicolle LE, Thomson MJ, Gray GJ

(1982) Long term antimicrobial prophylaxis for recurrent urinary infection in females. *Rev Infect Dis* 4: 438–43.

Hooton TM, Fihn SF, Johnson C, Roberts PL, Stamm WE (1989) Association between bacterial vaginosis and acute cystitis in women using diaphragms. *Arch Intern Med* 149: 1932–6.

Hooton TM, Hillier S, Johnson C, Roberts PL, Stamm WE (1991) *Escherichia coli* bacteriuria and contraceptive method. *JAMA* 265: 64–9.

Hooton TM, Roberts PL, Stamm WE (1994) Effects of recent sexual activity and use of a diaphragm on the vaginal microflora. *Clin Infect Dis* 19: 274–8.

Hooton TM, Scholes D, Hughes JP et al. (1996) A prospective study of risk factors for symptomatic urinary tract infection in young women. *N Engl J Med* 335: 468–512.

Leibovici L, Alpert G, Laor A, Kalter-Leibovici O, Danon YL (1987) Urinary tract infections and sexual activity in young women. *Arch Intern Med* 147: 345–7.

Meyhoff HH, Nordling J, Gammelgaard PA, Veilsgaard R (1981) Does antimicrobial ointment applied to urethral meatus in women prevent recurrent cystitis? *Scand J Urol Nephrol* 15: 81–3.

Mohler JL, Cower DL, Flanigan RC (1987) Suppression and treatment of urinary tract infection in patients with an intermittently catheterized neurogenic bladder. *J Urol* 138: 336–40.

Nicolle LE (1992) Prophylaxis: recurrent urinary tract infection in women. *Infection* 20 (suppl 3): S203–4.

Nicolle LE (1994) Screening for asymptomatic bacteriuria in pregnancy. In: *The Canadian Guide to Clinical Preventive Health Care* (ed. Canadian Task Force on the Periodic Health Care Examination), Health Canada, Canada Communication Group.

Nicolle LE (1997) Asymptomatic bacteriuria in the elderly. *Infect Dis Clin North Am* 11: 647–62.

Nicolle LE, Ronald AR (1987) Recurrent urinary tract infection in adult women: diagnosis and treatment. *Infect Dis Clin North Am* 1: 793–806.

Nicolle LE, Harding GKM, Preiksaitis J, Ronald AR (1982) The association of urinary tract infection with sexual intercourse. *J Infect Dis* 146: 579–83.

Nicolle LE, Harding GKM, Thomson M et al. (1988) Efficacy of five years of continuous low dose co-trimoxazole prophylaxis for prevention of urinary tract infection. *J Infect Dis* 157: 1239–42.

Nicolle LE, Harding GKM, Thompson M et al. (1989) A

prospective, randomized, placebo controlled trial of norfloxacin for the prophylaxis of recurrent urinary infection in women. *Antimicrob Agents Chemother* **33**: 1032–5.

Patterson TF, Andriole VT (1997) Detection, significance, and therapy of bacteriuria in pregnancy. *Infect Dis Clin North Am* **11**: 593–608.

Pfau A, Sacks TG (1991) Effective prophylaxis of recurrent urinary tract infections in premenopausal women. *Int Urogynecol J* **2**: 156–60.

Raz R, Boger S (1991) Long-term prophylaxis with norfloxacin versus nitrofurantoin in women with recurrent urinary tract infection. *Antimicrob Agents Chemother* **35**: 1241–2.

Raz R, Stamm W (1993) A controlled trial of intravaginal estriol in post-menopausal women with recurrent urinary tract infections. *N Engl J Med* **329**: 753–8.

Remis RS, Gurwith MJ, Gurwith D, Hargett-Bean NT, Layde PM (1987) Risk factors for urinary tract infection. *Am J Epidemiol* **126**: 685–94.

Rubin RH, Shapiro ED, Andriole VT, Davis RJ, Stamm WE (1992) Evaluation of new antiinfective drugs for the treatment of urinary tract infection. *Clin Infect Dis* **15** (suppl 1): S216–27.

Schulman CC, Corbusier A, Michiels H, Taenzer HJ (1993) Oral immunotherapy of recurrent urinary tract infections: a double-blind placebo-controlled multicenter study. *J Urol* **150**: 917–21.

Stamey RA, Condy M, Mehara G (1977) Prophylactic efficacy of nitrofurantoin macrocrystals and trimethoprim–sulfamethoxazole in urinary infections: biologic effects on the vaginal and rectal flora. *N Engl J Med* **296**: 780–3.

Stamm WE, Counts, GW, Wagner KF et al. (1980) Antimicrobial prophylaxis of recurrent urinary tract infections. A double-blind, placebo-controlled trial. *Ann Intern Med* **92**: 770–5.

Stapleton A, Latham RH, Johnson C, Stamm WE (1990) Postcoital antimicrobial prophylaxis for recurrent urinary tract infection. A randomized, double-blind placebo-controlled trial. *JAMA* **264**: 703–6.

Strom BL, Collins M, West SL, Kreisburg J, Weller S (1987) Sexual activity, contraceptive use, and other risk factors for symptomatic and asymptomatic bacteriuria: a case-control study. *Ann Intern Med* **107**: 816–23.

Uechling DT, Hopkins WJ, Dahmer LA et al. (1994) Phase I clinical trials of vaginal mucosal immunization for recurrent urinary tract infection. *J Urol* **152**: 2308–11.

Vosti KL (1975) Recurrent urinary tract infections: prevention by prophylactic antibiotics after sexual intercourse. *JAMA* **231**: 934–40.

Waites KB, Canupp KC, de Vivo MJ (1993) Epidemiology and risk factors for urinary tract infection following spinal cord injury. *Arch Phys Med Rehab* 74: 691–5.

Warren JW (1997) Catheter-associated urinary tract infections. *Infect Dis Clin North Am* **11**: 609–22.

Infants and children

Kate Bourdeaux and Kate Verrier Jones

6

Contents

I   Introduction

Urinary tract infections (UTIs) are among the commonest bacterial infections in paediatric practice (Miller, 1996), accounting for 4–10% of febrile children admitted to hospital. They are associated with acute morbidity, suffering and anxiety, as well as long-term renal damage if recurrent or untreated (Vernon, 1995). Renal damage or scarring, also referred to as chronic pyelonephritis or reflux nephropathy, is more likely and more severe following UTI in infancy or early childhood (Berg and Johansson, 1983; Winberg et al, 1982), particularly when vesicoureteric reflux is present or there is a delay in starting treatment (Smellie et al., 1994).

The presence of bacteria on direct microscopy and a colony count of >100,000 cfu/ml of a single strain of bacteria confirm the diagnosis of UTI. Unfortunately, underdiagnosis in children under two years old is common, due to a combination of contributing factors. Parents and health professionals are often unaware of the high risk of UTI in infancy or of the potential for permanent renal damage. Non-specific illness with fever may be caused by UTI, but symptoms related to the urinary tract are rarely observed before two years. Contamination rates are high in this age group and collection of samples and transfer to the laboratory is difficult and sometimes poorly organized from primary care.

Laboratories are often closed for routine work at nights and weekends when children are usually taken ill, and some GPs do not have access to emergency laboratory facilities. Direct phase contrast microscopy has been shown to be an excellent screening method for the diagnosis of childhood UTI. However, this method requires a suitable microscope and expertise (Vickers et al., 1991) and is not in widespread use.

Since UTI in infancy often leads to prolonged illness and long-term kidney scarring, provision for prompt diagnosis and appropriate management of UTIs is essential. At present these arrangements are only available in the minority of practices and underdiagnosis is a significant problem (Jadresic et al., 1993; van der Voort et al., 1997a).

II   Epidemiology

Epidemiological studies have demonstrated that childhood UTIs are common and the incidence of UTI varies by age and gender. The commonest age for the first symptomatic infection is during the first two years of life (Berg and Johansson, 1983). There is a progressive decline in the incidence of first infection with increasing age (Winberg et al., 1974). At least 7% of girls and 3% of boys will be affected by UTI at some time during childhood and recent studies have suggested that the incidence is even greater. During the first month, the incidence in boys is greater than in girls, whereas by six months girls predominate. In the neonatal period, the incidence has been shown to be inversely proportional to gestational age and is greater in low birthweight and preterm infants.

1. Recurrent infections

Recurrent infections are usually due to reinfection rather than relapse and are more common in girls, reoccurring in over 60%, with some having frequent reinfections over many years, often continuing into adult life. In boys, reinfection is less common but often develops quite soon after the presenting infection (Miller, 1996).

2. Asymptomatic bacteriuria

Some infections may give rise to minimal symptoms, where treatment and medical opinion is not sought. Asymptomatic bacteriuria is rare in males, except in infancy, but occurs in 1.7% of schoolgirls and 5% of adult women and can occur at any age, although evidence suggests chronic asymptomatic infection does not damage the kidneys (Verrier Jones, 1993). Asymptomatic bacteriuria may be detected in screening programmes and is common in girls who have previously had symptomatic infection. The high incidence of renal scarring in girls with asymptomatic bacteriuria is thought to be due

to earlier, unrecognized and untreated infections.

III Pathogenesis

In healthy children the urinary tract is normally sterile, although colonization of the perineum in girls and the foreskin in boys is common in susceptible children prior to the development of UTI. UTI may involve the urethra, bladder, ureters, renal pelvis, calyces or parenchyma. Infecting bacteria commonly ascend the urinary tract via the urethra. Usually, a single organism is present in uncomplicated infections. Severity of infection has been related to the adequacy of host defence mechanisms and virulence of the causative organism (Miller, 1996).

1. Host susceptibility factors

There are a variety of factors that predispose an individual to UTI (*Table 6.1*). Urinary stasis in a dilated or obstructed urinary tract and incomplete bladder emptying are important predisposing factors, since residual urine in the bladder provides an excellent culture medium for bacterial growth. Detrusor sphincter dyssynergia may contribute to UTI by forcing urine into the posterior urethra, allowing contaminated urethral urine to return to the bladder when the bladder contraction ceases. Naturally occurring antibacterial substances present in

Table 6.1
Examples of host susceptibility factors which influence the development of urinary tract infections in infants and toddlers

Type of factor	Examples of host variation	Effect on host susceptibility
Anatomical factors	Urethral length	Male > female, increases with age Shorter female and infant urethra provide easier access for ascending bacteria
Physiological factors	Bladder emptying	Incomplete in early childhood causes incomplete washout of ascending bacteria
Pathological factors	Constipation	Interferes with bladder emptying Bladder emptying improves with treatment of constipation
Congenital anomalies	Vesicoureteric reflux	Allows refluxing urine to return to the bladder after micturition and allows infected urine to reach the kidneys at high pressure
Immunological factors	Urinary IgA	Binds with invading bacteria, making them susceptible to phagocytosis Low urinary IgA in infants and susceptible individuals predisposes to recurrent UTIs

the urine vary with age and sex and may contribute to the observed epidemiology of this condition.

2. Route of entry

In the neonate, UTI often results from bloodborne spread of organisms. As the gut becomes colonized with *Escherichia coli*, some infants develop bacteraemia. In all other age groups bacteria reach the urinary tract via the urethra. A higher rate of infection in females may be attributed to a shorter urethra, with an increased chance of contamination from closer proximity to the anus. In boys, pathogens under the foreskin provide an important source.

3. Ascent to the bladder

Organisms ascend the urethra to the bladder as a result of bacterial multiplication, movement of bacteria in a film fluid or mucus, retrograde spread by turbulent flow during micturition or mechanical trauma during masturbation, sexual activity, scratching or secondary to threadworm infection. The organisms must be able to survive and multiply in urine and resist washout during micturition.

4. Pathogenic organisms

Escherichia coli is the commonest pathogen, accounting for more than 90% of straightforward UTIs, whilst *Proteus* accounts for 30% of UTI spp. in males but less than 5% in females. *Staphylococcus epidermidis, Staph. aureus, Streptococcus faecalis, Klebsiellas, Pseudomonas* and other gut organisms cause a small number of infections.

IV   Presentation (symptoms)

Severity of symptoms may vary from minimal upset to severe illness and symptoms may be local or systemic. Generally, the most severe illness occurs in the youngest infants.

1. Newborn infants

In the newborn, UTIs may be associated with prolonged jaundice, septicaemia and meningitis and may present with fits, dehydration, electrolyte disturbance and acute renal failure, and in premature infants, apnoea is common. The neonate is particularly prone to severe infection with Gram-negative organisms, often involving the meninges and bloodstream as well as the urinary tract. Delays in making the diagnosis and starting appropriate treatment contribute to the severity and duration of the illness as well as increasing the risk of renal scarring.

2. Infancy and early childhood

Symptoms referable to the urinary tract are seldom present in infants and toddlers and presenting symptoms are usually non-specific, including fever, malaise, vomiting, irritability, diarrhoea, screaming, abdominal distention, jaundice and failure to thrive. Fever is almost always present (Hoberman et al., 1993), but is a common manifestation in many childhood illnesses. UTI is also a common cause of febrile convulsions (Lee and Verrier Jones, 1991). For these reasons UTI must be considered in every febrile infant and toddler and those with chronic debility or failure to thrive.

3. Older children

The acute effects of UTI in older children and adults are mainly confined to the lower urinary tract, with minimal systemic upset. When acute pyelonephritis occurs, the classic symptoms of fever and loin pain are usually present at some stage but may not be obvious at initial presentation.

V Diagnosis of urinary tract infection

Urgent urine microscopy to note the presence of bacteria and pus cells (normal <25 white cells per mm³) is indicated in children under two years and all children with clinical evidence of fever or acute pyelonephritis, so that treatment is not delayed.

1. Laboratory criteria

Preliminary diagnosis is best made by microscopy (Vickers et al., 1991) of a fresh clean-catch urine sample whenever possible. Diagnosis is confirmed by culture showing a pure growth >100,000 cfu/ml after 24–48 hours. A normal urinary white cell count does not exclude infection. Occasionally the colony count is <100,000 cfu/ml in the presence of UTI. Techniques used vary from one laboratory to another and in many laboratories it is usual not to report the bacteria seen on microscopy to the clinician. There is no justification for this practice which is misleading and not in the interest of sick children. The judicious use of screening tests to reduce the workload on the laboratory is justified in selected cases provided both the clinicians and the laboratory staff are aware of the shortcomings of the screening test used.

2. Dipsticks

Stick tests for proteinuria and haematuria are of little predictive value in diagnosing or excluding UTI. Although proteinuria is present in advanced reflux nephropathy and sometimes in the presence of UTI and other febrile illnesses, it is often absent in cases of acute UTI (Working Group, 1991). However, new combination stick (*Figure 6.1*) have been developed so that urine can be tested for blood, protein, nitrites and leucocyte esterase (Bayer Multistix, Boehringer Nephurtest Leuco). They are useful for excluding UTIs in older children who are not severely ill as their negative predictive value has been shown to approach 100% when all the tests are taken together.

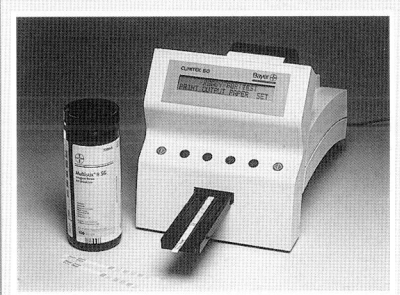

Figure 6.1
Clinitek machine and urinary dipsticks showing a positive (pink) reaction to nitrites. (Bayer Multistix 8SG reagent strips: by courtesy of Bayer plc, Newbury, UK.)

3.   Nitrite test

The nitrite test has been shown to be a
reliable sign of infection when positive in a
freshly voided urine sample, but has up to
a 48% false-negative rate in acutely ill
children when used in isolation (Powell et al.,
1987). The test depends on an assumption that
the urine has been in the bladder for at least an
hour, allowing time for bacterial conversion of
nitrate to nitrite. In infants and toddlers, the
bladder is often emptied more frequently,
reducing the sensitivity of the test in this age
group. Similarly, since UTIs cause frequency of
micturition, the test may be unreliable in
children with cystitis. In positive cases, culture
of urine is needed to demonstrate antibiotic
sensitivity and to confirm the diagnosis.

4.   Dipslides

Urinary dipslides containing culture media
(*Figure 6.2*) are very useful in the community,
eliminating the delay often incurred during
transport to the laboratory and therefore
reducing the contamination rate (Jewkes et al.,
1990). Despite their comparatively short shelf-
life, they have been shown to be an efficient and
reliable means of documenting bacteriuria
before initiation of treatment. Urine is plated
out immediately by dipping the slide into
freshly voided urine. The dipslide is then
replaced in a plastic bottle and sent to the
laboratory.

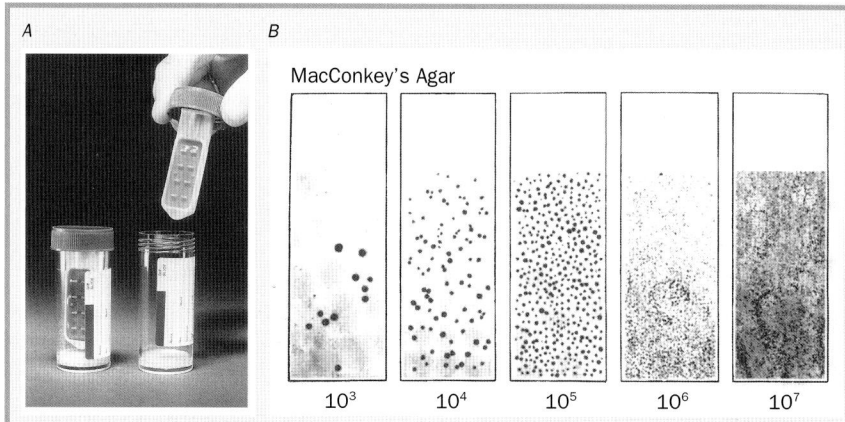

Figure 6.2
(A) Dipslide; (B) the colony count is estimated by comparing the density of the colonies with a chart provided.

5. Borate

The addition of a small amount of boric acid to a urine sample inhibits bacterial growth until plating out onto culture medium. However, there is some evidence that it renders some infected samples sterile because the inhibitory effect persists after plating out (M Coulthard, personal communication).

6. Urine collection methods

Diagnosis of UTI depends on the ability to examine a clean uncontaminated specimen of urine before initiation of antibiotic treatment. Several methods exist, depending on the age of the child. Samples collected in potties, poured from changing mats or squeezed from nappies carry a high rate of contamination.

(i) Clean-catch samples

Clean-catch samples, collected in a sterile foil bowl, have been advocated (Working Group, 1991) to provide an uncontaminated sample, although evidence of the superiority of these samples over bag samples is weak. The child is left without a nappy and a sterile container is available to catch the urine as soon as it is passed (*Figure 6.3*). Removal of the nappy and examination often stimulates micturition, although it may be time consuming. Alternatively, parents can sit with the baby following a feed and usually obtain a sample

in 30 minutes. Ideally, the vulval area or penis should be cleaned with normal saline or tap water and cotton wool prior to obtaining the specimen.

(ii) Midstream urine sample

In a toilet-trained child, urine can be collected as a midstream sample (MSU) after washing the perineum, although there is little evidence for the usefulness of washing in prepubertal children. Use of antiseptics to cleanse the perineum or sterilize the receiver may prevent bacterial growth, giving rise to a false-negative result (Verrier Jones, 1995). The child and parent need careful explanation of how to clean with sterile swabs, gently wiping the tip of the penis or between the labia. In older children the foreskin should be drawn back carefully or the labia held apart whilst passing urine. The middle of the specimen should be caught in a sterile container. Younger children will need assistance.

(iii) Urine bags

Adhesive bags are said to result in higher rates of contamination than clean-catch samples, but may be used if other methods fail. The bag should be attached to the perineum after careful cleaning with water. The adhesive rim should separate the urethral meatus and anal region. The nappy should be left off to obtain the sample as

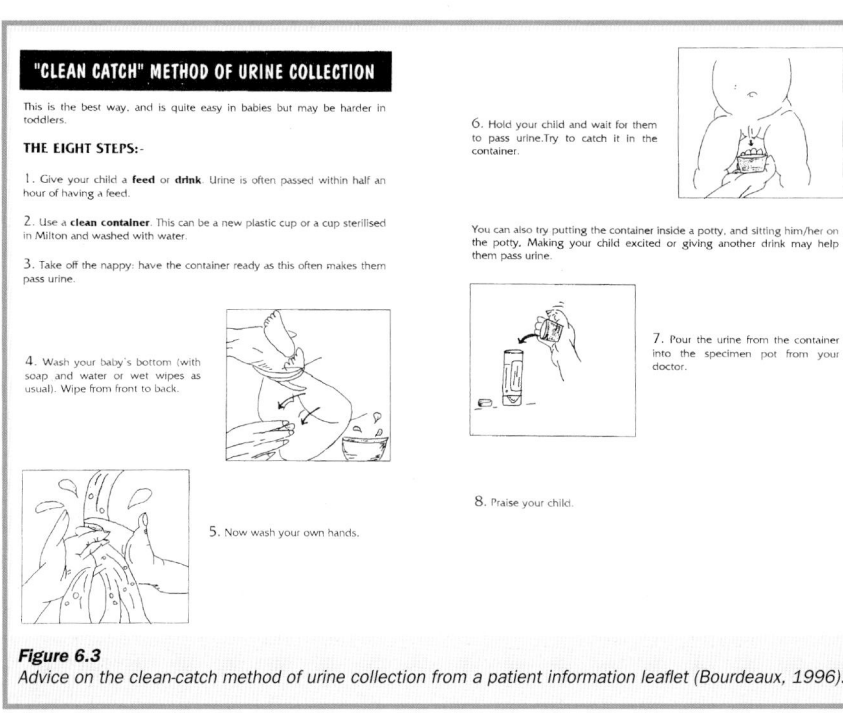

Figure 6.3
Advice on the clean-catch method of urine collection from a patient information leaflet (Bourdeaux, 1996).

soon as the child passes urine, reducing the risk of contamination. A negative result from a bag urine is reliable but a positive result should be confirmed by a clean-catch specimen or, in seriously ill infants, by a suprapubic aspiration (SPA) under ultrasound control or catheter specimen (Working Group, 1991). SPA is traumatic and therefore only indicated in very sick infants or when other methods fail to provide an uncontaminated sample.

(iv) Urine collection pads

Recently, a urine pad (Euron urine collection pads and the Newcastle urine collection pack by Ontex Hygienic Disposables) has been developed for urine collection in infants and toddlers, which is simple to use and preferred by parents and staff (Ahmed et al., 1991) (*Figure 6.4*).

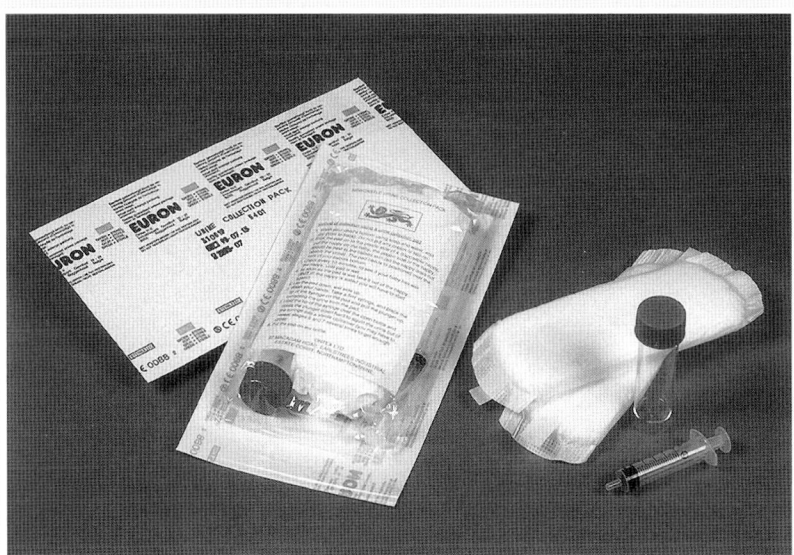

Figure 6.4
The Newcastle urine collection pack contains a sterile sanitary pad, syringe for aspiration of urine and a universal container for transfer to the laboratory (by courtesy of Ontex Hygienic Disposables, Ontex, Corby, UK).

(v)   Invasive methods of urine collection

Suprapubic aspiration of urine is preferable in newborn and sick infants in hospital due to the high contamination of bag samples and urgent need for accurate diagnosis. Alternatively, catheterization is an effective method which can be used prior to the start of antibiotic treatment.

7.   Storage and transport to the laboratory

Urine should be examined in the laboratory within two hours or chilled immediately to 4°C until transfer to the laboratory (Working Group, 1991). In practice, arrangements for storage and transfer are often inadequate, both in hospital and in the community, predisposing to multiplication of contaminating organisms.

8. Screening for urinary tract infection in acutely sick children under two years

UTI in sick children under two years is a condition which fulfils the criteria for screening, as the condition is common. Cheap, safe and non-invasive screening methods are available and short-term morbidity and long-term consequences may be prevented. This approach was recommended in published guidelines (Working Group, 1991).

VI Diagnostic difficulties

There are several reasons why the diagnosis of UTI in early childhood is difficult. Urinary symptoms are absent, infants cannot express their symptoms or co-operate with urine collection and the use of nappies often obscures changes in the appearance and smell of infected urine and pain or frequency of micturition.

1. Primary care

It has been demonstrated that UTI is frequently overlooked in primary care in the first two years of life. This age is when the risk of first UTI and of renal damage is highest. In addition, it appears also to be the age when children present in general practice most frequently with fever. In older children, UTI is often diagnosed in primary care because children present to the GP with acute urinary symptoms, whilst in contrast many infants and toddlers have UTI diagnosed only after admission to hospital. Furthermore, children with UTI appear to have visited their GPs with ill health significantly more often than controls before the diagnosis is established. This may be because some of these visits were due to the non-specific symptoms of unrecognized UTI (van der Voort et al., 1997b). Even when the diagnosis has been considered, urine is not always collected for confirmation. Contamination or inappropriate methods of collection have often been demonstrated. These observations lead to the conclusion that there is considerable scope to reduce the morbidity associated with UTI in the first two years of life in primary care.

GPs have reported a number of difficulties in diagnosis of UTI, including practical problems, such as engaging parental co-operation, shortage of time, lack of equipment, difficulty with specimen transport and lack of access to laboratory facilities (especially out of hours). There is wide variation in professional awareness of UTI in infants with non-specific symptoms. Most GPs would not routinely perform urine culture on a significantly febrile infant (van der Voort et al., 1997a).

2. Age and diagnosis

Clearly, before two years, children are unable to describe or localize urinary symptoms. In addition, they are unable to provide a urine sample on request or co-operate with urine collection. Difficulty in obtaining samples frequently results in high contamination rates; inappropriate methods for screening and culturing samples result in inaccurate interpretation of results. The non-specific nature of the presenting symptoms may account for underdiagnosis of UTI in young children and other diagnoses may be pursued. For these reasons, diagnosis of UTI may be unrecognized or overlooked by professionals and parents who are unaware of the usual presentation in this age group.

After two years, when children are toilet trained and are more able to localize their symptoms and describe their illness, diagnosis becomes less complicated. Symptoms resemble more closely the clinical picture seen in adults described as acute pyelonephritis (fever and loin pain) or cystitis. However, fever, vomiting and abdominal pain continue to be common presentations in children under 10 years.

3.   Parents' knowledge

Many parents are unaware of the importance of early detection of UTI, demonstrating a need to improve knowledge and awareness in the community. There is scope to modify parents' expectations and responses to undiagnosed fever and there is clearly a need to improve parental understanding and

awareness of possible UTI in their child through recognition of significant signs and symptoms. Increased parental involvement is essential to improve the number of urine cultures sent from febrile children and thus reduce the risk of overlooking UTIs. If parents feel that excluding UTI is important, they will request a urine sample when their child has a fever (van der Voort et al., 1997a). They may be more inclined to collect, store and return samples when requested by their GP if they have previously been appropriately informed and educated by members of the primary health care team. Parents could contact their GP, act appropriately and collect a urine sample using a satisfactory method in children under two years at home if they have been given appropriate advice and support.

The success of these educational objectives depends upon the successful implementation of a suitable programme by the primary health care team, particularly the health visitors and practice nurses.

4.   *Practical arrangements*

Measures to promote the importance of UTI in the first two years of life and improve collection methods at home and in surgery would be invaluable in reducing the duration of illness and hospital admission rate due to UTI in this age group (*Figure 6.5*). Universal containers, urine collection bags, pads and patient information leaflets should be

◆ HAS YOUR CHILD BEEN UNWELL?

● High Temperatures (over 38.5°C)
● Vomiting
● Weight Loss
● Diarrhoea
● Misery
● Excessive Screaming

◆ WHEN SHOULD I CALL THE DOCTOR?

IF YOUR CHILD HAS ONE OF THESE PROBLEMS, CONTACT YOUR DOCTOR, THEY ARE SOMETIMES CAUSED BY A URINE INFECTION.

◆ WHAT IS A URINE TEST?

Your doctor may suggest that a urine test is done. This is the only way to know if your child has an infection. Your doctor will give you a specimen pot to collect a urine sample.

◆ WHY IS URINE COLLECTION IMPORTANT?

Early detection of a urine infection means that it can be **treated quickly**. If it is not treated the illness will last longer, and there may be a risk of damage to the kidneys.

◆ HOW DO YOU COLLECT URINE FROM A BABY?

There are several ways. The main things you need are:
● Time (usually about half an hour), but maybe longer
● Patience
● A **clean** babies bottom
● A specimen pot (from your doctor)

Figure 6.5
Practical advice on the symptoms and importance of UTI for parents and health professionals (Bourdeaux, 1996).

routinely available to help parents in this difficult task. Advice in the parent-held child health record would be welcome, authoritative and available to a wide range of parents and professionals. All staff working in general practice should be aware of the need for urine collection in sick babies and toddlers so that it can be initiated while waiting to see the doctor.

5.   Risks and benefits

Renal complications have been shown to be rare in individual general practices and the effort required to screen for UTI may be perceived as not worthwhile (Stark, 1997). However, the observation by van der Voort et al. (1997b) that children with UTI and renal scarring attended their GPs twice as often as controls because of illness suggests that earlier diagnosis may reduce GP workload. In the UK, most children under two years only have UTIs diagnosed in hospital, often after the GP has failed to establish a diagnosis at home. This can lead to loss of confidence and dissatisfaction by the parents. The cost and trauma of hospital admission could have been avoided if UTI had been detected earlier at home.

Previous research suggests that the average GP sees one proven childhood UTI per year (Dighe and Grace, 1984), although this low rate may be due to poor collection technique or failure to suspect the diagnosis. Jadresic et al. (1993) found the incidence to be 10 times higher and showed that the rate of diagnosis was directly proportional to the number of samples collected. An audit of GPs in Wales showed that the number of samples sent each year varied between practices from 0 to 100, with a median of 3–4 and half the practices sending none (unpublished data). Concerns over the costs of urinalysis and dipsticks have been raised by GPs (van der Voort et al., 1997a).

When all these aspects are considered, the case in favour of better diagnostic facilities in primary care seems to be overwhelming.

6. Comparison between the UK and Sweden

In Sweden there is an active programme for the diagnosis and treatment of UTI in children under two years, where urine tests are routine in sick infants and toddlers. The median age of first diagnosis is four months for boys and nine months for girls, with low risk of previous undiagnosed infections. The prevalence of renal scarring is 4–7% and there were no cases of renal failure due to reflux nephropathy in a study by Helin and Winberg 1980.

In contrast, the UK median age of first diagnosis is 4–6 years (McKerrow et al., 1984), prevalence of scarring in studies is 5–25% of children investigated after UTI and reflux nephropathy accounts for up to 29% of children in the UK who have kidney transplants (UKTSSSHA, 1995). The primary care arrangements for infants and toddlers almost certainly account for these differences.

VII Management

1. Antibiotic treatment and prophylaxis

Following confirmation of a UTI, the child should be given an appropriate broad-spectrum antibiotic for 5–10 days depending on the severity of the illness. In early infancy and in children with vomiting or dehydration, the intravenous route is preferred initially. After completion of the course of treatment, prophylactic antibiotics are advised to reduce the risk of reinfection while completing imaging investigations of the urinary tract. Trimethoprim or nitrofurantoin given at a nightly dose of 1–2 mg/kg have been shown to reduce the risk of reinfection.

2. Imaging

It is recommended that all children should undergo renal imaging in case there is an underlying congenital anomaly (Rickwood, 1992), although evidence that this is effective is lacking and this strategy is under review. Vesicoureteric reflux (*Figure 6.6*) is present in one-third of children with UTI and renal scarring is present in 5–25%. Routine imaging after UTI may involve abdominal X-ray, ultrasound, static radioisotope scanning (*Figure 6.7*) and micturating cystography (McFarlane, 1993). It was recommended that all children should have ultrasound, those under seven years should also have a DMSA

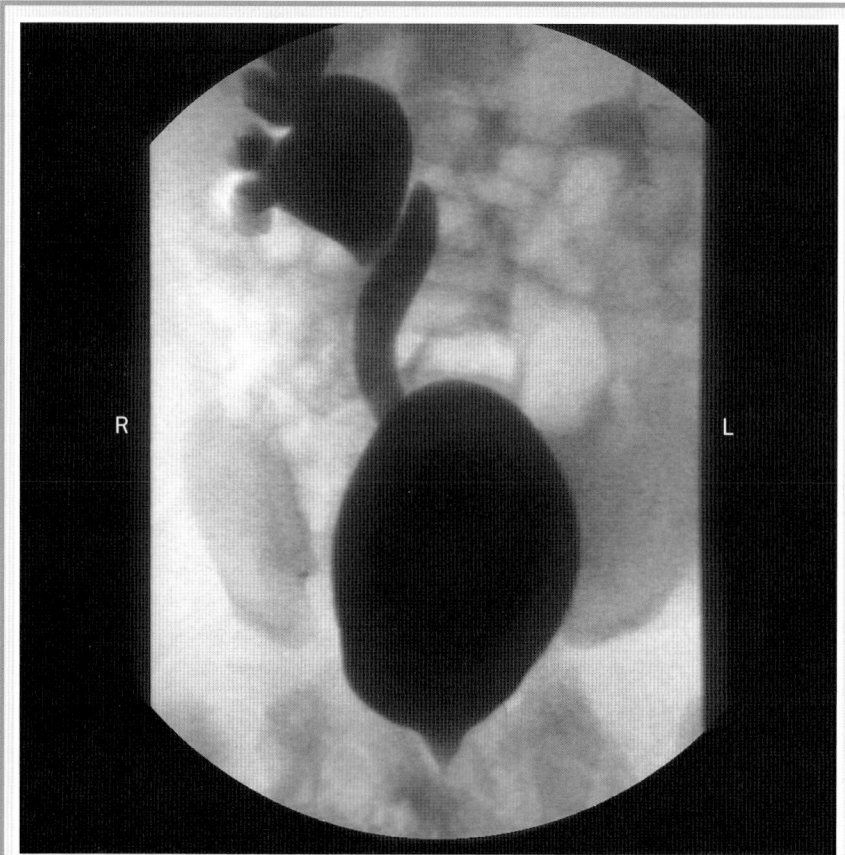

Figure 6.6
Micturating cysto-urethrogram in an infant showing bilateral severe vesico-ureteric reflux (right) grade 2/5, (left) grade 4/5 (international reflux grading system).

scan to look for renal scarring and infants under one year should have micturating cystography in addition (Working Group, 1991).

VIII   Guidelines

The development of good practice guidelines and consensus statements is an important step in the rationalization of treatment and

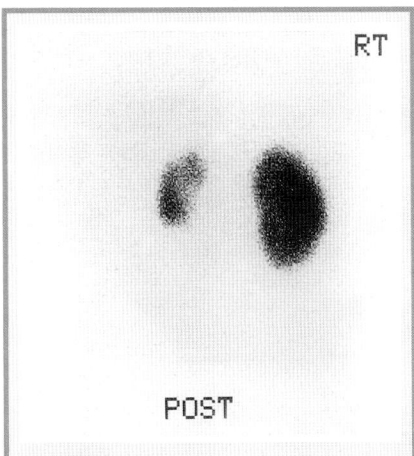

RT

POST

Figure 6.7
99m-Tc DMSA scan carried out after UTI in a toddler showing a normal right kidney and a severely scarred left kidney.

management. In 1991, the Royal College of Physicians published guidelines on the management of UTI in children. They recommended that all young children with a pyrexia greater than 38.5°C without an obvious cause should have urine collected for culture within 24 hours (Working Group, 1991). However, there was no specific process for dissemination of these guidelines to GPs and their implementation was not monitored (Grol, 1992), which may account for a lack of awareness of the guidelines in primary care and continued underdiagnosis of UTI in children under two years. In a survey of GPs in Wales, fewer than 1% were aware of the

existence of published guidelines or of the recommendation to collect a clean urine sample in infants and children with an undiagnosed fever of >38.5°C within 24 hours.

There should be locally developed procedures for urine collection, dipstick testing, transport to the laboratory, microscopy and urine culture appropriate for children in the first two years of life. Standards used for diagnosis of UTI should also be appropriate for the age of the child and method of urine collection.

1.   Patient information leaflets

There is clearly a need for information leaflets for parents to explain the important of this diagnosis (*Figure 6.8*) and the recommended methods for urine collection in children, particularly before they are toilet trained. Methods of urine collection include clean catch, bag sample, pad, catheter sample and suprapubic puncture. In primary care most samples are collected using the clean-catch method or into plastic urine bags. The success rate with both these methods is dependent on parental co-operation but parents can only co-operate if an adequate explanation is given.

Professionals have an important role in the preparation and distribution of written information. Health visitors have an education role and provide a direct contact point for the public. For information leaflets to be effective, it is essential that all health care workers

QUESTIONS ABOUT URINE INFECTION

◆ WHAT IS A URINE INFECTION?

Urine infections (UTI) are common in childhood. They are caused when bacteria enter the urinary system. Infection may occur in the upper or lower urinary tract, or both.

◆ DIAGRAM OF THE URINARY SYSTEM:

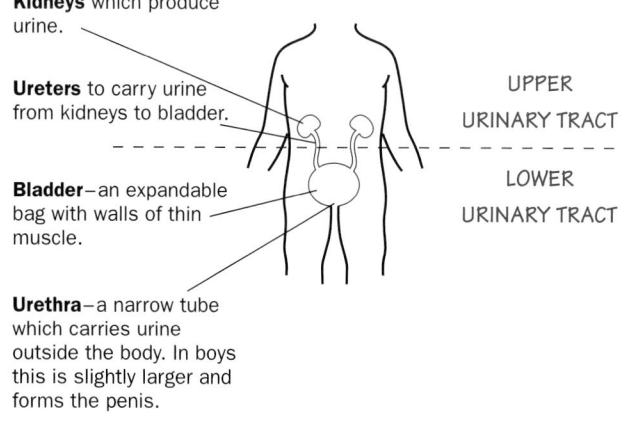

Kidneys which produce urine.

Ureters to carry urine from kidneys to bladder.

UPPER URINARY TRACT

LOWER URINARY TRACT

Bladder–an expandable bag with walls of thin muscle.

Urethra–a narrow tube which carries urine outside the body. In boys this is slightly larger and forms the penis.

◆ CAN THEY BE TREATED?

YES. It is important to know if your child has a urine infection **as soon as possible**. Treatment with antibiotics **is effective**.

Figure 6.8
Information about the kidneys and urinary tract from a patient information leaflet to help parents understand the importance of making the diagnosis of UTI in early childhood (Bourdeaux, 1996).

involved are aware of the diagnostic problem and perceive a useful and positive outcome from the diagnosis of UTI in infants. This can be achieved with staff training, locally agreed guidelines, access to appropriate equipment and a multidisciplinary approach to the problem. Leaflets have been shown to have the greatest benefit when they address a specific problem, are targeted at a vulnerable group and are used in conjunction with other resources (Bourdeaux, 1996). Co-ordination with a programme of education for staff is more likely to result in a positive outcome.

Information leaflets need to be sent to all families with children under two years since the difficulties in making the diagnosis and risk of renal scarring are greatest in this age group. They should also be available to all staff in the practice so that they are aware of the policy to exclude UTI in every sick infant and toddler.

Leaflets should outline the usual presenting symptoms, emphasizing the non-specific nature of illness and the absence of urinary symptoms in the majority of cases. There should be clear advice on what to do if an infant has a fever or other suggestive symptoms and advice on when to call the doctor or visit the surgery. There should also be advice on why urine collection is necessary, how to collect a sample, how to store urine and later transfer it to the laboratory. Some advice on treatment of the acute condition and long-term management plan is also helpful and puts the process into perspective.

IX Complications of urinary tract infection

Although many UTIs result in relatively trivial illness, in the acute situation they can cause electrolyte disturbances, septicaemia and occasionally acute renal failure. In the long term, renal scarring (see *Figure 6.7*) and poor renal growth are the main complications. Scarred renal tissue is non-functional and, as a consequence, the glomerular filtration rate of affected kidneys is reduced. If bilateral scarring is present the child is at risk of chronic renal failure. Renal scarring is also the commonest cause of hypertension and hypertensive encephalopathy in children. In pregnancy, there is an increased risk of pre-eclampsia. The incidence of renal scarring is increased in patients whose first UTI occurred during infancy (Miller, 1996) and in the presence of reflux and delays in treatment.

The infant kidney is particularly vulnerable to permanent damage. Infection often involves the renal parenchyma at this age, increasing the risk of renal scarring, 'chronic pyelonephritis' or 'reflux nephropathy' (Berg and Johansson, 1983). Kidney scarring has been reported following infection at all ages in childhood. However, in the UK, most scars are already present when the child is investigated following the first identified infection and new scars are rarely seen to develop, particularly after four years. This suggests that there have been unidentified infections earlier in childhood.

Once scarring has occurred, there is a small but significant risk of progression of kidney damage (Aggarwal et al., 1991). Delays in starting treatment with antibiotics, recurrent infections and vesicoureteric reflux all predispose to renal scar formation (Goldraich and Barratt, 1987; Smellie et al., 1985). Vesicoureteric reflux not only increases the risk of infection by interfering with bladder emptying but also enables bacteria to reach the upper tracts, predisposing to renal damage. Intrarenal reflux is present in infants with severe reflux and is closely associated with renal scarring even in the absence of UTIs. Vesicoureteric reflux is present in 30% of children with UTI and has a familial tendency with a dominant mode of inheritance (Aggarwal and Verrier Jones, 1989).

References

Aggarwal VK, Verrier Jones K (1989) Vesico-ureteric reflux: screening of first degree relatives. *Arch Dis Child* **64**: 1538–41.

Aggarwal VK, Verrier Jones K, Asscher AW, Evans C, Williams LA (1991) Covert bacteriuria: long term follow up. *Arch Dis Child* **66**: 1284–6.

Ahmed T, Vickers D, Campbell S, Coulthard MG, Pedler S (1991) Urine collection from disposable nappies. *Lancet* **338**: 674–6.

Berg UB, Johansson SB (1983) Age as a main determinant of renal functional damage in urinary tract infection. *Arch Dis Child* **58**: 963–9.

Bourdeaux KA (1996) A proposal for the development of new material for family teaching: urinary tract infections in children under two in primary care. BN Thesis, University of Wales College of Medicine.

Dighe AM, Grace JF (1984) General practice management of childhood urinary tract infection. *J Roy Coll Gen Pract* **34**: 324–7.

Goldraich N, Barratt TM (1987) Vesico-ureteric reflux and renal scarring. In: *Paediatric Nephrology*, 2nd edn (eds JM Barratt, M Holiday and R Vernier), Williams & Wilkins, Baltimore, pp 647–66.

Grol R (1992) Implementing guidelines in general practice care. *Quality Hlth Care* **1**: 184–91.

Helin I, Winberg J (1980) Chronic renal failure in Swedish children. *Acta Pardiatr Scand* **69**: 607–11.

Hoberman A, Chao H-P, Keller DM et al. (1993) Prevalence of urinary tract infection in februle infants. *J Paediatr* **123**(1): 17–22.

Jadresic L, Cartwright K, Cowie N, Witcombe B, Stevens D (1993) Investigations of urinary tract infection in childhood. *BMJ* **307**: 761–4.

Jewkes FEM, McMaster DJ, Napier WA, Houston IB, Postlewaite RJ (1990) Home collection of urine specimens: boric acid bottles of dipslides? *Arch Dis Child* 65: 286–9.

Lee P, Verrier Jones K (1991) Urinary tract infection in febrile convulsions. *Arch Dis Child* 66: 1287–90.

McFarlane K (1993) Primary vesicoureteric reflux in childhood. *Paediatr Nurs* 5(8): 20–2.

McKerrow W, Davidson-Lamb N, Jones PF (1984) Urinary tract infection in children. *BMJ* 289: 299–304.

Miller KL (1996) Urinary tract infections: children are not little adults. *Paediatr Nurs* 22(6): 473–80.

Powell HR, McCredie DA, Ritchie MA (1987) Urinary nitrite in symptomatic and asymptomatic urinary tract infection. *Arch Dis Child* 62: 138–40.

Rickwood A (1992) Current imaging of childhood urinary infections: prospective survey. *BMJ* 304: 663–5.

Smellie JM, Ransley PG, Normand ICS, Prescod N, Edwards D (1985) Development of new renal scars: a collaborative study. *BMJ* 290: 1957–60.

Smellie JM, Poulton A, Prescod NP (1994) Retrospective study of children with renal scarring associated with reflux and urinary infection. *BMJ* 308: 1193–6.

Stark H (1997) Urinary tract infection in girls: the cost effectiveness of currently recommended investigative routines. *Pediatr Nephrol* 11: 174–7.

United Kingdom Transplant Support Service Special Health Authority (1995) *Renal Transplant Audit 1984–1993*. UKTSSSHA, Bristol.

van der Voort J, Edwards A, Roberts R, Verrier Jones K (1997a) The struggle to diagnose UTI in children under two in primary care. *Fam Pract* 14(1): 44–8.

van der Voort J, Verrier Jones K, Edwards A (1997b) Can renal scarring be prevented by earlier diagnosis of urinary tract infection in infancy? *Kidney Int* 52: 1130.

Vernon S (1995) Urine collection from infants: a reliable method, *Paediatr Nurs* 7(6): 26–7.

Verrier Jones J (1993) Ask the expert – what is the current recommendation for the management of covert bacteriuria in infants and pre-school children? *Pediatr Nephrol* 7: 146.

Verrier Jones K (1995) What is the best way of achieving a urine specimen from a child under two years old? *Med Pract* 2(2): 2.

Winberg J (1982) Clinical pyelonephritis, focal renal scarring. A selected review of pathogenesis, prevention and prognosis. *Paediatr Clin North Am* 29: 801–14.

Winberg J, Anderson HJ, Bergstrom T, Jacobson B, Larson H, Lincoln K (1974) Epidemiology of symptomatic urinary tract infection in childhood. *Acta Paediatr Scand* **63** (suppl 252): 1–20.

Working Group of the Research Unit, Royal College of Physicians (1991) Guidelines for the management of acute urinary tract infection in childhood. *J Roy Coll Physicians London* **25**(1): 36–42.

Urinary tract infection: gynaecological aspects

Charlotte Chaliha and Stuart L Stanton

7

Contents

I   Introduction

Urinary tract infection is one of the most common infectious diseases seen in both community and hospital practice and a significant cause of morbidity in women. It is estimated to affect 50% of adult women at least once in their lives (Zielske et al., 1981) and accounts for 1–6% of consultations to general practitioners. The signs and symptoms of infection are diverse varying from asymptomatic bacteriuria to the more serious sequelae of acute pyelonephritis, bacteraemia and renal failure. Understanding the pathophysiology and aetiology of these infections will allow appropriate evaluation and classification of infection and so direct treatment more effectively and potentially reduce the distress and severity of symptoms for many women.

II   Terminology

Urinary tract infections encompass a wide spectrum of clinical and pathological conditions involving the whole or selected parts of the urinary tract. It is important to classify infection appropriately as the pathogenesis of these conditions may differ and distinguishing them has implications for both treatment and prognosis.

Cystitis is used to describe inflammation of the bladder. This can be bacterial or abacterial. The typical presenting symptoms are abdominal pain, dysuria, frequency and nocturia.

Urethritis indicates inflammation of the urethra and gives similar symptoms to cystitis. The term 'urethral syndrome' is used to describe the presence of dysuria, frequency and urgency in the absence of bacteriuria in the voided specimen. This may occur in combination with cystitis.

'Urinary tract infection' refers to the presence of bacteria in the urinary tract. There is no diagnostic requirement for this classification; however, most significant urinary tract infections are accompanied by bacteriuria.

'Bacteriuria' indicates the presence of bacteria in freshly voided urine or that obtained from suprapubic catheterization. This may occur as a result of infection or contamination of the urine specimen at the time of collection as bladder urine is usually sterile. Asymptomatic bacteriuria refers to significant bacteriuria in a patient without urinary tract symptoms. This is often seen in the elderly and pregnant patients (Andriole, 1975; Boscia et al., 1986). In those with symptoms this is called 'significant bacteriuria'. This term is used to distinguish the bacteriuria of 'infection' from that of 'contamination'. Traditionally, infection is distinguished from contamination at the threshold level of greater than 10^5 colony forming units (cfu) or organisms per mm^2 of voided urine. This definition proposed by

Kass (1956) is stringent and has come under scrutiny as it has low sensitivity though high specificity in symptomatic woman and more than 50% of women with acute symptomatic coliform infection have bacterial counts below this level. More recently, it has been suggested that a value of 10^2 cfu of coliform bacteria per millimetre of urine may be a more sensitive diagnostic criteria whilst being only slightly less specific than the former value (Stamm et al., 1982).

'Pyelonephritis' indicates infection of the kidney and can be acute or chronic. 'Acute' pyelonephritis is caused by infection of the renal parenchyma and collecting system and is often complicated by bacteraemia. 'Chronic' infection occurs from progressive inflammation of the renal interstitium and tubules. The sequelae include scarring and shrinkage of the kidney.

'Relapse of infection' is recurrence of bacteriuria with the same organism as originally isolated. It indicates persistence of the organism within the urinary tract. 'Reinfection' indicates acquisition of a new pathogen. 'Uncomplicated urinary tract' infections are bacterial infections in the bladder occurring in an otherwise healthy woman. These patients usually have a short duration of symptoms.

'Complicated urinary infections' are those in which there is also fever, flank pain and tenderness and occurs in men, pregnant women, those with recurrent infections, the immunocompromised, and those with structural and functional abnormalities of the urinary tract.

III Prevalence

Owing to the anatomically shorter urethra, women have a higher risk of urinary tract infection than men. The incidence of urinary tract infections increases with age. In the first year of life, the incidence is 1–2% and this is associated with congenital abnormalities of the urinary tract (Winberg et al., 1974). The incidence in women then decreases to 1% till puberty and then increases at about the age of 15 years, which corresponds with the initiation of sexual activity (Zielske et al., 1981). In non-pregnant women, the incidence is approximately 5% between the ages of 21 and 65 years (Kaye, 1980). In the elderly, urinary infections are far more common. The incidence rises markedly over 65 years (Brocklehurst et al., 1977) to 20% of women aged 65–70 years and up to 50% of women over the age of 80 years. This high prevalence in the elderly seems related to place of residence with the highest rates in those in nursing homes and extended care facilities compared to those in the community (Akhtar et al., 1972; Gladstone and Recco, 1976). This high prevalence in the elderly is suggested to be secondary to prior cerebrovascular accidents, decreased functional and mental capacity, bladder catheterization and prior antibiotic usage (Powers et al., 1988).

IV Microbiology

The majority of urinary tract infections are caused by bacteria though they can occasionally occur with fungi and viruses. The three postulated mechanisms for the development of infection are via haematogenous, lymphatic and ascending pathways. The majority of infections are secondary to Gram-negative aerobic organisms that originate from the faecal flora. *Escherichia coli* accounts for up to 85% of community acquired infections (Maskell et al., 1983; Bryan and Reynolds, 1984a). Other less common causative organisms are *Staphylococcus saprophyticus* which accounts for 10% of infections, *Klebsiella* for 5% of infections, and *Enterobacter* and *Proteus* species for approximately 2% each (Cunha, 1981).

Hospital-acquired infections have a different spectrum of causative organisms. *E. coli* accounts for 50% of cases and *Enterococcus faecalis* for approximately 15%. *Klebsiella, Enterobacter, Citrobacter, Serratia, Pseudomonas, Providencia, Enterococcus* and *Staphylococcus epidermidis* account for the rest (Bryan and Reynolds, 1984b). This altered spectrum of bacterial agents is owing to the use of indwelling catheters, cross-infection, urinary tract instrumentation and the selection of resistant organisms by antimicrobial agents. Fungal infections are also far commoner in hospital settings. In immunocompromised hosts, viral infection with HIV and the herpes virus accounts for a small number of infections.

Sexually transmitted agents such as *Trichomonas vaginalis, Chlamydia trachomatis, Neisseria gonorrhoea* and *Ureaplasma* may also cause urinary tract infection.

1. *Bacterial virulence factors*

These pathogenic organisms must override host defence systems to ascend and colonize the urinary tract and have specific virulence factors to facilitate this. The adherence of the bacteria to the uroepithelial cells is a prerequisite for infection to occur as they are most often washed away by the urine on entry to the urethra and bladder. Adherence is facilitated by bacterial surface structures called adhesins and complementary components on the uroepithelial cells or mucus. *E. coli* possess surface organelles called pili which act as adhesins. There are various adhesins that have been identified and are well documented in the pathogenesis of infection. The adherence of bacteria not only allows persistence at the site of infection but also has advantages in promoting growth and therefore toxin production (Zafriri et al., 1987). Other pathogens such as *Klebsiella* and *Proteus* have been shown to express pili that are important for adherence to urinary catheters (Mobley et al., 1987, 1988).

There are also factors specific to each bacterial pathogen that facilitate disease. Three specific antigens identified on the surface of pathogenic *E. coli* are O (lipopolysaccharide), K (capsular polysaccharide), and H (flagellar antigen) (Ofek et al., 1977; Brooks et al., 1980; Orskov and Orskov, 1983). The polysaccharide capsule of *E. coli* may aid resistance to phagocytosis by the host (Svanborg-Eden et al., 1987). The lipopolysaccharide present in the cell membrane of Gram-negative bacteria has been shown to reduce ureteric peristalsis, which may aid ascent of these organisms up the urinary tract (Thulesius and Araj, 1987). *E. coli* growth is strongly influenced by iron such that it produces virulence factors in the form of haemolysins that degrade cells and aerobactin that enhances iron uptake.

Virulence factors are most important for infectivity in a normal host as opposed to a host that has urinary tract abnormalities or is immunologically compromised. Strains that infect the normal host have multiple virulence factors compared to those infecting compromised hosts (Johnson et al., 1988).

2.   *Host factors*

There is evidence to suggest that impaired host factors predispose to urinary tract infection. These risk factors are most likely to be at the cellular or subcellular levels as anatomical abnormalities account for less than 5% of cases of recurrent cystitis (Fowler and Pulaski, 1981). Factors that may predispose to infection include local trauma such as after sexual intercourse, impaired bladder emptying so that wash-out of organisms does not occur and direct introduction of organisms during instrumentation of the urinary tract.

(i)   Systemic factors

Diabetic patients are particularly prone to urinary tract infections owing to neurogenic bladder dysfunction and the presence of glycosuria which is a potent culture medium for bacterial growth. Neurological disorders such as multiple sclerosis or after a cerebrovascular attack may result in impaired bladder emptying and predispose to infection. This can also occur with various anticholinergic medications. In the presence of stones or catheters, there is an increased likelihood of infection as these serve as a nidus for bacterial growth.

(ii)   Adherence factors

Uroepithelial and vaginal cells of women with a history of recurrent urinary tract infections show a stronger adherence to *E. coli* than control cells (Svanborg-Eden and Jodal, 1979; Schaeffer et al., 1981).

(iii) Sexual intercourse and method of contraception

There is a strong association with sexual activity and the development of infection (Kunin, 1978; Buckley et al., 1978; Foxman and Frerichs, 1985). Sexual activity can promote bacterial colonization not only by introducing rectal and vaginal bacteria into the urethral area, but also by disrupting the uroepithelial cells. There have been several prospective studies that have shown the onset of urinary infection occurs soon after sexual intercourse (Nicolle et al., 1982) such that a woman who has had sexual intercourse in the preceding 48 hours has a risk 60 times greater than one who has not. Cross-sectional data has shown that initiating sexual activity of any kind increases the risk of urinary infection 3.5-fold (Foxman et al., 1997).

This association of sexual activity and infection is strongly linked to contraceptive usage, specifically diaphragm and spermicide usage (Fihn et al., 1985; Hooton et al., 1991a, b). It had been thought that urethral obstruction from the diaphragm predisposed to urinary infection. However, it seems more likely from subsequent studies that it is an effect of spermicide on vaginal flora. Diaphragm–spermicide users have been noted to have an alteration of vaginal flora with an increase in *E. coli* colonization, an increase in vaginal pH, decrease in lactobacilli concentration and alteration in anaerobic flora. Urinating after sexual intercourse may decrease the risk of urinary infection by flushing out bacteria which have been introduced (Foxman and Frerichs, 1985; Strom et al., 1987).

(iv) Host defence factors

Regular voiding helps prevent infection by flushing out pathogens from the urinary tract. Urine of low and high osmolality combined with a low pH of urine is inhibitory to bacterial growth as it serves to decrease phagocytosis and complement reactions. There are also specific agents within the urine which may prevent attachment of the bacteria to the epithelial cells (Funfstuck et al., 1987). These include the immunoglobulins IgA, IgG (Svanborg-Eden and Svennerholm, 1978), and urinary oligosaccharides (Parkkinen et al., 1988). Other mechanisms to prevent adherence include the presence of lactobacilli (Chan et al., 1985) and uromucoid (Tamm–Horsfall protein) secreted by the loop of Henle, that interfere with binding of *E. coli* to uroepithelial cells (Orskov et al., 1980). Lactobacillus may also produce hydrogen peroxide that may inhibit vaginal colonization with uropathogens (Klebanoff et al., 1991). The glycosaminoglycans lining may prevent bacterial adherence and this layer has been shown to be reduced in patients with recurrent cystitis (Parsons et al., 1977; Parsons, 1982).

The vaginal pH and lactobacilli content

are important mechanisms to prevent infection. In premenopausal women, oestrogens promote the growth of lactobacilli within the vagina which maintains a low pH, inhibitory to the growth of many uropathogens (Molander et al., 1990). In menopausal women, the decrease in lactobacilli, and vaginal secretions with a high pH leads to a predisposition to growth of enterobacteria (Parsons and Schmidt, 1982).

V Clinical presentation

The signs and symptoms of urinary tract infection can vary widely. The typical symptoms of urinary tract infection are frequency, nocturia, dysuria, urgency and suprapubic pain. Haematuria may also be present though this is rarely frank haematuria. On examination, the patient is tender in the suprapubic region and generally looks unwell. If pyelonephritis is present the patient may also have loin pain and fever and usually feels systemically unwell. Signs of septicaemia such as tachycardia and postural hypotension may also be seen.

VI Diagnosis

A careful history is required to aid diagnosis and to indicate any predisposing features such as recent urinary tract instrumentation, recent intercourse, and a history of renal pathology or poor bladder emptying. A history of urinary tract infection in the past should be also noted, particularly if there was any microbiological confirmation of infection, and if so, what the organisms were, the treatment instituted and the response to treatment. This is particularly valuable if there is a history of recurrent infections. Contraceptive practice should be enquired about, particularly the use of the diaphragm and spermicide and whether sexual intercourse precipitates symptoms.

The fluid intake and voiding patterns of the patient should be recorded. Frequency itself may be solely due to a high fluid intake. In a woman who voids infrequently, there may be an increased risk of urinary infection if there is stasis of urine. The patient should be asked if her bladder feels empty after voiding, and if not, this may indicate a high residual urine.

The gynaecological examination should exclude a pelvic mass and pregnancy: any residual urine merits a neurological examination of the S2–4 nerve roots to exclude a neuropathy.

The differential diagnosis includes bladder conditions such as detrusor instability, interstitial cystitis, drug-induced cystitis, bladder calculi and other foreign bodies. Gynaecological conditions which may produce lower abdominal pain with some frequency and urgency, include endometriosis, ovarian torsion or cyst rupture, ectopic or early miscarriage.

VII   Investigation

1.   Stick tests

There are various commercial stick tests available for rapid analysis of urine. These are based on either photometry or bioluminescence and test for bacteriuria, pyuria and haematuria. The test most commonly used is the nitrite test which tests for urinary nitrite, formed by conversion of urinary nitrate by bacteria. This test can be combined with esterase which tests for pyuria. Ideally, these tests should be performed on the first voided urine of the day as false-negative results are more likely to occur with later samples (Wu et al., 1985).

Hurlbut et al. (1991) reviewed 51 articles, to assess the accuracy of these rapid dipstick tests. They found that the leukocyte esterase test was a better indicator of infection compared to the nitrite dipsticks. Whilst these tests provide a sensitive measure of bacteriuria, they are not sensitive enough to detect low count bacteriuria of 10^2–10^4 cfu/ml of urine (Johnson and Stamm, 1989) but they are useful in situations where laboratory facilities are not available (Olson et al., 1991). However, evaluation of reagent strips (blood, protein, nitrite and leukocyte esterase) in screening pregnant women for asymptomatic bacteriuria has too low a sensitivity to justify any cost savings as it has been estimated that up to 25% of cases of infected urine would be missed if reagent strips were used alone (Tincello and Richmond, 1998).

2.   Urine microscopy and culture

Traditionally, urine microscopy and culture have been the gold standard for the diagnosis of infection. Microscopy of a centrifuged urine sample assesses the presence of bacteria, pus and red blood cells. The presence of pus cells is seen in nearly all cases of women with urinary infection. The presence of pus cells when no organism is seen is called sterile pyuria and may indicate infection with tuberculosis.

Microscopy of urine has a high specificity of 90% and sensitivity of 80% in predicting infections at colony counts of greater than 10^4 cfu/ml (Fihn and Stamm, 1983). However, this is less reliable at lower colony counts and if the urine is not centrifuged adequately. Urine culture and sensitivity is advantageous since it allows detection of the organism as well as indicating appropriate antibiotic use. It should be performed in cases of complicated urinary infections such as patients with urinary tract abnormalities, pregnancy, diabetes, recurrent infections, those who have had recent instrumentation of the urinary tract, and if previous tests are not available or the diagnosis unclear. In these cases, there is the potential for serious sequelae if the incorrect antimicrobial regime is used.

Specimens for urine culture should be analysed as soon as possible and if necessary only stored for a few hours at 4°C, otherwise bacterial proliferation may occur leading to a falsely high count. Contamination of the specimen can also occur with skin flora during collection. This problem is avoided by use of a catheter specimen or one taken via suprapubic aspiration. Laboratories may differ in standardization of their reports, not always indicating the organisms present, nor the presence of any associated findings such as pus cells, and red cell casts. More importantly, the definition of infection may differ between laboratories. A cut-off level of 10^5 cfu/ml though standard in most but not all laboratories, may be too stringent and laboratories may report lower counts as negative specimens though as discussed this may miss early diagnosis of infection.

If a tuberculous cystitis is suspected, at least three early morning urine specimens should be sent for mycobacteria culture. Vaginal and urethral swabs should be sent for *Chlamydia*. If symptoms are recurrent, a renal ultrasound and abdominal (KUB) X-ray should be performed.

3.   Imaging studies

In the past, an intravenous urogram was a commonly requested investigation for women with recurrent urinary tract infections. This is not an ideal investigation in assessing this group of women who are often of childbearing age and in whom the possibility of pregnancy should always be considered, as it emits a large dose of radiation to the gonads. As well as this, the diagnostic yield is low and it is expensive to perform (Lieberman and Macchia, 1982; De Lange and Jones, 1983) and most importantly is associated with a high risk of allergy that may be fatal.

A combination of an ultrasound of the pelvis and plain abdominal X-ray (KUB) has been shown to be superior to an intravenous urography in the detection of abnormalities (Lewis-Jones et al., 1989; Spencer et al., 1990). A plain abdominal X-ray will detect the presence of stones and foreign bodies and the presence of calcification as seen with chronic infections. Ultrasound studies are useful in the assessment of the shape and contour of the kidneys and for the detection of any obstruction. If the bladder is full, calculi and diverticuli can be shown. It will also identify the presence of residual urine, assess bladder emptying and any co-existent pelvic pathology. It has the advantage over an intravenous urogram in that it is non-invasive and therefore more acceptable to the patient and does not utilize radiation. Should a pregnancy be detected on ultrasound, further investigation by means of a KUB, which involves radiation, can then be avoided.

VIII   Treatment

Patients should be advised to maintain a fluid intake of at least 2 litres of fluid per day and for those with a high residual urine, to void regularly to complete bladder emptying.

1. Prevention

Instructions on perineal hygiene are important to avoid further infections so that after defaecation or micturition, the perineum is wiped from front to back and not vice versa. For those women in whom sexual intercourse precipitates an attack, postcoital treatment combined with postcoital voiding is recommended. Women using spermicides and diaphragms for contraception should be counselled regarding the association of diaphragm–spermicide usage and infection and advised on alternative forms of contraception. Single doses of co-trimoxazole, nalidixic acid, and nitrofurantoin have been found to be effective in the treatment of recurrent urinary infections associated with sexual intercourse in young women (Pfau et al., 1983). The beneficial effects of cranberry juice are receiving increasing attention as a prophylactic measure that acts by reducing bacterial adherence to mucosal surfaces. At least 300 ml per day are recommended.

2. Antimicrobial therapy

The aim of treatment is to eradicate the pathogenic organism with minimal local and systemic side effects. Treatment should be tailored to the individual and be specific to the causative organism as well as accounting for antimicrobial resistance patterns. There is a high incidence of vulvovaginal candidiasis,

hypersensitivity and gastrointestinal disturbance with the use of antimicrobial agents. This can result in considerable morbidity, especially in elderly patients. Treatment should be balanced to minimize side effects which will increase patient compliance. The ideal antibiotic should have minimal effect on vagina and bowel flora as displacement of protective commensals predisposes to colonization with virulent resistant strains. This can occur if there is poor gastrointestinal absorption and high serum levels of the drug.

There are various properties that promote the effectiveness of an antimicrobial agent. The drug must be able to bind to the organism and interfere with its growth, be able to remain on the organism for a sufficient period of time to be effective and able to reach and penetrate the cell wall. To avoid high serum levels, rapid renal excretion of the antimicrobial is preferable. However, a drug that is excreted too rapidly may provide less therapeutic activity than one that is present at significant urinary concentrations for a longer time. The duration the drug remains within the circulation affects the dosing regime so one that remains at high concentrations can be given on a twice-daily basis which will aid patient compliance.

In the selection of the most suitable antimicrobial, various factors should be borne in mind. These include the site of infection, the aetiological agent, age of patient, complicating factors and the history of the infection.

Ampicillin and amoxycillin should be used with caution as there is a 20–50% resistance to *E. coli* and a high risk of allergic reaction and Stevens–Johnson syndrome. The addition of a β-lactamase inhibitor improves the effectiveness. Amoxycillin can also affect vaginal flora and lead to vaginal candidiasis in up to 25% of patients (Parsons, 1988). The cephalosporins cause less resistance amongst bowel flora than the penicillins and are excreted in high concentrations within the urine. They also affect vaginal flora, predisposing to candidiasis in 15% of women. Adverse reactions are rare, but there is a 10–20% cross-reactivity to cephalosporins in patients with a history of allergy to penicillin. Trimethoprim alone or in combination with sulfamethoxazole is effective against most urinary pathogens. Allergic reactions are common and include diarrhoea, nausea, vomiting and rashes. Five to fifteen percent of species are resistant to trimethoprim and the trimethoprim-sulfamethoxazole combination. Sulphonamides are also effective but associated with the emergence of resistant bowel flora. Nitrofurantoin is good first-line drug with only 15% drug resistance. It should be used with caution in the elderly and in patients with a poor glomerular filtration rate, as it is less effective, and in those with reduced renal function there is a risk of partially reversible peripheral neuropathy. The newer quinolone class of antibiotics, nalidixic acid derivatives, e.g. norfloxacin, ofloxacin and ciprofloxacin, are well tolerated and have a broad spectrum of activity. They are particularly effective against *Pseudomonas* species and multiple antibiotic-resistance infection. Side effects include dizziness, headaches, gastrointestinal disturbances, photosensitivity, and abnormal transaminases. They should be avoided in children under 13 years as there is a risk of osteochondritis, in pregnancy, patients on theophylline and those with a history of seizures. Only 5% of organisms are resistant to quinolones partially because these drugs have been in use a much shorter time (Inter-Nordic Urinary Infection Study Group, 1988; Johnson and Stamm, 1989; Wolfson and Hooper, 1989; Norrby, 1990).

The duration of antimicrobial therapy has come under much debate. The traditional 7- to 14-day regimes have largely been replaced by shorter duration regimes in the treatment of uncomplicated infection. Single-dose therapies are associated with better compliance, fewer side effects and are less expensive. However, large controlled trials have demonstrated that single-dose therapy is less effective than conventional therapy and more likely to result in recurrences (Schultz et al., 1984; Philbrick and Bracikowski, 1985; Fihn et al., 1988; Johnson and Stamm, 1989; Norrby, 1990). This is particularly so for patients with occult renal infection and when the urinary infection is complicated, e.g. in pregnancy, structural abnormalities of the urinary tract and diabetes (Fihn et al., 1988; Johnson and Stamm, 1989; Norrby, 1990). Single-dose therapy with fluoroquinolones is particularly prone to failure with infection with *Staphylococcus saprophyticus* (Norrby, 1990; Ronald et al., 1992). This recurrence of infection is thought to be secondary to persistent urethral colonization with the infective agent from the faecal and vaginal reservoirs from which the organism has not been eradicated. Higher cure rates of up to 95% are seen with trimethoprim and trimethoprim-sulfamethoxazole combinations compared to penicillins with cure rates of 50–85% (Johnson and Stamm, 1989; Norrby, 1990). This is probably secondary to the higher resistance rate of strains to penicillins and because penicillins are cleared from the urine more quickly.

Three-day regimes have been evaluated as an alternative to the relative poor efficacy of single-day regimes. Norrby (1990) in a review of trials comparing short-term treatment of acute cystitis, concluded that three-day courses of trimethoprim-sulfamethoxazole and penicillins were more effective than single-day regimes. Adverse side effects were commoner if treatment was extended past three days. In a comparison of three-day regimes using different antimicrobials, twice-daily trimethoprim-sulfamethoxazole was more effective than nitrofurantoin, cefadroxil or amoxycillin and was also the least expensive (Hooton et al., 1995). Therefore three-day regimes seem to be an optimal regime. Longer duration of therapy for 7–10 days should be considered in patients with systemic disease such as diabetes, those with a history of pyelonephritis, recurrent infection, childhood history of urinary infection, and those with known structural abnormalities of the urinary tract. In patients with acute cystitis whose symptoms persist beyond three days' therapy, a urine culture and sensitivity should be obtained to confirm the infecting organism and antibiotic sensitivities.

IX   Role of gynaecologists

Most initial attacks of urinary tract infection are dealt with by the primary physician or family doctor. The role of the gynaecologist is in the management of recurrent urinary tract infections including awareness of differential diagnosis, particularly from other bladder conditions such as detrusor instability, interstitial cystitis and drug-induced cystitis. The gynaecologist should be aware of the precipitating causes such as use of spermicides in condoms and diaphragms and compounded by infrequent voiding or inadequate fluid intake. In a postmenopausal woman, insufficient oestrogenization and occasionally an early bladder carcinoma will present as an infection. In a patient with a neuropathic bladder (e.g. multiple sclerosis) incomplete emptying and bladder or renal calculi and upper tract dilatation should be excluded.

During pregnancy, early detection of asymptomatic bacteriuria or overt urinary tract infection and its prompt treatment is necessary to avoid the development of acute pyelonephritis and premature labour.

Following bladder-neck surgery, management of any voiding difficulty may require indwelling or intermittent catheterization and clinical follow up to avoid the sequel of recurrent urinary tract infection.

X   Conclusions

Urinary tract infections are a significant cause of distress and morbidity in women. Effective management of these infections involves accurate diagnosis and treatment. Advice on prevention and prophylaxis of infection should be given as appropriate. Antimicrobial use must be tailored to the individual and be influenced by drug sensitivity, resistance patterns, patient compliance, side effects and cost-effectiveness. In cases of recurrent or persistent infection, referral to a specialist clinic for further investigation should be considered.

References

Akhtar AJ, Andrews GR, Caird FI et al (1972) Urinary tract infection in the elderly: A population study. *Age Ageing* 1: 48–54.

Andriole VT (1975) Urinary tract infections in pregnancy. *Urol Clin North Am* 2: 485.

Boscia JA, Kobasa WD, Knight RA et al (1986) Epidemiology of bacteriuria in an elderly ambulatory population. *Am J Med* 80: 208.

Brocklehurst JC, Bee P, Jones D, Palmer MK (1977) Bacteriuria in geriatric hospital patients; its correlates and management. *Age Ageing* 6: 240–5.

Brooks H, O'Grady F, Mcsherry A et al (1980) Uropathogenic properties of *Escherichia coli* in recurrent urinary tract infection. *J Med Microbiol* 13: 57.

Bryan CS, Reynolds KL (1984a) Community-acquired bacteremic urinary tract infection: Epidemiology and outcome. *J Urol* 132: 490.

Bryan CS, Reynolds KL (1984b) Hospital-acquired bacteremic urinary tract infection: Epidemiology and outcome. *J Urol* 132: 494.

Buckley RM Jr, McGuckin M, MacGregor RR (1978) Urine bacterial counts after sexual intercourse. *N Engl J Med* 298: 321–4.

Chan RCY, Reid G, Irvin RT et al (1985) Competitive exclusion of uropathogens from the human uroepithelial cells by *Lactobacillus* whole cells and cell wall fragments. *Infect Immun* 47: 84.

Cunha B (1981) Urinary tract infections. I. Pathophysiology and diagnostic approach. *Postgrad Med* 70: 141–58.

De Lange HE, Jones B (1983) Unnecessary intravenous urography in women with recurrent urinary tract infections. *Clin Radiol* 34: 551–3.

Fihn SD, Stamm WE (1983) Management of women with acute dysuria. In: Rund D, Wolcott BW, eds *Emergency Medicine Annual*, Vol. 2, p.225. Norwalk: Appleton-Century-Crofts.

Fihn SD, Latham RH, Roberts P, Running K, Stamm WE (1985) Association between diaphragm use and urinary tract infection. *JAMA* 254: 240.

Fihn SD, Johnson C, Roberts PL, Running K, Stamm WE (1988) Trimethoprim-sulfamethoxazole for acute dysuria in women: a single-dose or 10-day course. A double-blind randomised trial. *Ann Intern Med* 108: 350–7.

Fowler JE, Pulaski ET (1981) Excretory urography, cystography and cystoscopy in the evaluation of women with urinary tract infection: a prospective study. *N Engl J Med* 304: 462–5.

Foxman B, Frerichs RR (1985) Epidemiology of urinary tract infection: I. Diaphragm use and sexual intercourse. *Am J Public Health* 75: 1308–13.

Foxman B, Zhang L, Tallman P et al (1997) Transmission of uropathogens between sex partners. *J Infect Dis* 175: 989–92.

Funfstuck R, Stein G, Fuchs M, Bergner M, Wessel G, Keil E, Suss J (1987) The influence of selected urinary constituents on the adhesion properties of *Escherichia coli* to human uroepithelial cells. *Clin Nephrol* 28: 244–9.

Gladstone JL, Recco R (1976) Host factors and infectious diseases in the elderly. *Med Clin N Am* 60(6): 1225–40.

Hooton TM, Hillier S, Johnson C, Roberts PL, Stamm WE (1991a) *Escherichia coli* bacteriuria and contraceptive method. *JAMA* 265: 64–9.

Hooton TM, Fennell CL, Clark AM, Stamm WE (1991b) Nonoxynol-9: differential antibacterial activity and enhancement of bacterial adherence to vaginal epithelial cells. *J Infect Dis* 164: 1216–19.

Hooton TM, Winter C, Tiu F, Stamm WE (1995) Randomised comparative trial and cost analysis of 3-day antimicrobial regimen for the treatment of acute cystitis in women. *JAMA* 273: 41–5.

Hurlbut TA, Littenberg B and the Diagnostic Technology Assessment (1991) The diagnostic accuracy of rapid dipsticks to predict urinary tract infection. *Am J Clin Pathol* 96: 582–8.

Inter-Nordic Urinary Tract Infection Study Group (1988) Double-blind comparison of 3-day versus 7-day treatment with norfloxacin in symptomatic urinary infection. *Scand J Infect Dis* **20:** 619–24.

Johnson JR, Moseley SL, Roberts PL, Stamm WE (1988) Aerobactin and other virulence factor genes among strains of *E. coli* causing urosepsis: association with patient characteristics. *Infect Immun* **56:** 405–12.

Johnson JR, Stamm WE (1989) Urinary tract infections in women: diagnosis and treatment. *Ann Intern Med* **111:** 906.

Kass EH (1956) Asymptomatic infections of the urinary tract. *Trans Assoc Am Physicians* **69:** 56–64.

Kaye D (1980) Urinary tract infections in the elderly. *Bull NY Acad Med* **56:** 209–20.

Klebanoff SJ, Hillier SL, Eisenbach DA, Waltersdorph AM (1991) Control of the microbial flora of the vagina by H_2O_2-generating lactobacilli. *J Infect Dis* **164:** 94–100.

Kunin CM (1978) Sexual intercourse and urinary infections [Editorial]. *N Engl J Med* **298:** 336–7.

Lewis-Jones HG, Lang GHR, Hughes PL (1989) Can ultrasound replace the intravenous urogram in the preliminary investigation of urinary tract disease? *Br J Radiol* **62:** 977–80.

Lieberman E, Macchia RJ (1982) Excretory urography in women with urinary tract infection. *J Urol* **127:** 263–4.

Maskell R, Pead L, Sanderson RA (1983) Fastidious bacteria and the urethral syndrome: A 2-year clonical and bacteriological study of 51 women. *Lancet* **ii:** 1277.

Mobley HLT, Chippendale GR, Tenney JH et al (1987) Expression of type 1 fimbriae may be required for persistence of *Escherichia coli* in the catheterised urinary tract. *J Clin Microbiol* **25:** 2253.

Mobley HLT, Chippendale GR, Tenney GH et al (1988) MR/K haemagglutination of *Providencia stuartii* correlates with adherence to catheters and with persistence in catheter associated bacteriuria. *J Infect Dis* **157:** 264.

Molander U, Milsom I, Ekelund P, Mellstrom D, Eriksson O (1990) Effect of oral oestriol on vaginal flora and cytology and urogenital symptoms in the postmenopause. *Maturitas* **12:** 113–20.

Nicolle LE, Harding GKM, Preiksaitis J, Ronald AR (1982) The association of urinary tract infection with sexual intercourse. *J Infect Dis* **146:** 579–84.

Norrby SR (1990) Short-term treatment of uncomplicated lower urinary tract infections in women. *Rev Infect Dis* **12:** 458–67.

Ofek I, Mirelman D, Sharon N (1977) Adherence of *Escherichia coli* to human mucosal cells mediate by mannose receptors. *Nature* **265:** 623.

Olson ML, Shanholtzer CJ, Willard KE, Peterson LR (1991) The slide centrifuge Gram stain as a screening method. *Am J Clin Pathol* **96**: 454–8.

Orskov I, Orskov F, Birch-Anderson A (1980) Comparison of *Escherichia coli* fimbrial antigen F7 with type 1 fimbriae. *Infect Immun* **27**: 651.

Orskov I, Orskov F (1983) Summary of a workshop on the clone concept in the epidemiology taxonomy and evolution of the Enterobacteriaceae and other bacteria. *J Infect Dis* **148**: 346.

Parkkinen J, Virkola R, Korhonen TK (1988) Identification of factors in human urine that inhibit the binding of *Escherichia coli* adhesins. *Infect Immun* **56**: 2623.

Parsons CL (1988) Protocol for treatment of typical urinary tract infection: criteria for antimicrobial selection. *Urology* **32**(Suppl): 22–7.

Parsons DL, Schmidt JD (1982) Control of recurrent lower urinary tract infections in the postmenopausal women. *J Urol* **128**: 1224.

Parsons CL, Greenspan C, Moore SW et al (1977) Role of surface mucin in primary antibacterial defense of bladder. *Urology* **9**: 48–52.

Pfau A, Sacks T, Engelstein D (1983) Recurrent urinary tract infections in premenopausal women: prophylaxis based on an understanding of the pathogenesis. *J Urol* **129**: 1153–7.

Philbrick JT, Bracikowski JP (1985) Single-dose antibiotic treatment for uncomplicated urinary tract infections. *Arch Intern Med* **145**: 1672.

Powers JS, Tremaine Billings F, Behrendt D et al (1988) Antecedent factors in UTI among nursing home patients. *South Med J* **81**(6): 734–5.

Ronald AR, Nicolle LE, Harding GK (1992) Standards of therapy for urinary tract infections for adults. *Infection* **20**(Suppl 3): S164–S170.

Schaeffer AJ, Jones JM, Dunn JK (1981) Association of in vitro *Escherichia coli* adherence to vaginal and buccal epithelial cells with susceptibility of women to recurrent urinary tract infections. *N Engl J Med* **304**: 1062–6.

Schultz HJ, McCaffrey LA, Keys TF et al (1984) Acute cystitis: A prospective study of laboratory tests and duration of therapy. *Mayo Clin Proc* **59**: 391.

Spencer J, Lindsell D, Mastorakou I (1990) Ultrasonography compared with intravenous urography in the investigation of urinary tract infection in adults. *Br Med J* **301**: 221–4.

Stamm WE, Counts GW, Running KR et al (1982) Diagnosis of

coliform infection in acutely dysuric women. *N Engl J Med* **307**: 462.

Strom BL, Collins M, West SL, Kreisberg J, Weller S (1987) Sexual activity, contraceptive use, and other risk factors for symptomatic and asymptomatic bacteriuria. *Ann Intern Med* **107**: 816–23.

Svanborg-Eden C, Svennerholm AM (1978) Secretory immunoglobulin A and G antibodies prevent adhesion of *Escherichia coli* to human urinary tract epithelial cells. *Infect Immun* **22**: 790.

Svanborg-Eden C, Jodal U (1979) Attachment of *Escherichia coli* to urinary sediment epithelial cells from urinary tract in infection-prone and healthy children. *Infect Immun* **26**: 837–40.

Svanborg-Eden C, Hagberg L, Hull R et al (1987) Bacterial virulence versus host resistance in the urinary tracts of mice. *Infect Immun* **55**: 1224.

Thulesius O, Araj G (1987) The effect of uropathogenic bacteria on ureteral motility. *Urol Res* **15**: 273.

Tincello DG, Richmond DH (1998) Evaluation of reagent strips in detecting asymptomatic bacteriuria in early pregnancy: prospective case series. *BMJ* **316**: 435–7.

Winberg J, Anderson HJ, Bergstrom T et al (1974) Epidemiology of symptomatic urinary tract infection in childhood. *Acta Paediatr Scand* **252**(Suppl): 3–21.

Wolfson JS, Hooper DC (1989) Treatment of genitourinary tract infections with fluoroquinolones: activity in vitro, pharmacokinetics and clinical efficacy in urinary tract infections and prostatitis. *Antimicrob Agents Chemother* **33**: 1655–61.

Wu TC, Williams EC, Koo SY et al (1985) Evaluation of three bacteriuria screening methods in a clinical research hospital. *J Clin Microbiol* **21**: 796–814.

Zafriri D, Gron Y, Einstein BI et al (1987) Growth advantages and enhanced toxicity of *Escherichia coli* adherent to tissue culture cells due to restricted diffusion of products secreted by cells. *J Clin Invest* **79**: 1210.

Zielske JV, Lohr KN, Brook RH, Goldberg GA (1981) *Conceptualisation and the Measurement of Physiologic Health for Adults: Urinary Tract Infection.* Report R2262/16-HHS. Santa Monica: Rand Corporation.

Pregnancy

Allan B MacLean

8

Contents

I Introduction

Urinary tract infection is one of the most frequently seen 'medical' complications of pregnancy. It may be symptomatic or asymptomatic, it may be present at booking or appear acutely later in pregnancy and it may be persistent or recurrent.

II Definitions

Definitions are standard, whether the woman is pregnant or not; thus a urinary tract infection is the establishment and multiplication of micro-organisms within the urinary tract, whereas bacteriuria is the detection of bacteria in a voided urinary sample (Cattel, 1996). However, pregnancy requires that the definition of significant bacteriuria is equal to or more than 100,000 ($>1 \times 10^5$) of the same organism (or colony-forming unit) per millilitre of urine. Contamination from vulval skin or vaginal secretions (adding a mixture of organisms, mucus, vaginal cells and blood) may complicate dipstick analysis, microscopy and culture. Managing to catch a 'midstream' urine may be a problem during pregnancy, particularly in the third trimester, or difficult because of urgency, urinary leakage or the impossibility of stopping during micturition. Previously many antenatal clinics had a dedicated midwife to supervise the preparation and collection of midstream urines but such staff have disappeared in the drive for clinic economy, unless funded for research purposes. A single specimen may produce a false-positive rate of up to 40%, so that asymptomatic bacteriuria requires the identification of the same organism $>1 \times 10^5$ per millilitre in two consecutive samples.

Despite the obstetrician's enthusiasm for introducing needles into the amniotic sac, fetus or placenta, there is little or no interest in sticking a needle into distended bladders for confirmation by suprapubic aspiration.

Urinary tract organisms will be similar to those found in non-pregnant women, with 80% being *Escherichia coli* and the rest being from among *Enterococcus faecalis*, *Staphylococcus saprophyticus* or *Staph. epidermidis* group B streptococcus and various Gram-negative organisms including *Proteus*, *Klebsiella* and *Enterobacter* species (Bailey, 1990; Kass, 1962a; Wilkie et al., 1992). Recent research on *E. coli* has shown that only certain groups or strains (based on O antigens or serotypes) cause urinary tract infection (uropathogenic). Some of these strains may be characteristic in pregnant patients only and acute pyelonephritis during different trimesters of pregnancy may be associated with different though closely related *E. coli* isolates (Hart et al., 1996).

Earlier writers reported that the incidence of bacteriuria increased during pregnancy and was due to the pregnancy (Beard and Roberts, 1968; Kass, 1962a). However, it is likely that coitus is the important factor. Sleigh et al. (1964) found no cases of bacteriuria among pupil midwives in Edinburgh but an incidence of 8% among women attending an infertility clinic. Bailey (1972) described a rate of 1% among pupils leaving school and a rise to 10% when they returned to Student Health for contraception. Kunin and McCormack (1968) reported that the incidence of bacteriuria was lower in nuns than in working-class women, again suggesting that sexual activity and not pregnancy was responsible.

Many women will report urinary frequency and urgency as early symptoms of pregnancy. The differences between asymptomatic bacteriuria (strictly speaking, without urinary symptoms) and those women with cystitis, i.e. lower urinary tract infection, may be artificial. Abacterial cystitis is seen during pregnancy, perhaps as an hormonal association, and following delivery when urethral trauma and paraurethral bruising cause discomfort with micturition.

Acute pyelonephritis is the presence of fever, abdominal or loin pain, costovertebral angle tenderness, bladder and urethral symptoms during micturition but also at rest, and significant bacteriuria. It may be associated with preceding asymptomatic bacteriuria (see later) although the majority is not. Abdominal and back pain, tenderness and even fever occur during pregnancy for many reasons unrelated to the urinary tract.

Many patients admitted with a tentative diagnosis of acute pyelonephritis will have sterile urine, sometimes because antibiotics have been started prior to referral. Gilstrap et al. (1981a) found acute pyelonephritis in 2% of 24,000 obstetric patients reviewed.

The incidence is increased in the puerperium. Stray-Pedersen et al. (1990) found that 8% of 7000 postpartum patients had significant bacteriuria and Leigh et al. (1990) found that 34% of women in the first five days after caesarean section had symptomatic bacteriuria.

III Asymptomatic bacteriuria

On 25 January 1961, Dr Edward Kass participated in a panel discussion of the special committee on infant mortality for the Medical Society for the county of New York at the New York Academy of Medicine. Kass observed that bacteriuria was found in various patient groups in Boston City Hospital, including 6% of pregnant women presenting for their first antenatal visit. He described how patients with asymptomatic bacteriuria were divided into two groups, the first being treated with placebo and the second with either a long-acting sulphonamide or, if this failed (in approximately 20%) with nitrofurantoin. These patients were then followed at weekly intervals with urine cultures until they delivered. In the 48 patients who were given placebo, 20 developed pyelonephritis before term or during the first three months postpartum; 24% had prematurely born infants and there was 14% perinatal mortality rate. In the 43 patients who were treated there were no cases of pyelonephritis, there was no perinatal mortality and the prematurity rate was 10%. In 1000 non-bacteriuric control patients, there were no cases of pyelonephritis, perinatal mortality was 2% and prematurity rate was 9%. The untreated bacteriuric group had a greater likelihood of babies dying of prematurity, hyalinosis, pulmonary congestion or atelectasis, but not of sepsis. Kass urged that if asymptomatic bacteriuria was detected and treated, perinatal death could be reduced some 20–30% and that some 10–20% of premature births could be prevented.

In a subsequent report (Kass, 1962b), the number of patients was increased so that among 84 patients treated with antibiotics, only 7% had preterm delivery with no perinatal deaths, whereas in 95 patients treated with placebo only, there was a 27% preterm delivery and a 14% perinatal mortality rate. Thus asymptomatic bacteriuria produced a fourfold increase in prematurity and a significant association with perinatal mortality.

IV   Asymptomatic bacteriuria and pyelonephritis

Obstetricians have recognized for many years the dangers of pyelonephritis during pregnancy. The effect of progesterone produced in large quantities from the placenta is to alter ureteric activity, allowing organisms to ascend from the bladder into the renal pelvis and from there to infect the renal parenchyma. Many studies were performed before antibiotics were available but more recent epidemiological studies have linked acute urinary tract infection with increased fetal mortality and prematurity (Gilstrap et al., 1981b; McGrady et al., 1985). It is likely that systemic infection leads to prostaglandin release and the evidence that infection causes preterm labour is reviewed elsewhere (MacLean, 1991).

The progression of asymptomatic bacteriuria to symptomatic infection, i.e. pyelonephritis, ranges from 14% (Swapp, 1973) to 57% (McFadyen and Eykyn, 1968). Some of the variation is due to the lack of confirmatory microbiology in all patients presenting with typical symptoms or when treatment has commenced before the patient reached hospital. Little (1965) reported on 5000 antenatal patients from Charing Cross and Fulham Maternity Hospitals and showed that among those with asymptomatic bacteriuria, 36% progressed to acute pyelonephritis if they were not treated compared with only 5% developing pyelonephritis after treatment with antibiotics. Pyelonephritis was also more likely to develop if treatment failed to clear asymptomatic bacteriuria (Gruneberg et al., 1969).

What is more doubtful is whether screening for and treating asymptomatic bacteriuria is a useful way of preventing pyelonephritis during pregnancy. Some studies (Gilstrap et al., 1981a) found that the majority (66%) of those who presented with acute pyelonephritis had earlier asymptomatic bacteriuria while others (Dixon and Brant, 1967; Lawson and Miller, 1971) found this to be the case in only a third of patients. Lawson and Miller (1973) calculated that the test sensitivity of a single midstream urine to predict subsequent symptomatic infection was only 54%. Thus, of every 100 patients developing acute pyelonephritis during pregnancy, only 54 would have had asymptomatic bacteriuria, and of these only three-quarters were likely to have had infection prevented by treatment at the time of the initial screen. Similarly, Chng and Hall (1982) reported that screening for bacteriuria had a 33% sensitivity in predicting acute infection during pregnancy. The additional information of previous urinary tract infection was no more sensitive. The combination of asymptomatic bacteriuria on screening and a previous history of infection increased the likelihood of infection in pregnancy, but the sensitivity remained low at only 18%.

V   Asymptomatic bacteriuria and preterm labour

Early studies were inconsistent in their diagnosis of preterm labour or prematurity, usually relying on birth weight of less than 2.5 kg rather than gestational age. Nowadays preterm labour is defined as delivery before 37 weeks and it is recognized that infants may be inappropriately small for gestational age. It is interesting to note that the early Australian and American studies (Kincaid-Smith and Bullen, 1965; Savage et al., 1967; Stuart et al., 1965) showed increased prematurity rates among asymptomatic women with bacteriuria, but the majority of British studies (Sleigh et al., 1964; Little, 1966; Dixon and Brant, 1967; Swapp, 1973) did not. The study of Savage et al. (1967) only sustained significance if twins were included, a similar bias to that in the figures of Kass (1962b) which included three sets of twins in his placebo-treated group.

A large study from Kass's group in Boston (Elder et al., 1971) included more than 9000 patients, of whom 362 had asymptomatic bacteriuria. They used a definition of prematurity as a birth weight below 2.5 kg. Sulphonamides were used during their early experience of treating bacteriuria but, because a significant number of patients had persisting infection, tetracycline was prescribed (250 mg four times daily for six weeks). This study was performed before it was appreciated that using tetracyclines would lead to staining of dental enamel; interestingly, in the follow-up of infants delivered during this study, at the age of 5–6 years, there was no increase in dental caries or hypoplasia but one-third of the infants exposed had staining of their dental enamel. Of the patients with bacteriuria, 133 were given tetracyclines and 148 were given a placebo. Patients were also recruited who did not have asymptomatic bacteriuria; 147 of these were treated with tetracyclines and 132 were given placebo. Among the treated patients with asymptomatic bacteriuria the prematurity rate was 10% if the urine remained clear after treatment, and 21% if the patient subsequently developed acute pyelonephritis. Among those who were untreated, the prematurity was 9% providing the patient did not develop symptoms but 18% if she became symptomatic. Among those with no bacteriuria, the prematurity rate was 15.2% if given placebo but reduced to 5.4% among those treated with tetracyclines. These results suggest a close link between the development of asymptomatic infection and prematurity and that the use of antibiotic treatment may clear organisms from other sites, e.g. the genital tract, which will also have a beneficial effect on prematurity.

Two groups of authors have performed meta-analysis on the relationship between asymptomatic bacteriuria, preterm delivery and low birth weight. Romero et al. (1989) used a computer-assisted search of the English literature between 1966 and 1986 to identify 31 studies of bacteriuria during pregnancy. Twelve studies were rejected for various reasons and meta-analysis focused on the remaining 19. There were 17 cohort studies, i.e. studies where patients without bacteriuria and those with untreated bacteriuria were compared. From 13 studies analysed in depth, the relative risk of low birth weight in the presence of untreated bacteriuria was 0.65 (95% CI, 0.56–0.74), i.e. patients without bacteriuria had two-thirds the risk of having an infant with low birth weight. In four studies where there was information about preterm delivery, the relative risk was 0.50. In eight studies where there was randomization between treatment and no treatment, the relative risk of low birth weight was 0.56 (95% CI, 0.42–0.73), i.e. antibiotic treatment reduced the risk of low birth weight. In one case control study analysed, the prevalence of asymptomatic bacteriuria was significantly higher in the group delivering before 36 weeks compared with a matched control group delivering after 36 weeks.

Wang and Smaill (1990) reported an odds ratio of 0.89 in six case control studies. Their 95% confidence intervals transversed unity, suggesting that treatment did not influence preterm delivery or low birth weight. It is of interest that three of the eight randomized studies in the Romero et al. (1989) meta-analysis were included in the analysis by Wang and Smaill (1990) but the three other studies included one by Gold et al. (1966) which reversed the trend. In this study performed in Brooklyn, New York, two premature deliveries occurred among the 35 (5.7%) treated patients and none among the 30 control patients. The incidence of prematurity among 1216 non-bacteriuria patients was 13.9%. Whether these data are relevant to modern British practice, with preterm delivery rates between 3% and 7%, remains uncertain.

VI Asymptomatic bacteriuria and hypertension of pregnancy

Early studies of asymptomatic bacteriuria noted an association with hypertension (Kass, 1962a). Stuart et al. (1965), using the definition of hypertension as diastolic pressure greater than 100 mmHg, found that 40% bacteriuric patients aged 35 years or older developed hypertension, compared with only 5% of control non-bacteriuric patients. Kincaid-Smith and Bullen (1965), using a blood pressure recording of 140/90 mmHg plus oedema and proteinuria, found an increased association with bacteriuria, which was not reduced with antibiotic treatment. Savage et al. (1967) commented that their bacteriuric group was more likely to be hospitalized for various reasons including pre-eclamptic toxaemia.

Other studies have been unable to find an increased prevalence in hypertension developing among the bacteriuric patients (Little, 1966; Swapp, 1973). Norden and Kass (1968) reviewed the literature to that date and concluded that there was some relationship between bacteriuria and hypertension of pregnancy but that it might be indirect and might relate to other factors including socioeconomic group and patient population.

In an epidemiological study, a review was performed on patients delivered in the Boston Hospital for Women between 1977 and 1980 (Mittendorf et al., 1996). There were 386 cases of obstetrician diagnosed pre-eclampsia that were compared with randomly selected 2355 control patients. Multiple logistic regression was used to demonstrate that primigravida who had urinary tract infections during pregnancy were five times more likely (odds ratio 5.3, 95% CI 2.9–9.7) to have pre-eclampsia than were primigravida who did not have urinary tract infection during pregnancy. The women in the study were interviewed and information included the reporting of patients who had taken antibiotics for urinary tract infection during pregnancy. The authors admit that their definition of urinary tract infection lacked precision but felt that this would merely bias the relative risk towards a null value, i.e. the true association between pyelonephritis during pregnancy and pre-eclampsia could be much greater than what they identified. Unfortunately, in this study there is no knowing whether these patients had asymptomatic or symptomatic bacteriuria, whether the urine stayed sterile following the antibiotic course or indeed whether the antibiotics had been given for some other reason.

VII   Asymptomatic bacteriuria in early pregnancy loss

Early pregnancy loss occurs in some 15% of pregnancies and recurrent loss in less than 1%. The cause of such abortion is frequently unknown although there is a long list of organisms causing infection which sometimes may be implicated (MacLean, 1990). Such organisms are unlikely to cause recurrent loss although there is a link with bacterial vaginosis and second-trimester abortion. No studies have identified a link between asymptomatic bacteriuria and early pregnancy loss. A study from Salt Lake City, Utah (Mansfield et al., 1995), described the follow-up of women who in their childhood had undergone reimplantation of their ureters for vesicoureteric reflux. Among 62 women, 65% had experienced urinary tract infection during pregnancy but the spontaneous abortion rate was only 15%. Among 37 women who had not undergone surgery for a similar condition, 15% had experienced urinary tract infection in pregnancy with an 18% spontaneous abortion rate. The authors commented that the risk of spontaneous pregnancy loss with

bacteriuria was no higher than within the general population.

VIII   Management of urinary tract infection

Certain antibiotics are unsuitable for use during pregnancy (MacLean and McAllister, 1990). Sulphonamides cross the placenta and their use in late pregnancy may increase the risk of kernicterus by displacing bilirubin bound to albumin. Tetracyclines may be incorporated into teeth and bones to cause dysplasia and discolouration. Trimethoprim is an antifolate agent and its use should be avoided in early pregnancy during neural tube development. There is evidence that prolonged aminoglycoside use (streptomycin) may produce 8th-nerve damage in the fetus but this should not detract from the use of gentamicin for serious Gram-negative infection during pregnancy. Quinolones have been associated with alterations in the joint cartilage of puppies and should not be used in pregnancy. The addition of clavulanic acid to amoxycillin (Augmentin) has meant that use of this drug during pregnancy is not recommended unless essential; however, there was no evidence that clavulanic acid caused fetal toxicity when the drug was used to treat bacteriuria during pregnancy (Pedler and Bint, 1985). Care must be taken in the use of nitrofurantoin because of the risk of haemolysis in women with glucose-

6-phosphate dehydrogenase deficiency (but this occurs whether the woman is pregnant or not).

Recommended antibiotics for asymptomatic bacteriuria include amoxycillin, cephradine or a similar oral cephalosporin, nitrofurantoin, nalidixic acid or sulphonamide. Pyelonephritis should be treated with a second- or third-generation cephalosporin or a short course of an aminoglycoside (MacLean, 1996). Sanchez-Ramos et al. (1995) have shown that pyelonephritis can be treated effectively with a daily injection of ceftriaxone; one injection per day allows patients to be treated without hospital admission, with significant reduction in cost but equal efficacy compared with other cephalosporins.

Debate continues on the duration of therapy in pregnant women. Little and de Wardener (1966) described treatment of 53 pregnant women with acute pyelonephritis with either short-term treatment for 7–14 days or long-term treatment for up to 18 months and found that duration of therapy did not affect the rate of reinfection. There is now enthusiasm for single-dose treatment, because of the benefits of reduced fetal exposure and less chance of developing bacterial resistance (Bailey, 1990; McFayden et al., 1987). Comparisons with three-, five- and seven-day courses of the identical antibiotic show no advantage over single dose for cephalexin, cotrimoxazole and amoxycillin

(Bailey et al., 1983; Masterton et al., 1985; McFayden et al., 1987). Failure or reinfection rates of single-dose treatment may be as high as one in three (Harris et al., 1982; McFayden et al., 1987) but it appears that those who do not respond are more likely to have urinary tract abnormalities. Wilkie et al. (1992) suggested that short-course antimicrobial chemotherapy should not be used for pregnant women, but their statement was not supported by any evidence and has been challenged in the correspondence that followed this article. Those women who get recurrent bacteriuria during pregnancy should be given prophylactic nitrofurantoin 50 mg at night, until delivery.

Kass (1962a) found that about two-thirds of those with asymptomatic bacteriuria of pregnancy still had organisms present up to one year after delivery. This is perhaps not surprising following resumption of coital function. The need for follow-up has been stressed because of the association of subsequent renal failure (Parker and Kunin, 1973). Radiological abnormalities including calyceal changes with blunting or papillary necrosis, reduced cortical thickness and irregular renal contour, the presence of calculi, or congenital anatomical anomalies (Gilstrap et al., 1981a; Kincaid-Smith and Bullen, 1965; Leigh et al., 1968; Whalley et al., 1965) have been reported in up to 50% of patients. It is suggested that those who have symptomatic infection (Gower et al., 1968), evidence of upper urinary tract infection (Fairley et al., 1966), failure to respond to single-dose therapy (Bailey, 1990) or identification of an unusual organism (Wilkie et al., 1992) should have further investigation following delivery. Although earlier studies used intravenous pyelography or urography to investigate selected patients, it is suggested that they rarely provide information that is important in subsequent management (Engel et al., 1980; Fowler and Pulaski, 1981). An easier method of assessing these patients is renal ultrasound for length, shape and contour of each kidney.

IX   Should we continue to screen for bacteriuria?

The prevalence of asymptomatic bacteriuria ranges from 2% to 13% (Norden and Kass, 1968). It appears to rise with increasing age and parity (Savage et al., 1967; Stuart et al., 1965) and decrease with increasing social class. Thus the rates among the women confined in the Boston Lying-In Hospital were 1–2% lower than at the Boston City Hospital (Kass, 1962a; Norden and Kass, 1968). Bailey (1972) reported asymptomatic bacteriuria rates as low as 2% among antenatal patients attending a private clinic in New Zealand and as high as 18.5% among urbanized Maori patients. As many of these studies are more than 30 years old and during that time health has generally improved, it is

no longer appropriate to assume that all obstetric units will have patients at increased risk of asymptomatic bacteriuria.

A more recent study from North London (Campbell Brown et al., 1987) found that maximum prevalence of bacteriuria (using suprapubic aspiration catheterization to confirm bacteriuria after a first positive midstream urine sample) was only 2.6%. Studies confirm that more patients develop pyelonephritis among those who have sterile urine than those that have had asymptomatic bacteriuria. Lawson and Miller (1971, 1973) observed that only 19% of patients who developed acute pyelonephritis had asymptomatic bacteriuria and the other 81% had sterile urine when they were seen at the booking clinic.

Campbell Brown et al. (1987) noted that screening and treatment with antibiotics to prevent later acute pyelonephritis were expensive and suggested it was not worthwhile or cost effective for a population if there was a low prevalence and a small proportion who progressed to overt infection. The costs of screening include laboratory time and costs, the return of the patient to antenatal clinic and confirmatory tests, the costs of antibiotics and subsequent follow-up and more subtle consequences such as the effect of the antibiotic on the fetus (as shown in the study by Elder et al., 1971). Traditionally, urine has been screened by microscopy for pus cells and the culture in a quantity of urine followed by a colony count. Many hospitals, e.g. the Royal Free in London (MacLean, 1997), examine urine microscopically for pus cells in a microtitre tray and culture 0.3 μl of urine, the subsequent recognition of 30 colony-forming units being equivalent to 1×10^5 organism/ml; the cost of this procedure is about £4 per specimen. Other modern methods mix the urine specimen with a culture broth and subsequently monitor bacterial presence and proliferation by measuring optical density. An alternative approach is to test the urine before culture for the presence of nitrites (Gram-negative organisms present in the urine convert dietary nitrates to nitrites; the test is inexpensive at approximately £0.15 (UK) but will not detect Gram-positive organisms, e.g. group B streptococci), bacterial ATPase (using a bioluminescence test with purified firefly reagent) or catalase (Uriscreen) or leucocyte esterase (a marker of pyuria) (Brumfitt and Hamilton-Miller, 1990; Hagay et al., 1996). Although there is enthusiasm for using dipsticks in some situations, e.g. screening of the urine from children with acute abdominal pain (Woodward and Griffiths, 1993), there is recent published evidence that reagent strip testing for the presence of urinary protein, nitrite and leucocyte esterase is not sufficiently sensitive to be used in the screening for asymptomatic bacteriuria in early pregnancy (Tincello and Richmond, 1998). It must also be recognized that false-positive results can occur, e.g. the presence of certain antibiotics in the urine will give false-positive leucocyte esterase tests (Beer et al., 1996).

Rouse et al. (1995) performed a cost benefit analysis of screening and treatment of asymptomatic bacteriuria, although they were using North American costings. Only if the incidence of bacteriuria is greater than 9% does screening with culture methods become cost effective; if leucocyte esterase and nitrite dipstick screening is used, a prevalence of 6% is required for economical value.

If we are screening pregnant women for bacteriuria, such that appropriate treatment will reduce the risk of pyelonephritis and subsequent preterm labour, this can no longer be judged on 1960s standards. Effective treatment of acute pyelonephritis, reduced rates of preterm delivery and reduced perinatal mortality rates make it more difficult to justify the costs of screening for bacteriuria. Thus if an antenatal population has a low prevalence of asymptomatic bacteriuria, it may be more cost effective to save £4 by not analysing a midstream urine sample for each first-visit patient, but instead give each patient an information sheet advising them to present for a urine culture and treatment if during the pregnancy they develop chills, fever, loin pain and urinary symptoms (MacLean, 1997).

References

Bailey RR (1972) Urinary tract infection – some recent concepts. *Can Med Assoc J* **107**: 316–30.

Bailey RR (1990) Review of published studies on single dose therapy of urinary tract infections. *Infection* **18** (suppl 2): S53–6.

Bailey RR, Bishop V, Peddie BA (1983) Comparison of single dose with a five day course of co-trimoxazole for asymptomatic (covert) bacteriuria of pregnancy. *Aust NZ J Obstet Gynaecol* **23**: 139–41.

Beard RW, Roberts AP (1968) Asymptomatic bacteriuria during pregnancy. *Br Med Bull* **24**: 44–8.

Beer JH, Vogt A, Neftel K, Cottagnoud P (1996) False positive results for leucocytes in urine dipstick tests with common antibiotics. *BMJ* **313**: 25.

Brumfitt W, Hamilton-Miller JMT (1990) Urinary tract infection in the 1990s: the state of the art. *Infection* **18** (suppl 2): S34–9.

Campbell-Brown M, McFayden IR, Seal DV, Stephenson ML (1987) Is screening for bacteriuria in pregnancy worthwhile? *BMJ* **294**: 1579–82.

Cattell WR (1996) Urinary tract infection: definitions and classifications. In: *Infections of the Kidney and Urinary Tract* (ed. WR Cattell), Oxford University Press, Oxford, pp 1–7.

Chng PK, Hall MN (1982) Antenatal prediction of urinary tract infection in pregnancy. *Br J Obstet Gynaecol* **89**: 8–11.

Dixon HG, Brant HA (1967) The significance of bacteriuria of pregnancy. *Lancet* **i**: 19–20.

Elder HA, Santamarina BAG, Smith S et al. (1971) The natural history of asymptomatic bacteriuria during pregnancy: the effect of tetracycline on the clinical course and the outcome of pregnancy. *Am J Obstet Gynecol* **111**: 441–62.

Engel G, Schaeffer AJ, Grayhack JT, Wendel EF (1980) The role of excretory urography and cystoscopy in the evaluation and management of women with recurrent urinary tract infection. *J Urol* **123**: 190–1.

Fairley KF, Bond AG, Adey FD (1966) The site of infection in pregnancy bacteriuria. *Lancet* i: 939–41.

Fowler JE, Pulaski ET (1981) Excretory urography, cystography and cystoscopy in the evaluation of women with urinary tract infection. *N Engl J Med* **304**: 462–5.

Gilstrap LC, Cunningham FG, Whalley PJ (1981a) Acute pyelonephritis in pregnancy: an anterospective study. *Obstet Gynecol* **57**: 409–13.

Gilstrap LC, Leveno KJ, Cunningham FG et al. (1981b) Renal infection and pregnancy outcome. *Am J Obstet Gynecol* **141**: 709–16.

Gold EM, Traub FB, Daichman I, Terris M (1966) Asymptomatic bacteriuria during pregnancy. *Obstet Gynecol* **27**: 206–9.

Gower PE, Haswell B, Sidawar ME, de Wardener HE (1968) Follow-up of 164 patients with bacteriuria of pregnancy. *Lancet* i: 990–4.

Gruneberg RN, Leigh DA, Brumfitt W (1969) Relationship of bacteriuria in pregnancy to acute pyelonephritis, prematurity and fetal mortality. *Lancet* ii: 1–3.

Hagay Z, Levy R, Miskin A et al. (1996) Uriscreen, a rapid enzymatic urine screening test: useful predictor of significant bacteriuria in pregnancy. *Obstet Gynecol* **87**: 410–13.

Harris RE, Gilstrap LC, Pretty A (1982) Single-dose antimicrobial therapy for asymptomatic bacteriuria during pregnancy, *Obstet Gynecol* **59**: 546–9.

Hart A, Pham T, Nowicki S et al. (1996) Gestational pyelonephritis-associated *Escherichia coli* isolates represent a non-random closely related population. *Am J Obstet Gynecol* **174**: 983–9.

Kass EH (1962a) Maternal urinary tract infection. *New York State J Med* 2822–6.

Kass EH (1962b) Pyelonephritis and bacteriuria. A major problem in preventive medicine. *Ann Intern Med* **56**: 46–53.

Kincaid-Smith P, Bullen M (1965) Bacteriuria in pregnancy. *Lancet* i: 395–9.

Kunin CM, McCormack RC (1968) An epidemiologic study of bacteriuria and blood pressure among nuns and working women. *N Engl J Med* **278**: 635–42.

Lawson DH, Miller AWF (1971) Screening for bacteriuria in pregnancy. *Lancet* **i**: 9–11.

Lawson DH, Miller AWF (1973) Screening for bacteriuria in pregnancy. *Arch Intern Med* **132**: 904–8.

Leigh DA, Gruneberg RN, Brumfitt W (1968) Long term follow-up of bacteriuria in pregnancy. *Lancet* **i**: 603–5.

Leigh DA, Emmanuel FXS, Sedgwick J, Dean R (1990) Post-operative urinary tract infection and wound infection in women undergoing caesarean section: a comparison of two study periods in 1985 and 1987. *J Hosp Infect* **15**: 107–16.

Little PJ (1965) Prevention of pyelonephritis of pregnancy. *Lancet* **i**: 567–9.

Little PJ (1966) The incidence of urinary infection in 5000 pregnant women. *Lancet* **ii**: 925–8.

Little PJ, de Wardener HE (1966) Acute pyelonephritis – incidence of reinfection in 100 patients. *Lancet* **ii**: 1277–8.

MacLean AB (1990) Infection and the antenatal patient. In: *Clinical Infection in Obstetrics and Gynaecology* (ed. AB MacLean), Blackwell Scientific, Oxford, pp 21–38.

MacLean AB (1991) Infection and pre-term labour. *Curr Opin Obstet Gynaecol* **1**: 67–71.

MacLean AB (1996) Urinary tract infection and pregnancy. In: *Infections of the Kidney and the Urinary Tract* (ed. WR Cattell), Oxford University Press, Oxford, pp. 206–17.

MacLean AB (1997) Urinary tract infection in pregnancy. *Br J Urol* **80** (suppl 1): 10–13.

MacLean AB, McAllister T (1990) Antimicrobial therapy in obstetrics and gynaecology. In: *Clinical Infection in Obstetrics and Gynaecology* (ed. AB MacLean), Blackwell, Oxford, pp 210–23.

Mansfield JT, Snow BW, Cartwright PC, Wadsworth K (1995) Complications of pregnancy in women after childhood reimplantation for vesicoureteral reflux: an uptake with 25 years of follow-up. *J Urol* **154**: 787–90.

Masterton RG, Evans DC, Strike PW (1985) Single-dose amoxycillin in the treatment of bacteriuria in pregnancy and puerperium – a controlled clinical trial. *Br J Obstet Gynaecol* **92**: 498–505.

McFayden IR, Eykyn SJ (1968) Suprapubic aspiration of urine in pregnancy. *Lancet* **i**: 1112–4.

MacFayden IR, Campbell-Brown M, Stephenson M et al. (1987) Single-dose treatment of bacteriuria in pregnancy. *Eur J Urol* **13** (suppl 1): 22–5.

McGrady GA, Daling JR, Peterson DR (1985) Maternal urinary

tract infection and adverse fetal outcomes. *Am J Epidemiol* **121**: 377–81.

Mittendorf R, Lain KY, Williams MA, Walker CK (1996) Pre-eclampsia: a nested case control study of risk factors and their interactions. *J Reprod Med* **41**: 491–6.

Norden CW, Kass EH (1968) Bacteriuria of pregnancy – a critical appraisal. *Annu Rev Med* **19**: 431–70.

Parker J, Kunin C (1973) Pyelonephritis in young women. A 10 to 20 year follow-up. *JAMA* **224**: 585–90.

Pedler SJ, Bint AJ (1985) Comparative study of amoxycillin – clavulanic acid and cephalexin in the treatment of bacteriuria during pregnancy. *Antimicrob Agents Chemother* **27**: 508–10.

Romero R, Oyarzum E, Mazor M et al. (1989) Meta-analysis of the relationship between asymptomatic bacteriuria and preterm delivery/low birth weight. *Obstet Gynecol* **73**: 576–82.

Rouse DJ, Andrews WW, Goldenberg RL et al. (1995) Screening and treatment for asymptomatic bacteriuria of pregnancy to prevent pyelonephritis: a cost effectiveness and cost benefit analysis. *Obstet Gynecol* **86**: 119–23.

Sanchez-Ramos L, McAlpine KJ, Adair CD et al. (1995) Pyelonephritis in pregnancy: once a day ceftriaxone versus multiple doses of cefazolin. *Am J Obstet Gynecol* **172**: 129–33.

Savage WE, Hajj SN, Kass EH (1967) Demographic and prognostic characteristics of bacteriuria in pregnancy. *Medicine* **46**: 385–407.

Sleigh JD, Robertson JG, Isdale MH (1964) Asymptomatic bacteriuria in pregnancy. *J Obstet Gynaecol Br Cwlth* **71**: 74–81.

Stray-Pedersen B, Blakstad M, Bergan T (1990) Bacteriuria in the puerperium. Risk factors, screening procedures and treatment programmes. *Am J Obstet Gynecol* **162**: 792–7.

Stuart KL, Cummins GTM, Chin WA (1965) Bacteriuria, prematurity and the hypertensive disorders of pregnancy. *BMJ* **1**: 554–6.

Swapp GH (1973) Asymptomatic bacteriuria, birthweight and length of gestation in a defined population. In: *Urinary Tract Infection* (eds W Brumfitt and AW Asscher), Oxford University Press, London, pp 92–102.

Tincello DG, Richmond DH (1998) Evaluation of reagent strips in detecting asymptomatic bacteriuria in early pregnancy: prospective case series. *BMJ* **316**: 435–7.

Wang E, Smaill F (1990) Infection in pregnancy. In: *Effective Care in Pregnancy and Childbirth* (eds I Chalmers, M Enkin and MJNC Keirse), Oxford University Press, Oxford, pp 535–8.

Whalley PJ, Martin FG, Peters PC (1965) Significance of

asymptomatic bacteriuria detected during pregnancy. *JAMA* **193:** 107–9.

Wilkie ME, Almond MK, Marsh FP (1992) Diagnosis and management of urinary tract infection in adults. *BMJ* **305:** 1137–41.

Woodward MN, Griffiths DM (1993) Use of dipsticks for routine analysis of urine from children with acute abdominal pain. *BMJ* **306:** 1512.

Non-infective sensory disorders of the lower urinary tract

Anna Rosamilia and Peter L Dwyer

9

Contents

I   Introduction

Irritative bladder symptoms of frequency, urgency, pelvic pain and dysuria can have a number of causes other than urinary tract infection. In many cases the cause is obvious, e.g. malignancy, calculi, drug-induced cystitis, and the treatment is specific. In other women, the underlying cause is poorly understood, e.g. interstitial cystitis, urethral syndrome, and the treatment is frequently unsatisfactory. Typically, many women with lower urinary

tract sensory disorders present having had a number of courses of antibiotics for real or supposed urinary tract infection. It is only after a failure to respond to antibiotics and a failure to culture uropathogens that an alternative diagnosis is considered. This delay in diagnosis is frustrating and distressing for the patient and occasionally serious. Therefore, it is important for any clinician treating urinary infection to have a good knowledge of the diagnosis and treatment of non-infective sensory disorders of the lower urinary tract.

Table 9.1
Causes of non-infective sensory disorders of the lower urinary tract

Non-infective cystitis	*Interstitial cystitis*
	Drug-induced cystitis, e.g. cyclophosphamide, tiaprofenic acid
	Eosinophilic cystitis
	Granulomatous cystitis – postsurgical, bacille Calmette–Guérin, malakoplakia
	Radiation cystitis
Proliferative and metaplastic bladder lesions	*Proliferative cystitis – Brunn's nests, cystitis cystica, cystitis glandularis*
	Squamous metaplasia – non-keratinizing (pseudomembranous cystitis), leukoplakia
	Intestinal metaplasia
Bladder and urethral tumours	*Bladder and urethral papillomas, polyps*
	Carcinoma in situ, bladder and urethral carcinoma
	Non-epithelial bladder tumours, nephrogenic adenoma, endometriosis, primary localized amyloidosis
Miscellaneous	*Bladder and urethral calculi, intravesical foreign bodies*
	Urethral diverticulum
	Acute and chronic urethral syndromes including atrophic urethritis
	Reiter syndrome

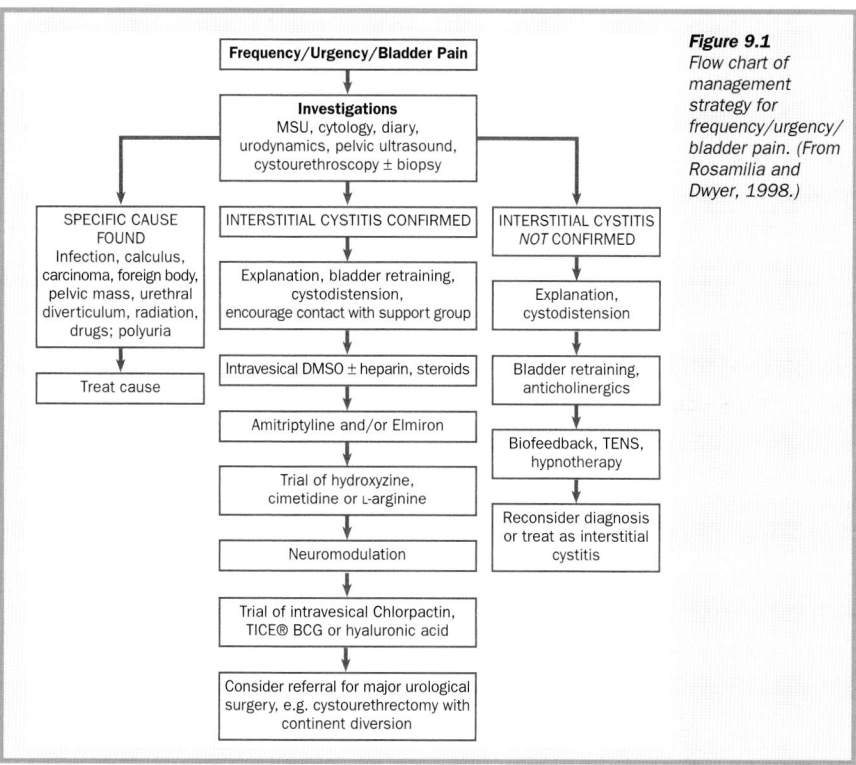

Figure 9.1
Flow chart of
management
strategy for
frequency/urgency/
bladder pain. (From
Rosamilia and
Dwyer, 1998.)

Irritative symptoms of the lower urinary tract may be caused by: interstitial cystitis; urethral syndrome; allergic, radiation- or drug-induced (e.g. cyclophosphamide) cystitis; benign, premalignant and malignant tumours; calculi, foreign bodies or urethral diverticulum (*Table 9.1*). Irritative bladder symptoms can also be caused by functional abnormalities of the lower urinary tract such as detrusor instability or voiding dysfunction. These conditions need to be differentiated from other causes of frequency and urgency symptoms which do not originate in the lower urinary tract such as polydipsia, pregnancy, diabetes mellitus, diabetes insipidus, cervicitis, vaginitis, chemical irritants (e.g. vaginal foams, douches, diaphragm use), vulvar, vaginal and cervical carcinoma, diuretics, pelvic mass or renal disorders. Women presenting with irritative urinary symptoms should be assessed both generally and gynaecologically (*Figure 9.1*).

II Non-infective cystitis

1. Interstitial cystitis

The prevalence of interstitial cystitis has been estimated to be 30 to 500 cases per 100 000 (Jones and Nyberg, 1997). The criteria for the diagnosis of interstitial cystitis are symptoms of frequency, urgency and often pain; the findings of a low bladder capacity on urinary diary or urodynamic assessment and the cystoscopic appearance of mucosal fissuring, tearing (*Figure 9.2a*) or glomerulations (petechial haemorrhages) seen during or after bladder distension. The National Institute of Arthritis, Diabetes, Digestive and Kidney Diseases (NIDDK) criteria for interstitial cystitis, which were developed for the purposes of research and clinical trials, include the urodynamic findings of no bladder instability, a capacity less than 350 ml with urgency at less than 150 ml and cystoscopic evidence of a classic Hunner's ulcer, mucosal tearing or glomerulations (Gillenwater and Wein, 1988). Exclusion criteria according to this definition are age younger than 18 years, symptom duration less than 9 months, nocturia less than one and frequency less than eight, the presence of urinary or genital tract infection, tumour, radiation effect or cyclophosphamide cystitis (Hanno, 1994).

In an epidemiological study of 500 patients, Koziol (1994) found that the main symptoms in women with interstitial cystitis were frequency (92%), urgency (92%) and

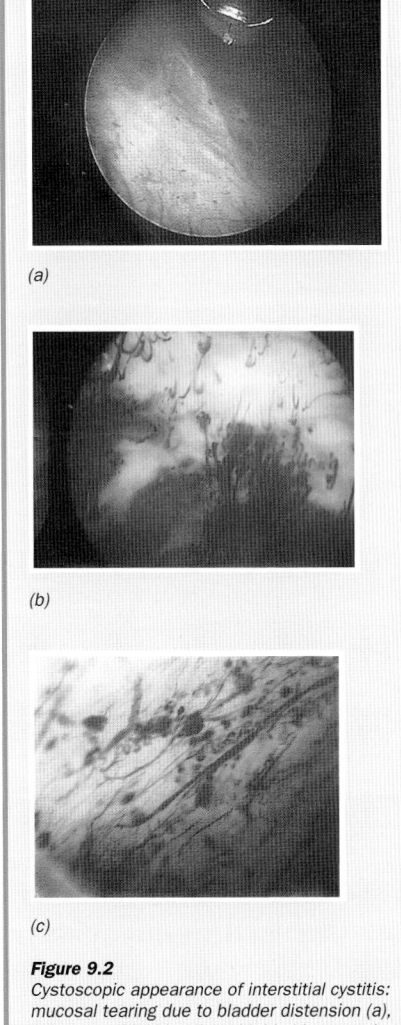

(a)

(b)

(c)

Figure 9.2
Cystoscopic appearance of interstitial cystitis: mucosal tearing due to bladder distension (a), filling petechial bleeding with bladder emptying (b), and splotchy mucosal haemorrhages on bladder refilling (c).

pelvic pain (70%); physical examination was generally unrevealing apart from the possible presence of vaginal or suprapubic tenderness. Women with interstitial cystitis charted an average number of 21 voids in 24 hours with an average interval of 2.6 hours between voids overnight.

Cystourethroscopy in women with interstitial cystitis is very painful and should be performed under general or regional anaesthesia. Cystodistension is part of the diagnostic procedure and provides short-term symptomatic relief in 20–30% of patients (Hanno, 1994). The most common diagnostic finding in interstitial cystitis are glomerulations, generalized petechiae which ooze fresh blood often in cascades (***Figure 9.2b***) when the bladder is being emptied following distension (Messing and Stamey, 1978). On reinspection of the bladder, these glomerulations coalesce to become splotchy haemorrhages (***Figure 9.2c***). As the bladder is emptied, the fluid becomes increasingly blood stained which produces the characteristic terminal haematuria.

Biopsy for histological analysis is performed to exclude carcinoma in situ (Utz and Zincke, 1974) or carcinoma of the bladder rather than to diagnose interstitial cystitis. The histological findings in women with interstitial cystitis are non-specific and may include mucosal denudation, leukocytic and plasma cell infiltration, vascular congestion and haemorrhage, and fibrosis

(Lynes et al., 1990; Johansson and Fall, 1994). Histological assessment of bladder biopsies from women with interstitial cystitis were abnormal in less than 50% of cases (Rosamilia et al., 1999a).

Hunner described the condition of interstitial cystitis in 1914, but the aetiology remains unclear. Theories of pathogenesis are infection, an abnormal glycosaminoglycan layer, nitrofurantoin use (Ruggieri et al., 1994) or an immunological disorder. Light microscopy and culture, electron microscopy studies, serology and molecular biologic techniques have not to date consistently isolated a microorganism or viral agent in interstitial cystitis (Duncan and Schaeffer, 1997). It is not known whether the abnormal glycosaminoglycan layer is the cause of interstitial cystitis (Parsons, 1994; Wilson et al., 1995; Hurst et al., 1993) or is the effect of another pathologic process such as reduced subepithelial microvasculature (Rosamilia et al., 1999b). No consistent evidence for an immunological mechanism in interstitial cystitis has been found (Ratliff et al., 1995). The interaction between mast cell activation, sensory nerve fibre proliferation and altered neuropeptide and inflammatory mediator expression is the basis for the current hypothesis that the important underlying mechanism in interstitial cystitis is neurogenic inflammation (Steers and Tuttle, 1997; Elbadawi 1997).

In view of the poorly understood pathogenesis of interstitial cystitis, it is not surprising that the treatment is frequently unsuccessful. Women with interstitial cystitis need a clear explanation of this condition and their treatment options. Other important issues are the provision of easy toilet access, family and professional support, stress reduction and bladder training techniques. The placebo effect in women with interstitial cystitis for oral or intravesical therapy is of the order of 20–30% (Hanno and Wein, 1994) and a 50% incidence of temporary remission with an average duration of eight months independent of therapy has been reported (Jones and Nyberg, 1997). Anticholinergic, non-steroidal anti-inflammatory agents and steroids are of limited value. Amitriptyline was shown in an uncontrolled trial to result in symptomatic improvement in about half the patients treated but about one in four subjects could not tolerate the side effects (Hanno et al., 1989). Pentosan polysulfate sodium (PPS or Elmiron), a heparin analogue was shown to produce symptomatic improvement in 32% of patients with severe disease compared with 16% for placebo (Parsons et al., 1993). Adverse events of reversible alopecia, diarrhoea, nausea, rash and dyspepsia are uncommon (< 4%) (Hanno, 1997).

Dimethylsulfoxide (DMSO) is the drug most widely used for interstitial cystitis either as single therapy or in combination with heparin, steroids and/or local anaesthetic agents. The treatment regimens vary with once or twice weekly instillations for 4 to 12 treatments commonly used. A response rate to DMSO of 50–90% has been reported. Relapse rate can be as high as 40% although 75% of relapsers respond to further instillations. Reported side effects are a garlic-like breath odour and taste, and transient bladder spasm and irritability due to a chemical cystitis in 10% (Sant and La Rock, 1994). Both objective and subjective improvement over placebo has been demonstrated (Perez-Marrero et al., 1988). DMSO is cheap, and self-instillation using ISC can be taught if required. Other intravesical agents include sodium oxychlorosene (chlorpactin), heparin, TICE® bacille Calmette–Guérin (BCG) (Peters et al., 1997), pentosan polysulfate sodium (Bade et al., 1997) and hyaluronic acid (Morales et al., 1997). Recent reports of randomized placebo-controlled trials in the treatment of interstitial cystitis have demonstrated significant beneficial effect (generally double the response rate of placebo) with oral L-arginine, a nitric oxide synthase inhibitor (Korting et al., 1999); open label trials of the oral histamine antagonists hydroxyzine (Theoharides and Sant, 1997) and cimetidine (Seshadri et al., 1994) demonstrated some efficacy. Transcutaneous electrical nerve stimulation (TENS) also has been of beneficial effect in 25–50% of patients studied (Fall and Lindstrom, 1994). The role of neuromodulation has not yet been established but holds promise.

Major open surgery should be reserved for the small percentage of women with severe symptoms who have not responded to conservative therapies. Supratrigonal cystectomy and substitution cystoplasty is thought to produce most benefit in those with small capacity, contracted bladders (Irwin and Galloway, 1994) but a better alternative in those with significant urethral pain may be total cystourethrectomy and urinary diversion (Lotenfoe et al., 1995).

2. Drug-induced cystitis

The term 'drug-induced cystitis', as compared with 'drug-associated cystitis', is used where the causality has been proven by assessment of a large number of patients or by rechallenging with the same drug. This diagnosis requires a high index of suspicion and careful drug history. The time interval between drug administration and the onset of symptoms can be quite variable, ranging up to many years. Confirmation of the diagnosis occurs when the symptoms and cystoscopic appearance resolve on drug withdrawal and recur on drug rechallenge.

The Australian Adverse Drug Reactions Advisory Committee has received 127 reports of drugs potentially causing cystitis (most would fall in the drug-associated classification) since its establishment in November 1972 until September 1998 (personal communication). Ninety-two of these were

due to tiaprofenic acid (Surgam™). Other drugs reported independently include (number of cases in brackets): alendronate sodium (1), allopurinol (1), α-tocopherol, intravesical BCG (6), chlorhexidine gluconate (1), cisapride (1), clindamycin (1), cyclophosphamide (2), fenfluramine (1), fluoxetine (2), flupenthixol (1), frusemide (2), gemfibrozil (3), ketoprofen (1), loratadine (1), naproxen (3), nitrazepam (1), paroxetine (1), piroxicam (2), sertraline (1), simvastatin (2), sulindac (1) and sulphasalazine (1).

Tiaprofenic acid was described as a cause of cystitis in 1991 by Ahmed and Davison and has resulted in major surgery in at least 17 patients because the drug was not suspected or known; there is one reported fatality (Bramble and Morley, 1997). In 1997, Henley et al. found 108 reported cases in the UK; the mean duration of drug treatment prior to the onset of symptoms was 14 months with a range of 6 days to 4 years. Usually, withdrawal of the drug results in symptom resolution with a mean time to resolution of 6 to 14 weeks. In 10% there are residual symptoms and in some cases evidence of fibrosis and reduced capacity.

Dysuria and cystitis has been described in association with a number of non-steroidal anti-inflammatory drugs (NSAIDs) (O'Brien, 1986). Danazol has been associated with haemorrhagic cystitis in patients with hereditary angioneurotic oedema; Trilast, an anti-asthma drug, has been reported to cause eosinophilic cystitis (Okada et al., 1992). Cyclophosphamide and ifosfamide are used to treat lymphoproliferative disorders, some solid tumours, systemic lupus erythematosus and nephrotic syndrome and induce a sterile haemorrhagic cystitis in 2–40% of patients. The metabolite responsible for this is acrolein which causes death of urothelial cells. Clinically, haemorrhagic cystitis occurs three weeks to six months after the commencement of therapy and can have a presentation which varies from asymptomatic haematuria to fulminating ulcerating inflammation with life-threatening haemorrhage. Treatment is supportive with hydration and withholding the chemotherapy (Relling and Schunk, 1986).

3.   Eosinophilic cystitis

Allergic cystitis is an uncommon condition and is thought to be a type 1 hypersensitivity reaction in women usually with a strong allergic history or asthma. Food, inhalants, drugs, alcohol, contact allergens possibly due to organisms or topical agents have been incriminated. The clinical course may be acute or chronic with remissions and exacerbations. There is usually spontaneous resolution and steroids are useful only for symptomatic relief. Cystitis symptoms with proteinuria, pyuria and microscopic or gross haematuria is a common presentation. Eosinophiluria occurs in 10–30% and blood eosinophilia in one-third to one-half of cases. It may result in markedly reduced bladder capacity. Cystoscopically it may be a diffuse or localized process with 5–10-mm sized yellow velvety erythematous plaques, bullous oedema, verrucous or polypoidal folds, trabeculation, ulcers and a thickened bladder wall. Microscopically, the lamina propria has a heavy infiltrate of eosinophils as well as some plasma cells, lymphocytes and macrophages (Sidh et al., 1980).

4.   Granulomatous cystitis

Granulomatous cystitis is characterized by necrobiotic, foreign body or epitheloid granulomas, or diffuse histiocytic inflammation. It may occur following surgery (bladder biopsy or resection) or be secondary to intravesical BCG instillation or bacterial infection; tuberculous cystitis needs to be excluded.

Malakoplakia (soft plaque) is an uncommon condition which occurs predominantly in women over fifty. The patient may be asymptomatic or present with haematuria, frequency, urgency, dysuria or pain. The duration of symptoms can range from weeks to years with a median of six months. At cystoscopy, multiple raised discrete plaques or firm, thickened and granular nodules may be present. The lesions are yellow, raised and soft in 25% but may be grey, tan, red or brown, ulcerated, haemorrhagic, firm or plaque-like. They may appear as filling defects on contrast bladder imaging. Histologically, the lesions are composed of aggregates of large histiocytic cells which are pathognomonic of malakoplakia with the granulomatous reaction occurring only in the epithelium and superficial submucosa (Long and Althausen, 1989).

5.   Radiation cystitis

Radiation cystitis of variable severity may be an early or late complication in patients undergoing radiotherapy for female genital tract or urinary tract cancer. Haemorrhagic cystitis after pelvic radiotherapy for bladder and cervical carcinoma occurs in 7–9% of patients and is related to the type of regimen used and the dose–time–volume relationship. A single dose greater than 2000–2500 rads or a complete course of 5000–6000 rads carries a definite risk of late subacute reaction. Biological factors are also important; the type of pre-existing carcinoma, post-operative irradiation, infection, previous radiotherapy and racial differences increase susceptibility (DeVries and Freha, 1990).

Clinically, radiotherapy complications can be divided into acute (less than six months), subacute (six months to two years) or chronic (two to five years). Acute radiation cystitis presents with dysuria, urgency, frequency and nocturia four to six weeks after radiotherapy. Usually the symptoms improve two to six weeks after the completion of radiotherapy. Bladder perforation, fistulas or ureteritis may also occur. The cystoscopic appearance is of diffuse hyperaemia with occasional petechiae; in severe cases, partial desquamation with or without superficial ulceration may occur. Subacute cystitis is heralded by painless haematuria indicating chronic radiation cystitis with trigonal ulcers: its recurrence and severity are not always related to the occurrence of the acute symptoms previously or the radiation dose. Healing of ulcers may take weeks to months. The cystoscopic appearance is of areas of atrophic pale mucosa with central telangiectasia, bleeding ulcers, bladder wall necrosis, bullous oedema and tortuous blood vessels.

Chronic radiation cystitis may result in a contracted fibrotic bladder (Noorkool et al., 1993) which develops insidiously and can be progressive especially if infection, prior radionecrosis, surgery or extensive carcinoma is present. Symptoms may include frequency, nocturia, dribbling and haematuria with the cystoscopic appearance of mucosal atrophy.

III   Proliferative and metaplastic lesions of the bladder

1.   Proliferative cystitis

Brunn's nests, cystitis cystica and cystitis glandularis are found in up to 90% of both sexes, increasing with age, and are located in the trigone and anterior wall of the bladder (Ito et al., 1981). Therefore, in most cases, they should be regarded as variations of normality. If symptoms of frequency, dysuria and suprapubic pain are present, they are related to associated inflammatory conditions, such as chronic and recurrent infection, calculi, obstruction, foreign body or neoplasia. Brunn's nest, the simplest form of proliferative cystitis, is a reaction to inflammation and is a precursor for cystitis cystica and cystitis glandularis. The morphology reveals nodular thickening of the urothelium resulting in nests of cells in the lamina propria.

The cystoscopic appearance of cystitis cystica is usually of cysts which are regular and rounded, 1–5 mm in diameter and are translucent, pearl or yellow in colour, or they may be present as a localized solid intravesical soft-tissue mass in the trigone which must be differentiated from carcinoma. Histologically cystitis cystica is formed by dilatation of Brunn's nests. Cysts, located in the lamina propria are lined by flat or stratified transitional epithelium. In cystitis glandularis, the cysts are lined by columnar cells which may exfoliate into urine as glandular cells and fragments.

2. Squamous metaplasia

(i) Non-keratinizing metaplasia or pseudomembranous trigonitis

This is commonly found in the trigone of females during oestrogen production. It is found in 36–80% of apparently normal bladders and most likely represents a normal variant under hormonal influence (Weiner et al, 1979; Ito et al., 1981). Cystoscopically, it is characterized by a well-demarcated, often irregular white patch on the trigone, frequently with a rim of vascularity (***Figure 9.3***). Microscopically, it resembles vaginal epithelium and is frequently associated with Brunn's nests, cystitis cystica or cystitis glandularis on the trigone.

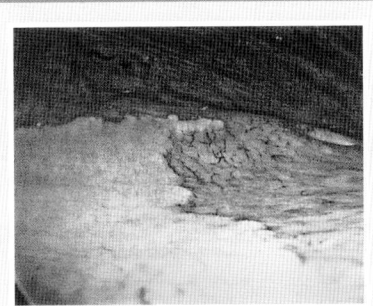

Figure 9.3
Icing sugar coating appearance of squamous metaplasia on the trigone clear of left ureteric orifice.

(ii)   Keratinizing squamous metaplasia or leukoplakia

This is rarely confined to the trigone and is usually a result of long-term irritation or chronic infection, or is found in association with calculi or diverticula. At cystoscopy, the appearance is grey–white leathery, parchment or coral-like, often floating on an inflamed urothelium which characteristically spares the ureteric orifices. The microscopic appearance is that of keratinized mature stratified squamous epithelium. There is evidence that leukoplakia is premalignant and needs careful and frequent follow-up (Benson et al., 1984).

3.   Intestinal metaplasia

Columnar cell metaplasia may occur as focal surface change usually in association with chronic irritation or infection, or as a component of cystitis glandularis. It is potentially premalignant.

IV   Bladder and urethral tumours

1.   Carcinoma in situ

Carcinoma in situ can be asymptomatic or can cause severe urgency, frequency and dysuria (Utz and Farrow, 1984). Cystoscopically, the bladder mucosa may be normal or have an inflamed reddened appearance. The histology is that of abnormal pleomorphic transitional cells confined to the urothelium. Urine cytology is positive in 80–90% of cases. Carcinoma in situ is more common in men and occurs in 25% of patients with high-grade malignancy but rarely in those with well-differentiated superficial tumours. The recurrence rate and progression to muscle invasion occurs in 40–80% where the initial treatment is surgical excision alone. The natural history is not well understood and is variable, ranging from a protracted course of greater than ten years, to rapid progression to invasive bladder cancer with a poor prognosis. Patients with marked urinary symptoms generally have a shorter interval to muscle-invasive cancer. Currently, intravesical therapy with bacille Calmette–Guérin (BCG) is the preferred treatment, producing complete regression in approximately 50–65% of patients (Coplen et al., 1990).

2.   Bladder tumours

Ninety-five percent of bladder tumours are epithelial with the commonest presenting symptom being painless haematuria. Symptoms of bladder irritability such as urinary frequency, urgency and dysuria are the second most common presentation and are usually associated with diffuse carcinoma in situ or invasive bladder cancer. Urinary tract infection is commonly present in women with bladder tumours (La Vecchia et al., 1991) and in addition is a frequent complication following transurethral resection. Risk factors include cigarette smoking, occupational exposure (in, for example, dry-cleaning workers), schistosomiasis infections and possibly alcohol and coffee consumption. Iatrogenic causes include cyclophosphamide exposure and pelvic radiotherapy (van der Poel et al., 1999).

In Western societies transitional cell carcinoma make up more than 90% of bladder tumours and are further graded on growth pattern (papillary (70%), nodular (10%), mixed (20%)), the histological grade and degree of differentiation and the extent of spread. The majority (75–80%) are superficial bladder tumours at presentation, including papillary tumours involving only mucosa (stage T_a) (*Figure 9.4*) or submucosa (stage T_1) and flat carcinoma in situ. Squamous cell carcinoma accounts for approximately 5% bladder tumours in the United States but more than 75% in Egypt, the great majority of which are associated with schistosomal infection. Other associations include chronic irritation from calculi, long-term catheterization, chronic infection, and diverticula. Adenocarcinoma accounts for less than 2% of primary bladder cancers. They are classified into: (a) primary vesical which develop in response to chronic inflammation; (b) urachal; or (c) metastatic from sites such as rectum, stomach, endometrium, breast and ovary. The majority are poorly differentiated and invasive.

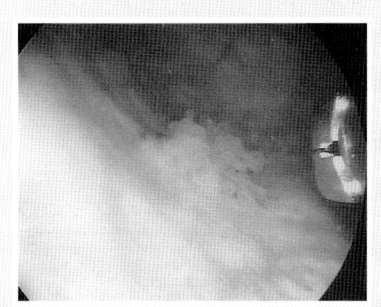

Figure 9.4
Transitional carcinoma diagnosed on routine cystoscopy at Burch colposuspension. This lesion was completely excised by the biopsy forceps.

Other types of bladder carcinoma are small-cell carcinoma and carcinosarcoma. Non-epithelial bladder tumours include neurofibroma, phaeochromocytoma, primary lymphoma, leiomyosarcoma and rhabdomyosarcoma. Lastly, there is a group of uncommon miscellaneous pseudotumours which include inflammatory pseudotumours described as fibromyxoid pseudosarcomatous lesions, endometriosis and primary localized amyloidosis (Messing and Catalona, 1998).

3. Urethral carcinoma

Urethral carcinoma is more prevalent in women with the majority being older than fifty years. There is an association with chronic irritation or infection. Sixty percent are squamous cell carcinoma, 20% are transitional cell carcinoma, 10% are adenocarcinoma, and the remainder are undifferentiated, sarcoma or melanoma. Most patients have non-specific symptoms such as frequency, hesitancy and obstruction. A palpable urethral mass or induration may be present; if advanced, examination may reveal a perineal mass with palpable inguinal nodes (Klein, 1994).

4. Nephrogenic adenoma

This condition, named for its resemblance to primitive renal tubular strucures (*Figure 9.5*) is a form of immature urothelial metaplasia which occurs in the bladder (82%), the urethra (13%) and ureter (5%) usually in the setting of acute or chronic cystitis. The clinical presentation is of macroscopic or microscopic haematuria, frequency, dysuria, nocturia and other irritative symptoms. At cystoscopy, 60% are papillary, 15% polypoidal with the remainder sessile, often raised yellow nodules. These lesions are usually solitary but may be multiple in approximately 20% of cases and usually occur in the trigone (Gonzales et al., 1988).

V   Bladder calculi

Vesical calculus is predominantly a disease of men and is associated with outlet obstruction. In women, calculi are commonly secondary to structural abnormalities such as bladder diverticulum, urethrocoele or foreign body (*Figure 9.6*) and frequently present with

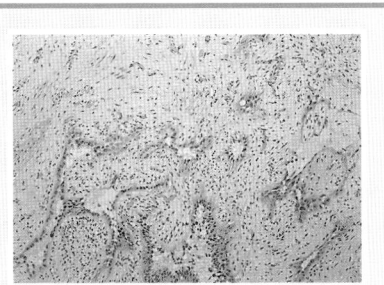

Figure 9.5
Nephrogenic adenoma in a 41-year-old woman who presented with urinary frequency, urgency and urinary leakage and had a 3-cm paraurethral mass. Histology shows irregularly branching tubules set in an oedematous stroma. The tubule is lined by cells with regular nuclei. (Haematoxylin & Eosin × 10.)

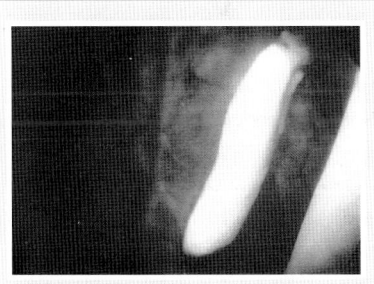

Figure 9.6
Bladder calculus attaching to intravesical suture (late complication of Burch colposuspension) in a woman with recurrent UTI. (From Dwyer et al., 1999.)

urinary tract infection or irritable bladder symptoms (Dwyer et al., 1999). Most bladder calculi are composed of uric acid, or struvite, in the presence of infected urine. Calcium oxalate or cystine stones are usually renal in origin (Douenias et al., 1991).

VI   Urethral diverticulum

Women with urethral diverticulum are usually asymptomatic until ductal obstruction and infection intervene. Presenting symptoms are urethral pain aggravated by voiding or coitus, an anterior vaginal wall mass, frequency or recurrent UTI. Stress incontinence is commonly reported. Postmicturition dribbling is frequently cited as a cardinal symptom but in our experience is rarely of diagnostic value. Urethral diverticulum has been estimated to be present in 1–5% of women with urinary symptoms (Leach and Bavendam, 1987). On vaginal examination, the urethra is very tender if infection is present and a mass is palpable between the vaginal examining finger and the back of the pubic symphysis in 90% of cases (Ganabathi et al., 1994). Urethral compression may express urine, or a purulent or bloody (beware cancer) discharge from the urethra. Histologically, the diverticulum is lined with inflamed fibrous tissue although a muscular layer is frequently present (Moran et al., 1998) suggesting, at least in some cases, a congenital abnormality of Mullerian origin.

Another widely accepted theory is that urethral diverticulum results from the infection and rupture of periurethral glands which are situated along the distal two-thirds of the urethra. Cystourethroscopy (***Figure 9.7a, b***), a micturating cystourethrogram or retrograde positive-pressure urethrogram using a Tratner double-balloon catheter will confirm the diagnosis, reveal the number and location of the diverticula and the presence of

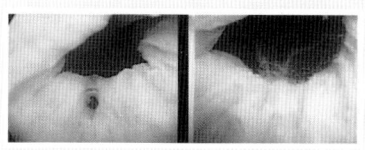

Figure 9.7
Cystourethroscopy using a 0° telescope and Sache sheath reveals a urethral orifice (A) and cloud of pus on urethral compression (B).

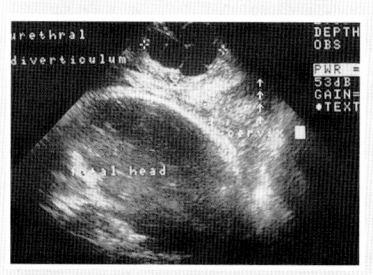

Figure 9.8
Transvaginal ultrasonography demonstrating a multilocular urethral diverticulum adjacent the fetal head. (From Moran et al., 1998.)

any filling defect suggestive of a calculus or tumour. Transvaginal ultrasound is useful particularly if radiological assessment is inappropriate, i.e. pregnancy (*Figure 9.8*). Urodynamic assessment will detect any co-existing genuine stress incontinence although the value of urethral pressure profiles to detect small diverticulum orifices is controversial.

Recurrent symptomatic urethral diverticulum are treated by transvaginal excision following wide dissection and layered closure without tension. Reported surgical complications are urethrovaginal fistula (4%), recurrence (12%), stress incontinence (9%), urethral stricture (2%) and recurrent UTI (23%) (Ganabathi et al., 1994).

VII   Urethral syndrome

Urethral syndrome is a non-specific constellation of lower urinary tract symptoms of urethral pain aggravated by voiding, suprapubic discomfort, with or without frequency and urgency, where no objective cause can be found. It is therefore a diagnosis of exclusion where urogenital infection has been ruled out, as have been non-infectious causes of urethritis secondary to chemical irritants (soaps, douches, spermicidals), trauma (foreign bodies), structural abnormalities (urethral strictures, diverticulum, tumours), and systemic disease (Steven–Johnson syndrome, Reiter syndrome).

In 1980, Stamm et al. found that women with recent onset dysuria and frequency (acute urethral syndrome) and a midstream urine (MSU) specimen of $< 10^5$ microorganisms per ml, frequently had an infective cause for their symptoms, especially in the presence of pyuria (> 8 leukocytes/ml urine). In their study, 42 of 59 women with the acute urethral syndrome had pyuria; cultures revealed coliforms in 24 (57%), *Chlamydia* in 10 (24%), and *Staphylococcus sacrophyticus* in 3 (7%). However the role of infection has been disputed; no difference in pyuria or culture of fastidious organisms was found between a group of patients with acute urethral syndrome and asymptomatic controls (Gillespie et al., 1989). Nevertheless the presence of pyuria in sexually active women with the acute urethral syndrome should suggest an infective cause. Cultures for *Neisseria gonorrhoea* and *Chlamydia trachomatis* should be performed, and even if cultures are negative, empirical treatment with an antibiotic such as doxycycline be considered possibly in combination with sulphamethoxazole/trimethoprim (Latham and Stamm, 1984).

In chronic urethral syndrome an infective cause is less likely. Infective and non-infective causes of urethral pain and frequency need to be excluded along the same lines as in interstitial cystitis (*Figure 9.1*). Bonica in 1990 states that 'the aetiology of the chronic pelvic pain syndrome is unknown, but is a result of a complex, poorly understood, abnormal physiological interaction among noxious stimuli, both visceral and somatic; actual dysfunction with the nervous system itself; and adverse interplay with psychologic, family and social relationships and interactions'. Not surprisingly, there are no proven pharmacological or surgical treatments for the chronic urethral syndrome. Urethral dilatation has traditionally been used based on the belief that there is distal urethral constriction. Rutherford et al. (1988) found an 80% improvement with urethral dilatation to French 36–42 which was identical to the response to cystoscopy alone. Repeated urethral dilatation can cause urethral fibrosis and stress incontinence. Prazosin and diazepam have been used based on the presumed effect to reduce spasm of the urethral smooth and striated muscle. Amitriptyline is used in the treatment of chronic pain and has an added beneficial anticholinergic action. Nevertheless the primary goal of management is patient and family education and support with the alleviation of suffering rather than the elimination of pain.

References

Ahmed M, Davison OW (1991) Severe cystitis associated with tiaprofenic acid. *BMJ* **303**: 1376.

Bade JJ, Laseur M, Nieuwenburg A, van der Weele LT, Mensink HJ (1997) A placebo-controlled study of intravesical pentosan polysulfate for the treatment of interstitial cystitis. *Br J Urol* **79**: 168–71.

Benson RC Jr, Swanson SK, Farrow GM (1984) Relationship of leukoplakia to urothelial malignancy. *J Urol* **131**: 507–11.

Bonica JJ Cause and mechanism of chronic pain. In: Bonica JJ, ed. *Management of Pain*, 2nd edn, Vol I. Philadelphia: Lea & Febiger, 1990: 183.

Bramble FJ, Morley R (1997) Drug-induced cystitis: the need for vigilance. *Br J Urol* **79**: 3–7.

Coplen DE, Marcus MD, Myers JA, Ratliff TL, Catalona WJ (1990) Long-term follow-up of patients treated with 1 or 2, 6-week courses of intravesical bacillus Calmette-Guérin; analysis of possible predictors of response free tumor. *J Urol* **144**: 652–7.

deVries CR, Freha FS (1990) Hemorrhagic cystitis: a review. *J Urol* **143**: 1–7.

Douenias R, Rich M, Badlani G (1991) Predisposing factors in bladder calculi: review of 100 cases. *Urology* **37**: 240–3.

Duncan JL, Schaeffer AJ (1997) Do infectious agents cause interstitial cystitis? *Urology* **49**(Suppl 5A): 48–51.

Dwyer PL, Carey MP, Rosamilia A (1999) Suture injury to the urinary tract in urethral suspension procedures for stress incontinence. *Int Urogynec J* **10**: 15–21.

Elbadawi A (1997) Interstitial cystis: a critique of current concepts with a new proposal for pathologic diagnosis and pathogenesis. *Urology* 49(Suppl 5A): 14–40.

Fall M, Lindstrom S (1994) Transcutaneous electrical nerve stimulation in classic and nonulcer interstitial cystitis. *Urol Clin North Am* 21: 131–9.

Ganabathi K, Leach GE, Zimmern PE, Dmochowski RR (1994) Experience with the management of urethral diverticulum in 63 women. *J Urol* 152: 1445–52.

Gillenwater JY, Wein AJ (1988) Summary of the National Institute of Arthritis, Diabetes, Digestive and Kidney Diseases Workshop on Interstitial Cystitis. *J Urol* 140: 203–6.

Gillespie WA, Henderson EP, Unton KB, Smith PJB (1989) Microbiology of the urethral frequency and dysuria syndrome. A controlled study with 5 year review. *Br J Urol* 64: 270–4.

Gonzales JA, Watts JC, Alderson TP (1988) Nephrogenic adenoma of the bladder: report of 10 cases. *J Urol* 139: 45–7.

Hanno PM (1994) Diagnosis of interstitial cystitis. *Urol Clin North Am* 21: 63–6.

Hanno PM (1997) Analysis of long-term Elmiron therapy for interstitial cystitis. *Urology* 49(Suppl 5A): 93–9.

Hanno PM, Wein AJ (1994) Interstitial cystitis. Part I and II. *Urol Clin North Am* 21: 124–41.

Hanno PM, Buehler J, Wein AJ (1989) Use of amitriptyline in the treatment of interstitial cystitis. *J Urol* 141: 846–8.

Henley MJ, Harriss D, Bishop MC (1997) Cystitis associated with tiaprofenic acid (Surgam): a survey of British and Irish urologists. *Br J Urol* 79(4): 585–7.

Hurst RE, Parsons CL, Roy JB, Young JL (1993) Urinary glycosaminoglycan excretion as a laboratory marker in the diagnosis of interstitial cystitis. *J Urol* 149: 31–5.

Irwin PP, Galloway NTM (1994) Surgical management of interstitial cystitis. *Urol Clin North Am* 21: 145–51.

Ito N, Hirose M, Shirai T, Tsuda H, Nakanishi K et al. (1981) Lesions of the urinary bladder epithelium in 125 autopsy cases. *Acta Pathol Jpn* 31: 545–57.

Johansson SL, Fall M (1994) Pathology of interstitial cystitis. *Urol Clin North Am* 21: 55–62.

Jones CA, Nyberg L (1997) Epidemiology of interstitial cystitis. *Urology* 49(Suppl 5A): 2–9.

Klein EA Urethral carcinoma. In: Seidmon EJ, Hanno PM, eds *Current Urologic Therapy*. London: WB Saunders, 1994: 432–4.

Korting GE, Smith SD, Wheeler MA, Weiss RM, Foster HE Jr (1999) A randomized double-blind trial of oral L-arginine for treatment of interstitial cystitis. *J Urol* **161**: 558–65.

Koziol JA (1994) Epidemiology of interstitial cystitis. *Urol Clin North Am* **21**: 7–20.

Latham RH, Stamm WE (1984) Urethral syndrome in women. *Urol Clin North Am* **11**: 95–101.

La Vecchia C, Negri E, D'Avanzo B, Savoldelli R, Franceschi S (1991) Genital and urinary tract diseases and bladder cancer. *Cancer Res* **51**: 629–31.

Leach GE, Bavendam TG (1987) Female urethral diverticula. *Urology* **30**: 407–15.

Long JP, Althausen AF (1989) Malacoplakia: a 25 year experience with a review of the literature. *J Urol* **141**: 1328–31.

Lotenfoe RR, Christie J, Parsons A, Burkett P, Helal M et al. (1995) Absence of neuropathic pelvic pain and favorable psychological profile in the surgical selection of patients with disabling interstitial cystitis. *J Urol* **154**: 2039–42.

Lynes WL, Flynn SD, Shortliffe LD, Stamey TA (1990) The histology of interstitial cystitis. *Am J Surg Pathol* **14**: 69–76.

Messing EM, Stamey TA (1978) Interstitial cystitis, early diagnosis, pathology, and treatment. *Urology* **12**: 381–92.

Messing EM, Catalona W (1998) Urothelial tumors of the urinary tract. In: Walsh PC, Retik AB, Darracott Vaughan E, Wein AJ, eds *Campbell's Textbook of Urology*, 7th edn. Philadelphia: WB Saunders, 1998: 2327–83.

Morales A, Emerson I, Nickel JC (1997) Intravesical hyaluronic acid in the treatment of refractory interstitial cystitis. *Urology* **49**(Suppl 5A): 111–13.

Moran PA, Carey MP, Dwyer PL (1998) Urethral diverticula in pregnancy. *Aust NZ J Obstet Gynaec* **38**: 102–6.

Norkool DM, Hampson NB, Gibbons RP, Weissman RM (1993) Hyperbaric oxygen therapy for radiation-induced hemorrhagic cystitis. *J Urol* **150**: 332–4.

O'Brien WM (1986) Adverse reactions to non-steroidal anti-inflammatory drugs. *Am J Med* **80**(Suppl 4B): 70–80.

Okada H, Minayoshi K, Goto A (1992) Two cases of eosinophilic cystitis induced by Tranilast. *J Urol* **147**: 1366–8.

Parsons CL Interstitial cystitis. In: Kursh ED, McGuire EJ, eds *Female Urology*. Philadelphia: JB Lippincott, 1994: 421–38.

Parsons CL, Benson G, Childs SJ, Hanno P, Sant GR et al. (1993) A quantitatively controlled method to prospectively study interstitial cystitis and demonstrate the efficacy of pentosan polysulfate. *J Urol* **150**: 845–8.

Perez-Marrero R, Emerson LE, Feltis JT (1988) A controlled study of dimethyl sulfoxide in interstitial cystitis. *J Urol* **140**: 36–9.

Peters K, Diokno A, Steinert B, Yuhico M, Mitchell B et al. (1997) The efficacy of intravesical TICE strain bacillus Calmette-Guérin in the treatment of interstitial cystitis: a double-blind, prospective, placebo controlled trial. *J Urol* 157: 2090–4.

Ratliff TL, Klutke CG, Hofmeister M, He F, Russell JH et al. (1995) Role of the immune response in interstitial cystitis. *Clin Immunol Immunopathol* 74: 209–16.

Relling MV, Schunk JE (1986) Drug-induced hemorrhagic cystitis. *Clin Pharmacy* 5: 590–7.

Rosamilia A, Dwyer PL (1998) Interstitial cystitis and the gynecologist. *Obstet Gynec Surv* 53: 309–19.

Rosamilia A, Cann L, Dwyer P, Scurry J, Rogers P (1999a) Bladder microvasculature in women with interstitial cystitis. *J Urol* 161: 1865–70.

Rosamilia A, Dwyer P, Kende M, Clements J, Campbell D (1999b) Activation of urinary kinin system in interstitial cystitis. *J Urol* 162: 129–34.

Ruggieri MR, Chelsky MJ, Rosen SI, Shickley TJ, Hanno PM (1994). Current findings and future research avenues in the study of interstitial cystitis. *Urol Clin North Am* 21: 163–76.

Rutherford AJ, Hinshaw K, Essenhigh DM, Neal DE (1988) Urethral dilatation compared with cystoscopy alone in the treatment of women with recurrent frequency and dysuria. *Br J Urol* 61: 500–4.

Sant GR, LaRock DR (1994) Standard intravesical therapies for interstitial cystitis. *Urol Clin North Am* 21: 73–83.

Seshadri P, Emerson L, Morales A (1994) Cimetidine in the treatment of interstitial cystitis. *Urology* 44: 614–16.

Sidh SM, Smith SP, Silber SB, Young JD (1980) Eosinophilic cystitis; advanced disease requiring surgical intervention. *Urology* 15: 23–6.

Stamm WE, Wagner KF, Amsel R, Alexander ER, Turck M et al. (1980) Causes of the acute urethral syndrome in women. *N Engl J Med* 303: 409–15.

Steers WD, Tuttle JB Neurogenic inflammation and nerve growth factor: possible roles in interstitial cystitis. In: Sant GR, ed. *Interstitial cystitis*. Philadelphia: Lippincott-Raven, 1997: 67–75.

Theoharides TC, Sant GR (1997) Hydroxyzine therapy for interstitial cystitis. *Urology* 49(Suppl 5A): 108–10.

Utz DC, Zincke H (1974) The masquerade of bladder cancer in situ as interstitial cystitis. *J Urol* 111: 160–1.

Utz DC, Farrow GM (1984) Carcinoma in situ of the urinary tract. *Urol Clin North Am* 11: 735–40.

Van der Poel HG, Mungan NA, Witjes JA (1999) Bladder cancer in women. *Int Urogynecol J* 10: 207–12.

Wiener DP, Koss LG, Sablay B, Freed SZ (1979) The prevalence and significance of Brunn's nests, cystitis cystica, and squamous metaplasia in normal bladders. *J Urol* 122: 317–21.

Wilson CB, Leopard J, Nakamura RM, Cheresh DA, Stein PC et al. (1995) Selective type IV collagen defects in the urothelial basement membrane of interstitial cystitis. *J Urol* 154: 1222–6.

Sex and recurrent urinary tract infection

Phillip Hay

10

Contents

I Introduction

An association between sexual intercourse and urinary tract infection (UTI) in women has long been recognized. This is reflected in the well-known term 'honeymoon cystitis'. Both men and women can develop cystitis after sexual intercourse but women are considerably more vulnerable. Approximately half of all women had experienced UTI by their late 20s and the incidence rises progressively from the age of sexual maturity (Zielske et al., 1981). Approximately 25% of women have another infection within six months of their first. In the USA estimates have been made of 7 million cases per year, with costs of more than 1 billion dollars (Hooton et al., 1996a). For the individual, recurrent bouts of cystitis may mean pain, lost sleep and days off work and can lead eventually to sexual dysfunction.

II Diagnosis and differential diagnosis

Cystitis needs to be distinguished from urethritis, 'urethral syndrome' and interstitial cystitis. This is not always straightforward. Cystitis is confirmed conventionally by finding a pure growth of an organism at a concentration $\geq 10^5$/ml in a midstream urine (MSU). Maskell (1995) reminds us that Kass (1957), comparing bacterial counts taken from catheter specimens (CSUs) and MSUs collected in the early morning from symptom-free women, defined this figure. Most, but not all, of the women in whom bacteria were present had counts $\geq 10^8$/l. This probably reflects multiplication of bacteria in the favourable environment of urine collecting in the bladder overnight for several hours. Lower concentrations of organisms in MSUs collected under other conditions are likely to be significant.

Stamm and colleagues (1980) investigated the urethral syndrome in women attending a STD clinic. Those who reported dysuria and/or frequency but did not fulfil the conventional criteria for cystitis (bacterial counts $\geq 10^8$/l) were assessed. Many of them had low count bacteriuria with coliforms or *Staphylococcus saprophyticus* at concentrations $> 10^5$ per litre, with pyuria. Their symptoms resolved with appropriate antibiotic therapy (Stamm et al., 1981). In addition, 10 of 16 women with pyuria who had sterile bladder urine had *Chlamydia trachomatis* detected. Overall, 42 of 59 women with urethral syndrome and pyuria had either low count bacteriuria or *C. trachomatis* detected. These authors also demonstrated that women with pyuria in association with urethral syndrome had a good response to antibiotic therapy whilst those without pyuria did not.

Most women with chlamydial or gonococcal infections are asymptomatic. Some present with symptoms of dysuria and urinary frequency, due to urethritis. Such symptoms often resolve spontaneously but these infections should always be considered, particularly if sterile pyuria is found. Postcoital or intermenstrual bleeding should raise suspicion of mucopurulent cervicitis or endometritis, whilst pelvic pain and deep dyspareunia are most probably due to pelvic inflammatory disease. Bacteriuria and STDs often coexist in sexually active women. An excess of polymorphonuclear cells (more than 10 per high-power field) can often be demonstrated in Gram-stained urethral smears from women with urethral infections. Chlamydia and gonorrhoea can only be excluded reliably by taking appropriate diagnostic tests from urethral and cervical swabs (Horner et al., 1995); Wallin et al., 1981). Interstitial cystitis, a condition seen more commonly in postmenopausal women, may produce similar symptoms to bacterial cystitis. The diagnosis is confirmed on cystoscopy, with a small bladder volume, haemorrhagic areas and sometimes a 'Hunner's ulcer'. Mast cell infiltration may be seen on histological examination of bladder biopsies. There is continuing debate as to whether this has an infective or other aetiology.

In clinical practice, women with cystitis present with dysuria and urinary frequency. In more severe cases there is fever, haematuria and lower abdominal pain. Loin pain and tenderness might indicate pyelonephritis. Ideally, sexually active women should be screened for chlamydia, gonorrhoea,

Trichomonas vaginalis and bacterial vaginosis before treatment is prescribed for cystitis. Many broad-spectrum antibiotics might suppress but not eradicate chlamydia and gonorrhoea, making the diagnosis more difficult subsequently. A urine test such as Nephur test shows the presence of leucocyte esterase (LE), indicating the presence of polymorphonuclear cells. This is sensitive but not specific for bacteriuria, as it is often positive in women with urethritis. The presence of nitrite is sensitive and specific for detecting *E. coli* bacteriuria.

If the symptoms are suggestive of a UTI and either the LE or the nitrite test is positive, treatment should be prescribed for a presumptive UTI, whilst microscopy and culture results are awaited. The choice of antibiotic depends on local resistance patterns and previous exposure of the individual. In general, three-day courses of an antibiotic which does not inhibit lactobacilli are preferable. These include trimethoprim, nitrofurantoin and quinolones.

III Pathophysiology

Escherichia coli, which cause urinary tract infections in women, originate usually from the bowel flora. In one study, half of all paired first and second UTI isolates from the same subject were apparently the same (Foxman et al., 1995a). A crucial first step is for uropathogenic bacteria to colonize the vagina, particularly the periurethral area (Stamey, 1973). During subsequent vaginal intercourse, trauma and mechanical distortion of the urethra might assist the ascent of organisms pushed into the bladder. Thus, in one study, the concentration of bacteria in the urine was increased following intercourse in 30% of women (Buckley et al., 1978). Another study documented that both asymptomatic and symptomatic bacteriuria were found more commonly the day after intercourse (Nicolle et al., 1982).

In 1973 Stamey described a prospective longitudinal study in which women took swabs regularly from the vaginal vestibule and the urethra. Twenty-seven of 30 women, who had never had a urinary tract infection tended to have persistent colonization with higher colony counts during the period when they suffered from recurrent UTIs. When the introital flora reverted to normal, the urinary tract infections ceased. Following short courses of antibiotics, the organism tends to remain in the periurethral area with the women remaining vulnerable to a repeat episode. Such organisms are occasionally transmitted to male partners. In the longitudinal study, there was a mean of 34 days from periurethral colonization with coliforms to the next symptomatic UTI. In some women, however, the onset was less than seven days. Pfau and Sacks (1981) confirmed these findings. They reported that the appearance of Gram-negative enterobacteria

in normal women was rare and transitory. Urinary tract infections were preceded by persistent Gram-negative vulval, vaginal and urethral colonization.

Stamey (1973) concluded that we need to determine the nature of the biological defect that allows pathogenic introital colonization to occur. By doing so we might intervene to return the introital bacteriology to normal. This observation remains as valid today as it was in 1973.

Abnormal vaginal colonization might be due to several factors.

- virulence of the pathogens,
- host susceptibility,
- the quality of the endogenous lactobacillus flora,
- disturbance to the vaginal flora.

Virulence factors such as possession of fimbriae and other adherence mechanisms are well recognized for *E. coli*. Host susceptibility factors include ABO blood group non-secretor status, which was associated with increased binding of *E. coli* to vaginal epithelial cells in vitro (Stapleton et al., 1992).

Control of the vaginal microflora is complex and involves factors such as the resident lactobacilli, vaginal pH, hormonal status and the adherence of enterobacteria to the epithelium. Lactobacilli produce lactocins, bacteriocins, lactic acid and hydrogen peroxide which together inhibit the growth of other bacterial species and help to maintain a vaginal pH of less than 4.5. Factors that disturb the normal flora, such as broad-spectrum antibiotics, menstruation, sexual intercourse and use of spermicides, might favour colonization by uropathogens.

Several studies have documented the association of spermicide with disturbed vaginal flora. Early studies documented that women using spermicides and diaphragms were at an increased risk of urinary tract infection, being between two and 3.5 times more likely to have one than sexually active women not using diaphragms. Initially, this was attributed to a mechanical effect of the diaphragm distorting the urethra, leading to incomplete voiding. However, it is now thought that alteration of the vaginal flora in response to the spermicide is more important (Fihn et al., 1996; Hooton et al., 1994). Women using diaphragms with spermicides with no history of UTIs typically have levels of periurethral colonization with uropathogenic organisms similar to those seen in women with recurrent UTIs.

In vitro, nonoxynol-9, the most commonly used spermicidal agent, inhibits the growth of lactobacilli but not uropathogenic *E. coli*. The adherence of *E. coli* to vaginal cells may also be increased (Hooton et al., 1991). A prospective study performed by Fihn and colleagues (1996) similarly demonstrated that women who used a spermicide-coated condom had a greatly increased risk of UTI compared to women not doing so. If they used such condoms more than once a week, the odds ratio was 3.34 rising to 5.65 for more than twice weekly, in a multivariate analysis.

It is likely that the cyclical changes in female sex hormones influence the vaginal flora significantly. Hootton and colleagues (1996b) found that the peak incidence of symptomatic cystitis was between the eighth and 15th day of the menstrual cycle in women infected with either *E. coli* or *Staphylococcus saprophyticus* (**Figure 10.1**). This could be related to the peak of coital frequency that occurs soon after menstruation finishes (James, 1971) but is more likely to be due to hormonal influences.

In vitro the attachment of *E. coli* to HeLa cells is increased in the presence of oestrogen. Progesterone had no such effect (Sugarman and Epps, 1982). Lactobacilli that produce high levels of hydrogen peroxide can inhibit the growth of anaerobic organisms implicated in bacterial vaginosis (Klebanoff et al., 1991). When bacterial vaginosis develops the lactobacilli may disappear. The development of bacterial vaginosis is also linked to the menstrual cycle, developing around the time of menstruation and spontaneously regressing in midcycle (Hay et al., 1997). One study has reported an association between bacterial vaginosis and recurrent urinary tract infection (Hooton et al., 1989). If clindamycin or other broad-spectrum antibiotics are used as

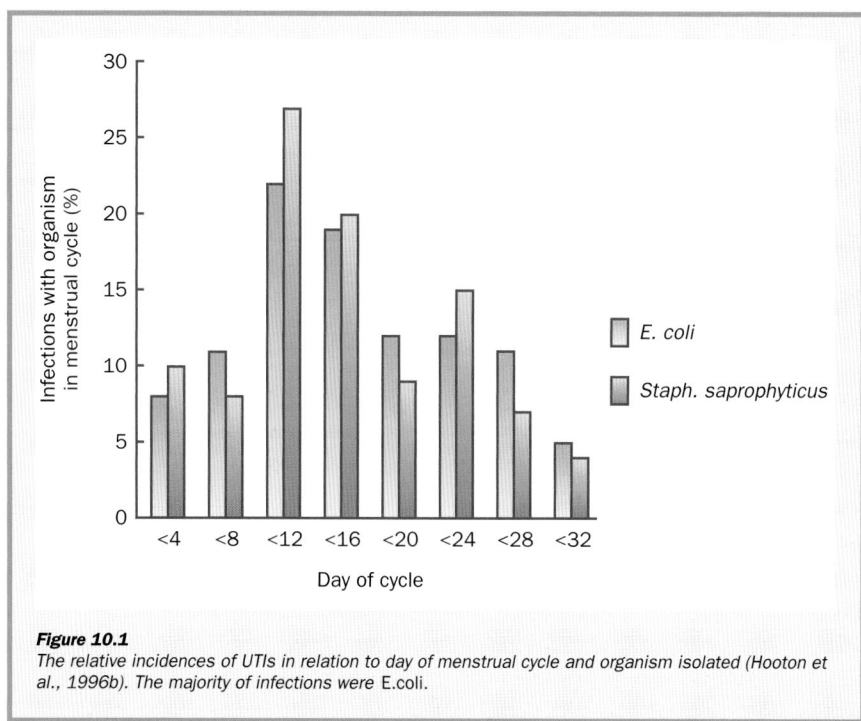

Figure 10.1
The relative incidences of UTIs in relation to day of menstrual cycle and organism isolated (Hooton et al., 1996b). The majority of infections were E.coli.

treatment for bacterial vaginosis, lactobacilli may be eradicated, leading to a usually transient overgrowth of Gram-negative organisms in the vagina (Hill and Livengood, 1994). This would predispose such women to developing urinary tract infections.

The possible role of sexual transmission of a virulent uropathogenic *E. coli* is difficult to assess. Stamey (1973) reported that *E. coli* could be transmitted to a male sex partner and has occasionally produced an episode of cystitis in the male partner. Foxman was able to isolate identical strains of *E. coli* from four of 19 male partners of women with urinary tract infections (Foxman et al., 1997). Krieger and colleagues (1993) looked at UTIs in healthy men attending a university health service. The incidence was very low at 5 per

10,000 man-years. Ninety percent of them were sexually active. Only one of the 38 men presenting with urinary tract infection had prostatitis and the symptoms usually cleared with short courses of treatment.

1. Adherence of E. coli

Further in vitro experiments have shown that the adherence of *E. coli* to vaginal epithelial cells rises with increasing pH which may be an additional factor for an association with bacterial vaginosis. There is competitive inhibition from lactobacilli. For many years cranberry juice has been a folk remedy for urinary tract infections and in vitro *E. coli*. Adherence was decreased by 80% in the presence of cranberry juice (Avorn et al., 1994). This is partly explained by the presence of fructose but also a specific polymer, which appears to interfere with binding. This has yet to be characterized. The apparent protective effect of cranberry juice is interesting but its role in treatment has not been assessed in prospective studies of premenopausal women.

IV Prospective clinical studies

Two well-designed studies have recently examined the relationship between intercourse and UTI. Foxman and colleagues (1995b) studied risk factors for first-time, urinary tract infections in young women. They argued that

women with recurrent UTIs may alter their behaviour in response to the problem and that good information could therefore only be obtained by studying women with a first episode. Their study recruited women from a university health centre who had never married, had no history of UTI and who had engaged in sexual activity at least once. The study group consisted of 86 female students who presented with UTI and 288 controlled women. *E. coli* was isolated from 86% of women with a UTI. A multiple logistic regression analysis identified several factors associated with increased risk of UTI. These are summarized in *Table 10.1*.

A high frequency of vaginal intercourse was associated strongly with UTI. Partner change might be important in two ways: intercourse may be more frequent during a 'honeymoon' period but also may involve exposure to new genital pathogens. This might be because trauma, increased secretions and manipulation of the urethra occur during sexual activity. This would help to move uropathogens to the urethral opening and into the urinary tract. Birth control methods such as diaphragm and condom use might exacerbate these factors, with the additional effects of spermicides on the vaginal flora.

The association with black race has not been looked for in most studies. Other genital infections including bacterial vaginosis, chlamydia and gonorrhoea have also been associated with black race in recent studies.

Table 10.1
Risk factors for first episode of UTI in sexually active women (Foxman et al., 1995b)

Risk factor	Odds ratio for UTI	95% CI
Partner change within one year	2.10	1.12–4.32
Receptive anal intercourse within last two weeks	2.2	1.8–18.5
Condom use > four times in last two weeks	6.5	2.16–26.12
Black race	5.1	1.89–24.63
Habitual cranberry juice drinker	0.5	0.19–1.02
No intercourse in last two weeks	1.0	Comparator
Intercourse 1–5 times in last two weeks	21.04	8.39–62.22
Intercourse >5 times in last two weeks	34.47	12.59–106.23

Hooton and colleagues (1996a) performed a prospective study of 796 healthy, sexually active non-pregnant women from two populations. The incidence of UTI was 0.7/person-year in university students requesting a new method of contraception and 0.5/year in slightly older women, attending a health maintenance organization (HMO). The mean age of university students was 23 years, compared to 29 years for the HMO attendees. *E. coli* was the pathogen in 93% of cases.

Again, there was a strong correlation between frequency of intercourse and UTI, with spermicide use, condoms and diaphragms adding increased risk (*Table 10.2*). There was a trend for increasing age to be associated with reduced incidence of UTI. A history of two or more previous UTIs was also associated with an increased incidence of UTI. A woman having intercourse daily, without spermicide or diaphragm, was nine times more likely to develop a UTI than a woman having no intercourse. There was no detectable association with ABO blood group non-secretor status or with time interval to voiding after intercourse, two factors that have been associated with increased risk in prior case

Table 10.2
Risk factors for UTI in a multivariate model. Risk relative to women having no intercourse during the previous week (Hooton et al., 1996a).

	Relative risk for university students (mean 6.4 episodes intercourse/month)			Relative risk for women attending an HMO (mean 5.0 episodes intercourse/month)		
Married	0.48 (p < 0.09)			0.44 (p < 0.002)		
≥2 prior UTIs	5.58 (p < 0.001)			2.10 (p < 0.006)		
Number of episodes, in last week, of	**One**	**Three**	**Five**	**One**	**Three**	**Five**
Sexual intercourse	1.37	2.56	4.81[1]*	1.24	1.91	2.96[2]†
Diaphragm and spermicide use	1.42	2.83	5.68[1]*	1.29	2.14	3.54[3]†

* p < 0.001
[†] p = 0.04
[‡] p = 0.002

control studies. The authors concluded that at least two-thirds of UTIs in this population could be attributed to intercourse.

V Treatment and prevention

1. Hormonal manipulation

Postmenopausal women are vulnerable to UTI, which affects more than 10% of women over the age of 60. This has been attributed to atrophic change occurring as a consequence of diminished oestrogen levels. There are also changes in vaginal fluid with a rise in pH, decreased lactobacillus concentrations and increased colonization with faecal flora (Cardozo, 1996). Oestrogen therapy can reverse these changes (Molander et al., 1990). No prospective studies have assessed the role of intercourse in triggering UTI in this group of women. Treatment studies have generally focused on the role of oestrogen replacement therapy, either topical or systemic.

Raz and Stamm (1993) enrolled 93

Table 10.3
A double-blind placebo-controlled study of oestriol cream in postmenopausal women with recurrent UTIs (Raz and Stamm, 1993)

	Treatment group (50)	Placebo
Number of UTIs/year	0.5	5.9*
Mean vaginal pH	3.8	5.5*
Colonized by lactobacilli after one month	61%	0%*
Colonized by enterobacteria after one month	31%	63%*
* p < 0.005		

postmenopausal women with a history of recurrent UTI into a double-blind, placebo-controlled trial. Sixty women completed eight months of follow-up. The results, summarized in *Table 10.3*, showed a dramatic reduction in the incidence of UTI in those receiving oestriol cream, associated with favourable changes in the vaginal ecosystem.

Some studies of systemic hormone replacement therapy (HRT) have reported less benefit. In a case control study women who were taking HRT had a slighter greater incidence of UTI than those who had never taken it (Oliveria et al., 1998). In a prospective study, Cardozo and colleagues (1998) studied 72 postmenopausal women (mean age 73 years). Oral oestriol at a dose of 3 mg/day was not shown to be superior to placebo in the prevention of recurrent UTIs, although urinary symptoms improved in both

groups. A smaller placebo-controlled study of 40 women used oestriol 3 mg/day for four weeks, followed by 1 mg/day for eight weeks (Kirkengen et al., 1992). The incidence of UTI fell in both groups but during the latter eight weeks there was a significant lower incidence of UTI in the oestriol group. This was associated with a reduction in the vaginal pH.

2.   Biotherapeutics

Lactobacilli play an important role in maintaining a healthy vaginal flora. Natural yoghurt, which usually contains *L. acidophilus*, is often ingested or applied topically to the vagina by women with vaginitis, although there are no good randomized trials to support this approach. In a small study, 10^9 lactobacillus organisms (a combination of

L. caseii subsp. *Rhamnosus* and *L. fermentum*) were inserted into the vagina daily for one year. The incidence of UTI fell from >4/year before treatment to 1.3/year during treatment (Reid and Bruce, 1995). A similar approach is to use a hydrogen peroxide-producing strain of *L. crispatus* for the treatment of bacterial vaginosis (Klebanoff et al., 1991).

3.   Self-help

Women with recurrent UTIs are often encouraged to void soon after intercourse. There are no prospective studies to demonstrate a benefit from such a 'common sense' approach. The rationale of flushing the urethra and emptying the bladder after intercourse is, however, biologically plausible and most physicians recommend it. Similarly, women are encouraged to wipe from 'front to back' after defaecation to reduce the exposure of the vagina to faecal flora.

Regular drinking of cranberry juice was associated with a reduced risk of first-episode UTI in Foxman et al.'s (1995b) prospective study, as was regular ingestion of vitamin C. A randomized, double-blind, placebo-controlled trial was performed in 153 postmenopausal women (mean age 78.5 years) (Avorn et al., 1994). They received 300/per day of a standard cranberry juice drink or a synthetic placebo drink that was indistinguishable in taste, appearance and vitamin C content but lacked cranberry content. The incidence of bacteriuria (>10^5/ml) with pyuria in those receiving cranberry juice was 42% of that in the control group ($p = 0.004$). They were also nearly four times more likely to clear bacteriuria spontaneously when it did occur ($p = 0.006$).

4.   Antibiotic therapy

Although many broad-spectrum antibiotics are effective against coliforms, those that have low activity against lactobacilli are favoured, as they are thought least likely to disturb the vaginal microflora. A short course of antibiotics for cystitis may clear organisms from the bladder but rarely from the vaginal introitus. Many women with recurrent UTIs require antibiotic therapy for symptomatic infections, and for many regular antibiotic therapy nightly or following intercourse offers relief from the constant threat of cystitis. The value of such treatment is now well established by randomized controlled trials. Early studies established a role for co-trimoxazole, nalidixic acid or nitrofurantoin (Pfau et al., 1983) and for postcoital trimethoprim–sulphamethoxazole (Stapleton et al., 1990).

Recent studies have focused on the role of quinolone antibiotics, to which resistance is currently uncommon. Three-day courses of most antibiotics including ciprofloxacin are sufficient to treat acute episodes of cystitis but not to prevent recurrences (Iravani et al.,

1995). Thus, Pfau and Sacks (1994) studied 33 sexually active women who had experienced a mean of more than four UTIs in eight months prior to treatment. They were randomized to receive postcoital treatment with ofloxacin 100 mg or norfloxacin 200 mg or ciprofloxacin 125 mg. Over 15 months of mean follow-up, only one woman had a UTI. The mean antibiotic use was 117 doses/year. Improvement in vaginal microbiology was documented by enterobacteria being cultured from introital swabs of 74% of women prior to treatment, but only 11% following treatment.

A study of 135 women in Greece compared the use of 125 mg ciprofloxacin as daily prophylaxis with its use as postcoital treatment, in sexually active young women (Melekos et al., 1997). The mean incidence of UTI before treatment was 3.7/year. With treatment, the incidence was reduced to 0.043 per patient-year in the daily treatment group and 0.031 in the postcoital group ($p < 0.0001$). Similarly, enterobacteria were cultured from the introitus of 86% of women before treatment and 2.5% and 5.6% of the treatment groups respectively.

VI Clinical management

Most young sexually active women who develop recurrent UTIs do so for the reasons discussed above. However, those with chronic pyelonephritis, stones or other underlying causes may present in a similar manner. It is prudent therefore to arrange an ultrasound scan of the urogenital tract to screen for any underlying abnormality. Consider the possibility of concomitant STDs such as chlamydia and gonorrhoea as well as bacterial vaginosis, which might predispose a woman to UTIs. Screening of both the woman and her partner is necessary to exclude STDs.

As both postcoital and daily low-dose antibiotic therapy are equally effective in preventing recurrences, either can be used. If intercourse is relatively infrequent, postcoital treatment may be preferred. If coitus occurs four or more times per week, daily treatment may be simpler. There are no trials to assess the optimum duration of therapy, but it is reasonable to prescribe treatment for six months in the first instance. If STDs have been excluded it may be helpful to see a couple together to explain the nature of the condition. As Ronald (1996) remarked: 'Couples need to understand that sexually associated infections are not necessarily sexually transmitted and that neither partner is responsible for their occurrence. Guilt and fear must not be allowed to interfere with sexual fulfilment'.

VII Conclusion

Sexual intercourse is a powerful trigger for the development of UTIs in young sexually active women. For cystitis to develop, the vaginal introitus and periurethral area must be colonized by uropathogenic bacteria, which is *E. coli* in >90% cases. Physical trauma during intercourse may assist organisms to enter the bladder. The use of spermicide with diaphragms or condoms enhances the risk, probably through altering the vaginal flora. Relapse is common and often an identical bacterium is responsible for subsequent infections. Whilst three days of antibiotic therapy is optimal for uncomplicated cystitis, elimination of vaginal carriage and subsequent prevention of relapse requires longer courses of low-dose daily or postcoital therapy. The possible roles of regular consumption of cranberry juice or application of lactobacilli to the vagina have not yet been elucidated. Many women with recurrent UTIs have vaginal infections reflecting a disturbed flora in the form of recurrent vaginal candidiasis and bacterial vaginosis as well as increased susceptibility to sexually transmitted infections. Improved understanding of the mechanisms by which such conditions develop in susceptible women may yet lead to improved means of prevention.

References

Avorn J, Monane M, Gurwitz JH et al. (1994) Reduction of bacteriuria and pyuria after ingestion of cranberry juice. *JAMA* **271**: 751–4.

Buckley RM Jr, McGuckin M, MacGregor RR (1978) Urine bacterial counts after sexual intercourse. *N Engl J Med* **298**: 321–4.

Cardozo L (1996) Postmenopausal cystitis. *BMJ* **313**: 129.

Cardozo L, Benness C, Abbott D (1998) Low dose oestrogen prophylaxis for recurrent urinary tract infections in elderly women. *Br J Obstet Gynaecol* **105**: 403–7.

Fihn SD, Boyko EJ, Normand EH et al. (1996) Association between use of spermicide-coated condoms and *Escherichia coli* urinary tract infection in young women. *Am J Epidemiol* **144**: 512–20.

Foxman B, Zhang L, Tallman P et al. (1995a) Virulence characteristics of *Escherichia coli* causing first urinary tract infection predict risk of second infection. *J Infect Dis* **172**: 1536–41.

Foxman B, Geiger AM, Palin K, Gillespie B, Koopman JS (1995b) First-time urinary tract infection and sexual behaviour. *Epidemiology* **6**: 162–8.

Foxman B, Zhang L, Tallman P et al. (1997) Transmission of uropathogens between sex partners. *J Infect Dis* **175**: 989–92.

Hay PE, Ugwumadu A, Chowns J (1997) Sex, thrush and bacterial vaginosis. *Int J STD AIDS* **8**: 603–8.

Hill GB, Livengood CH 3rd (1994) Bacterial vaginosis-associated microflora and effects of topical intravaginal clindamycin. *Am J Obstet Gynecol* **171**: 1198–204.

Hooton TM, Fihn SD, Johnson C, Roberts PL, Stamm WE (1989)

Association between bacterial vaginosis and acute cystitis in women using diaphragms. *Arch Intern Med* **149**: 1932–6.

Hooton TM, Fennel CL, Clark AM et al. (1991) Nonoxynol-9 differential antibacterial activity and enhancement of bacterial adherence to vaginal epithelial cells. *J Infect Dis* **164**: 1216–19.

Hooton TM, Roberts PL, Stamm WE (1994) Effects of recent sexual activity and use of a diaphragm on the vaginal microflora. *Clin Infect Dis* **19**: 274–8.

Hooton TM, Scholes D, Hughes JP et al. (1996a) A prospective study of risk factors for symptomatic urinary tract infection in young women. *N Engl J Med* **335**: 468–74.

Hooton TM, Winter C, Tiu F, Stamm WE (1996b) Association of acute cystitis with the stage of the menstrual cycle in young women. *Clin Infect Dis* **23**: 635–6.

Horner P, Hay PE, Thomas BJ, Renton AM, Taylor-Robinson D (1995) The role of *Chlamydia trachomatis* in urethritis and urethral symptoms in women. *Int J STD AIDS* **6**: 31–4.

Iravani A, Tice AD, McCarty J et al. (1995) Short-course ciprofloxacin treatment of acute uncomplicated urinary tract infection in women. The minimum effective dose. *Arch Intern Med* **155**: 485–94.

James WH (1971) The distribution of coitus with the human intermenstruum. *J Biosoc Sci* **3**: 159–71.

Kass EH (1957) Bacteriuria and the diagnosis of infections of the urinary tract. *Arch Intern Med* **100**: 709–14.

Kirkengen AL, Andersen P, Gjersoe E et al. (1992) Oestriol in the prohylactic treatment of recurrent urinary tract infections in postmenopausal women. *Scand J Prim Health Care* **10**: 139–42.

Klebanoff SJ, Hillier SL, Eschenbach DA, Waltersdorf AM (1991) Control of the microbial flora of the vagina by H_2O_2-generating lactobacilli. *J Infect Dis* **164**: 94–100.

Krieger JN, Ross SO, Simonsen JM (1993) Urinary tract infections in healthy university men. *J Urol* **149**: 1046–8.

Maskell R (1995) Broadening the concept of urinary tract infection. *Br J Urol* **76**: 2–8.

Melekos MD, Asbach HW, Gerharz E et al. (1997) Post-intercourse versus daily ciprofloxacin prophylaxis for recurrent urinary tract infections in premenopausal women. *J Urol* **157**: 935–9.

Molander U, Milson I, Ekelund P, Mellstrom D, Eriksson O (1990) Effect of oral oestriol on vaginal flora and cytology and urogenital symptoms in the post menopause. *Maturitas* **12**: 113–20.

Nicolle LE, Harding GK, Periksaitis J, Ronald AR (1982) The

association of urinary tract infection with sexual intercourse. *J Infect Dis* 146: 579.

Oliveria SA, Klein RA, Reed JL et al. (1998) Estrogen replacement therapy and urinary tract infections in postmenopausal women aged 45–89. *Menopause* 5: 4–8.

Pfau A, Sacks T (1981) The bacterial flora of the vaginal vestibule, urethra and vagina in premenopausal women with recurrent urinary tract infections. *J Urol* 126: 630–4.

Pfau A, Sacks T (1994) Effective postcoital quinolone prophylaxis of recurrent urinary tract infections in women. *J Urol* 152: 136–8.

Pfau A, Sacks T, Engelstein D (1983) Recurrent urinary tract infections in premenopausal women: prophylaxis based on an understanding of the pathogenesis. *J Urol* 129: 1153–7.

Raz R, Stamm WE (1993) A controlled trial of intravaginal estriol in postmenopausal women with recurrent urinary tract infections. *N Engl J Med* 329: 753–6.

Reid G, Bruce AW (1995) Low vaginal pH and urinary-tract infection. *Lancet* 346: 1704.

Ronald A (1996) Sex and urinary tract infections. *N Engl J Med* 335: 511–12.

Stamey TA (1973) The role of introital enterobacteria in recurrent urinary tract infections. *J Urol* 109: 467–8.

Stamm WE, Wagner KF, Amsel R et al. (1980) Causes of the acute urethral syndrome in women. *N Engl J Med* 303: 409–15.

Stamm WE, Running K, McKevitt WH et al. (1981) Treatment of the acute urethral syndrome. *N Engl J Med* 304: 956–8.

Stapleton A, Latham RH, Johnson C, Stamm WE (1990) Postcoital antimicrobial prophylaxis for recurrent urinary tract infection. A randomized, double-blind, placebo-controlled trial. *JAMA* 264: 703–6.

Stapleton A, Nudelman E, Clausen H, Hakomori S, Stamm WE (1992) Binding of uropathogenic *Escherichia coli* R45 to glycolipids extracted from vaginal epithelial cells is dependent on histo-blood group secretor status. *J Clin Invest* 90: 965–72.

Sugarman B, Epps LR (1982) Effect of estrogens on bacterial adherence to HeLa cells. *Infect Immun* 35: 633–8.

Wallin JE, Thompson SE, Zaidi A, Wong K-H (1981) Urethritis in women attending an STD clinic. *Br J Vener Dis* 57: 50–4.

Zielske JV, Lohr KN, Brook RH, Goldberg GA (1981) *Conceptualization and Measurement of Physiologic Health for Adults: Urinary Tract Infection.* Report R2262/16-HHS. Rand Corporation.

Management of the elderly

Eric Knight and Jerry Avorn

11

Contents

I   Introduction

With advancing age there is an increase in the number of urinary tract infections (UTI), and their clinical and biological significance is different from UTI in younger patients. In a longitudinal study of 61 older women at community housing sites and a long-term care facility, we found that bacteriuria alone ($\geq 10^5$ organisms) in the absence of white blood cells occurred in 17% of all urine samples, bacteriuria with pyuria in 15%, and bacteriuria with symptoms in 3% (Monane et al., 1995). Other studies have reported rates of asymptomatic bacteriuria ranging from 5 to 43% in older women (Nicolle, 1997). The rates in men are generally lower, and range from less than 5% in younger community dwelling men to 5–20% in men over 70 (Nicolle, 1997). The most commonly isolated organisms in our study were: *Escherichia coli* (76%), *Klebsiella* spp. (10%), and *Proteus mirabilis* (2%) (Monane et al., 1995). Generally, the organisms that affect older patients are similar to those affecting younger patients. However, older patients may be more likely to have resistant strains of bacteria, possibly because of repeated antibiotic exposure or acquisition of resistant organisms in the institutional setting. In a large study in Finland, there was a significant correlation between age and the incidence of *E. coli* resistance, but this correlation only occurred among catheterized patients

(Arstial et al., 1994). *Proteus mirabilis* and *E. coli* are common in ambulatory patients but appear with greater frequency in the institutional setting, and enterococcal infections are much more likely to occur in the setting of prior antimicrobial use (Lloyd et al., 1998).

Older patients may be at greater risk for urinary tract infections because of changes in the urinary tract with age. For example, older persons have a decrease in overall bladder contractility (Resnick, 1998). This can result in an increased residual volume of urine after voiding and a predisposition to bacterial colonization, which may be especially important in men with prostatic enlargement and resulting urodynamic obstruction.

In women, with age, there is a decline in urethral pressure. This decline in urethral pressure could potentially result in increased bacterial colonization of the bladder. In addition, the urethral length declines in women with age, and this may predispose to bacterial colonization. Vaginal atrophy and loss of the oestrogenic effect on the vaginal mucosa may also result in increased risk of infection. A controlled trial of topical oestrogen in postmenopausal women with recurrent urinary tract infections demonstrated a decreased frequency of infections in the oestrogen-treated group, although the exact mechanism for this effect is not known (Raz and Stamm, 1993).

II   Assessment

The first issue to resolve in evaluating an older woman for possible urinary tract infection is to determine whether or not bacteriuria is present. The most convenient method for assessing the presence of bacteria in the urine is the urine dipstick. In a study of adult patients in the emergency department, Jou and Powers (1998) examined whether or not urine dipstick results could effectively guide therapy. They examined 118 urine samples for possible infection, and the treatment decision was guided by the presence or absence of leukocyte esterase or nitrites. The results of microbiological results resulted in six changes in therapy for UTI, and one decision to withhold therapy. Another study in incontinent nursing home residents examined the utility of dipstick testing for nitrite and leukocyte esterase, and the utility of a rapid, enzyme-based screening test for bacteriuria (Ouslander et al., 1995). The enzyme-based screening had the highest sensitivity (90%), but the lowest specificity. Leukocyte esterase had fairly good sensitivity (85%), but low specificity (51%). Nitrite testing had low sensitivity (69%), but high specificity (90%). When all of these tests were used together there was high sensitivity if any of the tests were positive (97%), and high specificity if all three of the tests were positive. Leukocyte esterase and nitrite together had high sensitivity (94%), and good specificity (93%).

The positive and negative predictive values of these diagnostic tests will vary depending on the prevalence rates of bacteriuria in the population being evaluated. Nonetheless, leukocyte esterase and nitrite, which are both present on commonly used dipstick testing, may be useful tools to identify bacteriuria. One problem that may arise in the care of frail older women is the inability to obtain a voluntarily voided urine specimen. This may occur because of chronic urinary incontinence, physical frailty, or dementia. In a study comparing bacteriuria in urine samples from pressed disposable diapers to urine samples from catheterization, it was found that there was excellent correlation (kappa = 0.84) for the diagnosis of bacteriuria (Belmin et al., 1997). This suggests that urine samples from diapers may be an acceptable alternative to catheterized samples, and this methodology could potentially avoid the discomfort and physical trauma associated with the use of bladder catheterization for determining the presence or absence of infection.

Studies have also been done to determine who is at risk for developing persistent bacteriuria in patients without urinary catheters (the management of bacteriuria in catheterized patients will be discussed separately), although the clinical significance of persistent bacteriuria is debatable. In a study of risk factors in a nursing home setting, Eberle et al. (1993) found incontinence of bladder or bowel, dementia, and functional disability were each highly associated with chronic bacteriuria. The physiological changes that predispose to urinary incontinence, as stated earlier, may also predispose to bacteriuria.

1.   Whether to treat

After a probable diagnosis of bacteriuria is made, the next step is to determine whether or not to treat, since not all bacteriuria in the elderly requires intervention. Many studies provide evidence that patients with asymptomatic bacteriuria may do just as well if not treated. For example, Nicolle et al. (1987, 1993) studied the treatment of asymptomatic bacteriuria in the long-term care setting and found no improvement in clinical outcomes with treatment. In fact, among the treated women, there was an increased incidence of adverse drug reactions and increased bacterial resistance. Some have hypothesized that treating asymptotic bacteriuria could have other beneficial effects such as improving chronic urinary incontinence. However, this notion has been refuted in the literature. Ouslander et al. (1995) performed a trial to test whether eradicating bacteriuria would improve bladder control in nursing home residents with chronic incontinence. They found that in patients with chronic bacteriuria treatment was moderately effective in eradicating

bacteriuria but had no effect on the severity of chronic urinary incontinence.

When should a clinician treat bacteriuria in the elderly? Treatment is suggested in older patients if both symptoms and bacteriuria are present. Unfortunately, as in many conditions in geriatric medicine, the symptoms of urinary tract infection may present differently in older patients. For example, classic symptoms such as dysuria, frequency, and urgency may be absent. Instead, UTI in older patients may present as confusion, falls, fever, or a myriad of non-specific symptoms. Therefore, when the clinical status of an older person changes, one needs to think of the possibility of a urinary tract infection.

2.   Treatment

The approach will depend on many variables including age, antimicrobial resistance patterns, and clinical status. Traditionally, urinary tract infections can be divided into uncomplicated UTI and complicated UTI (Nicolle, 1997). Complicated infections are defined as occurring in patients with functionally, metabolically or anatomically abnormal urinary tracts, or with organisms resistant to conventional antibiotic therapy (Stamm and Hooton, 1993).

Fluoroquinolones are generally not advocated as first-line agents for uncomplicated UTI because of increasing resistance and cost concerns (Arstial et al.,

1994). In older patients, a longer course of antibiotic therapy is recommended for symptomatic urinary tract infections, rather than the short courses currently preferred in younger patients, but there is limited data on the optimal length of therapy in older patients (Lacey et al., 1981). A recent review of the management of urinary tract infections in geriatrics recommends treating older women with uncomplicated UTI for 10 days (Yoshikawa, 1996).

An interesting study of how cost influences physician prescribing practices was performed by Hart et al. (1997). These investigators examined the effect of antibiotic cost awareness on treatment of uncomplicated urinary tract infections. When physicians were unaware of the cost of antibiotics, 56% of the physicians prescribed trimethoprim-sulfamethoxazole and 40% of the physicians prescribed quinolones. When physicians were aware of costs, 83% prescribed trimethoprim-sulfamethoxazole and 13% prescribed quinolones.

The treatment of complicated urinary tract infections is more variable and depends on resistance patterns and clinical status. Generally, if there is mild-to-moderate illness with no nausea or vomiting, then an oral fluoroquinolone is recommended (Nicolle, 1997). A study comparing lomefloxacin with trimethoprim-sulfamethoxazole for complicated urinary tract infections found bacteriologic cure rates at 5–9 days to be greater for lomefloxacin compared with trimethoprim-sulfamethoxazole (Nicolle et al., 1994). However, cure rates at four to six weeks were not significantly different, except lomefloxacin was superior for Gram-negative organisms. There is no evidence, though, that one fluoroquinolone is superior to another (Naber and Sigl, 1993; McCue et al., 1995; Naber et al., 1998).

If patients are more seriously ill then hospitalization is necessary for treatment with parenteral antibiotics. Usually, empiric therapy is necessary until urine culture and sensitivity results are available. Recommended parenteral therapy includes ampicillin and gentamicin, ciprofloxacin, ofloxacin, ceftriaxone, aztreonam, ticaracillin–clavulanate or imipenem–cilastatin. Single agent coverage may be used unless the patient's condition worsens or does not improve. Potential infecting organisms include *E. coli, Proteus, Klebsiella, Pseudomonas, Serratia, Enteroccocus* and *Staphylococcus.*

One study has compared the efficacy of an intravenous fluoroquinolone, fleroxacin, with ceftazadine for complicated UTI (Naber and Sigl, 1993). The cure rates were similar between the two medications. Patients with UTI who are more seriously ill or septic require dual antibiotic therapy (Hattan et al., 1994). After parenteral therapy, when patients become clinically stable, then oral therapy is initiated based on antimicrobial susceptibility.

Typically, patients are treated with antibiotics for at least two weeks (Nicolle, 1997).

The choice of empiric antimicrobial therapy for complicated UTI may also be influenced by cost awareness. In a study of physician prescription decisions, physicians were given a choice of antimicrobial agents for complicated UTI (Hart et al., 1997). When physicians were unaware of the cost of antibiotic therapy, they chose gentamicin 63% of the time compared with 33% of the time for ceftriaxone/cefotaxime. When physicians were aware of the cost of antibiotic therapy they chose gentamicin 86% of the time compared with 10% of the time for ceftriaxone/cefotaxime.

The use of cranberry juice-containing products has been a time-honoured approach in popular culture to the prevention and even management of urinary tract infections, but for many years there was very little in the way of rigorous scientific data to substantiate this practice. Initially, it was thought that cranberry-containing products rendered the urine more acidic, and thus reduced the likelihood of an infection, but this belief proved to be groundless. In the late 1980s, reports began to appear of a substance unique to cranberries (and to their close botanical cousins, blueberries) that was capable of inhibiting the capacity of some bacteria to adhere to mucosal surfaces (Sobota, 1984; Zafriri et al., 1989; Ofek et al., 1991). However, clinical trial data to substantiate

such an effect in humans was still lacking. To address this issue, our group conducted a randomized double-blind placebo controlled trial of standard cranberry juice beverage compared to an identical appearing and tasting placebo drink, administered to 153 elderly women (mean age, 75.5 years) (Avorn et al., 1994). Subjects were randomly assigned to consume 300 ml per day of either beverage for a period of six months. A baseline urine sample and six clean-voided study urine samples were collected at approximately one-month intervals and tested for bacteriuria and the presence of white blood cells.

We found that the older women randomized to the cranberry group had a risk of bacteriuria in any given sample that was only 42% of the risk seen in women randomized to the placebo group. For samples in which bacteriuria and pyuria were present, the odds of continuing in this state (versus conversion to a non-infected state) in the subsequent month were reduced by about three-quarters in the cranberry group compared to the placebo group. However, it is important to point out that it is not clear how such effects seen in women with primarily asymptomatic bacteriuria would relate to the management of symptomatic urinary tract infections in older women, or to the treatment or prevention of urinary tract infections in younger patients.

III Catheter-associated urinary tract infections

Urinary catheters are often overused in the care of elderly patients. In response to this overuse, The United States Center for Disease Control and Prevention has published guidelines for using indwelling urinary catheters (McLaughlin and Scinto, 1996). These include the following indications: to relieve urinary tract obstruction, to permit urinary drainage in patients with neurogenic bladder dysfunction and urinary retention, to obtain accurate intake and output in critically ill patients, and to aid in urologic surgery or other surgery in contiguous structures. A fifth, vaguer indication has also been added which allows the clinician to determine whether the risk of infection related to the use of the catheter is less than the potential complications if the catheter is not used. Possible examples which would fall into the latter category would include patients with pressure sores or patients undergoing major surgery. In our experience, catheters are often used merely for staff convenience in patients with urinary incontinence. In a study of 4259 older patients in 53 random nursing homes in the state of Maryland, 15% of men and 10% of women used a urine collection device (Hebel and Warren, 1990). Among patients confined to bed, 58% of men and 47% of women used a urine collection device.

Urinary catheters predispose to urinary tract infection through multiple mechanisms (Warren, 1997). First, catheters enable bacteria to enter the bladder from outside the urethra. Second, catheters have an external biofilm, and bacteria contained within this biofilm appear to be protected from normal host defences. Third, there is improved bacterial adhesion to the bladder in the presence of an indwelling catheter. Fourth, the catheter may impair white blood cell function. Fifth, the catheter may not completely drain the bladder, and therefore may enable bacterial colonization of the residual urine.

Several risk factors for catheter-associated bacteriuria have been identified (Platt et al., 1986). These include: duration of catheterization, absence of use of a urinemeter, microbial colonization of the drainage bag, diabetes, no antibiotic use, female gender, indications other than surgery or measurement of urinary output, decreased renal function, and errors in catheter care. Length of time of catheterization also contributes to the risk of infection. In nursing home patients with chronic, indwelling catheters, virtually all patients have bacterial colonization with multiple organisms (Frykland et al., 1997). These bacteria may differ from usual urinary pathogens because of the unique microenvironment. *Providencia* spp. and *Morganella morganii* may be seen in this setting, in addition to common organisms such as *E. coli*. *Candida* infections are also common in this setting.

As with older patients without catheterization, treatment is indicated only if symptoms develop. However, there may be certain exceptions to this general rule such as the treatment of clusters of infections by specific organisms, or the treatment of patients at high risk of systemic complications (such as neutropenic patients) (Warren, 1997). If symptomatic infection is present, the choice of antibiotic therapy should be guided by known resistance patterns and by urine culture. A Gram stain of the urine may also be helpful to rule out enterococcal infection, and catheter obstruction should be ruled out. Once the infection is cleared, preventive measures should be considered. Most important, the necessity of chronic indwelling catheterization should be assessed. A trial of intermittent catheterization can be tried. There is also some evidence to suggest that patients with urinary catheters should not share rooms due to the risk of cross-infection (Frykland et al., 1997).

IV   Conclusion

Urinary tract infections are very common in older individuals and increase linearly with age. Older women are more likely to have resistant organisms, possibly because of repetitive antibiotic exposure or acquisition of resistant organisms in the institutional setting. As in younger ages, women are more likely to acquire UTI than men. Anatomic changes in the urinary tract predispose older patients to infection. Simple measures such as oestrogen treatment of vaginal atrophy may decrease UTI frequency.

Commonly available tests such as leukocyte esterase and nitrite may be helpful in identifying bacteriuria, but treatment of bacteriuria is usually not indicated unless symptoms are present. There is also no evidence that treating asymptomatic bacteriuria improves urinary incontinence. When treatment is necessary, older women should be treated for at least 10 days for uncomplicated urinary tract infections. Generally, trimethoprim-sulfamethoxazole is the first agent of choice. The treatment of complicated urinary tract infections is more variable and depends on the clinical setting. For mild-to-moderate illness, a fluoroquinolone may be indicated, and for more severe illness parenteral antibiotics are recommended.

Urinary catheters should only be used for specific indications, and are not recommended for management of chronic urinary incontinence. Such catheters predispose to urinary tract infections through multiple mechanisms. Patients with indwelling catheters should only be treated if symptoms develop. Efforts should be made to avoid indwelling catheter use.

References

Arstial T, Huovinen S, Lager K, Lehtonen A, Huovinen P (1994) Positive correlation between the age of patients and the degree of antimicrobial resistance among urinary strains of *Escherichia coli*. *J Infect* **29**: 9–16.

Avorn, J, Monane M, Gurwitz JH et al. (1994) Reduction of bacteriuria and pyuria after ingestion of cranberry juice. *JAMA* **271**: 751–4.

Belmin J, Hervias Y, Avellano H, Oudart O, Durand I (1993) Reliability of sampling urine from disposable diapers in elderly incontinent women. *J Am Geriatr Soc* **41**: 1182–6.

Eberle CM, Winsemius D, Garibaldi RA (1993) Risk factors and consequences of bacteriuria in non-catheterized nursing home residents. *J Gerontol (Med) Sci* **48**(6): 266–71.

Frykland B, Haeggman S, Burman LG (1997) Transmission of urinary bacterial strains between patients with indwelling urinary catheters – nursing in the same room and in separate rooms compared. *J Hosp Infect* **36**: 147–53.

Hart J, Salman H, Bergman M et al. (1997) Do drug costs affect physicians' prescription decisions? *J Intern Med* **241**: 415–20.

Hattan J, Hughes M, Raymond CH (1994) Management of bacterial urinary tract infections in adults. *Ann Pharmacother* **28**: 1264–72.

Hebel JR, Warren JW (1990) The use of urethral, condom, and suprapubic catheters in aged nursing home patients. *J Am Geriatr Soc* **38**: 777–84.

Jou WW, Powers RD (1998) Utility of dipstick urinalysis as a guide to management of adults with suspected infection or hematuria. *South Med J* **91**(3): 266–9.

Lacey RW, Simpson MHC, Lord VL et al. (1981) Comparison of single-dose trimethoprim with a five-day course for treatment of urinary tract infections in the elderly. *Age Ageing* 10: 179–85.

Lloyd S, Zervos M, Mahayni R, Lundstrom T (1998) Risk factors for enterococcal urinary tract infection and colonization in a rehabilitation facility. *Am J Infect Control* 26: 35–9.

McCue JD, Gaziano P, Orders D (1995) A randomized controlled trial of ofloxacin 200 mg four times daily or twice daily in elderly nursing home patients with complicated UTI. *Drugs* 49(Suppl 2): 368–73.

McLaughlin A, Sciuto D (1996) Catheter patrols: a unique way to reduce the use of convenience urinary catheters. *Geriatric Nursing* 17(5): 240–4.

Monane M, Gurwitz JH, Lipsitz LA et al. (1995) Epidemiologic and diagnostic aspects of bacteriuria: a longitudinal study in older women. *J Am Geriatr Soc* 43: 618–22.

Naber KG, Sigl G (1993) Fleroxacin versus ofloxacin in patients with complicated urinary tract infection: a controlled clinical study. *Am J Med* 94(Suppl): 114–17.

Naber KG, Well M, Hollauer K, Kirchbauer D, Withe W (1998) In vitro activity of enoxacin versus ciprofloxacin, fleroxain, lomefloxacin, efloxacin, pefloxacin, and nufloxacin against unopathogens. *Chemotherapy* 44: 77–84.

Nicolle LE (1997) Asymptomatic bacteriuria in the elderly. *Infect Dis Clin North Am* 11(3): 647–63.

Nicolle LE, Mayhew JW, Bryan L (1987) Prospective randomized comparison of therapy and no therapy for asymptomatic bacteriuria in institutionalized women. *Am J Med* 83: 27–33.

Nicolle LE, Bjornsen J, Harding GK, MacDonell JA (1993) Bacteriuria in elderly institutionalized men. *N Engl J Med* 309: 1420–5.

Nicolle LE, Louie TJ, Dubois J et al. (1994) Treatment of complicated urinary tract infections with lomefloxacin compared with that with trimethoprim-sulfamethoxazole. *Antimicrob Agents Chemother* 38: 1368–73.

Ofek I, Golhar J, Zafriri D et al. (1991) Anti-*Escherichia* adhesin activity of cranberry and blueberry juices. *N Engl J Med* 324: 1599.

Ouslander JG, Schapira M, Schnelle JF et al. (1995) Does eradicating bacteriuria affect the severity of chronic urinary incontinence in nursing home residents? *Ann Intern Med* 122: 749–54.

Ouslander JG, Schapira M, Fingold S, Schnelle J (1995) Accuracy of rapid urinary screening tests among incontinent nursing home residents with asymptomatic bacteriuria. *J Am Geriatr Soc* **43**: 772–5.

Platt R, Polk BF, Murdock B, Rosner B (1986) Risk factors for nosocomial urinary tract infection. *Am J Epidemiol* **24**: 977–85.

Raz R, Stamm WE (1993) A controlled trial of intravaginal estriol in postmenopausal women with recurrent urinary tract infections. *N Engl J Med* **329**: 753–6.

Resnick NM (1996) Geriatric incontinence. *Urol Clin North Am* **23**(1): 55–2.

Sobota AE (1984) Inhibition of bacterial adherence by cranberry juice: potential use for the treatment of urinary tract infections. *J Urol* **131**: 1013–16.

Stamm WE, Hooton TM (1993) Management of urinary tract infections in adults. *N Engl J Med* **329**: 1328–34.

Warren JW (1997) Catheter-associated urinary tract infections. *Infect Dis Clin North Am* **11**(3): 609–22.

Yoshikawa TT, Nicolle LE, Norman DC (1996) Management of complicated urinary tract infection in older patients. *J Am Geriatr Soc* **44**: 1235–41.

Zafriri D, Ofek I, Adar R, Pocino M, Sharon N (1989) Inhibitory activity of cranberry juice on adherence of type 1 and P fimbriated *Escherichia coli* to eukaryotic cells. *Antimicrob Agents Chemother* **33**: 92–8.

Management in primary care

Adrian GK Edwards

12

Contents

I Introduction

Urinary tract infection (UTI) in women is common. The clinical syndrome of frequency and dysuria is very well recognized and includes up to a half of these women who have no evidence of infection by standard microbiological criteria (urethral syndrome) (Jolleys, 1991). Between 10% and 20% of women have a confirmed UTI at some time in their life (Brucker, 1990) and the frequency–dysuria syndrome accounts for an appreciable proportion of the general practitioner's workload: 6 per 100 women in the general population per year (Jolleys, 1991) or 2–3% of all consultations (Brooks, 1990).

Despite its importance, there is enormous variation in clinical practice (Berg, 1991; Carlson and Mulley, 1985; Olesen and Oestergaard, 1995). There are probably three contributions to this. The first is genuine uncertainty amongst practitioners about the most appropriate management – the hallowed gap between research findings and clinical implementation. The second is that there may also be a lack of clear and relevant evidence to guide management, as will be discussed below (Carlson and Mulley, 1985) but the third contribution is likely to arise from the wide variation in clinical contexts for treatment of UTI (Stamm and Hooton, 1993).

Berg (1991) asked 137 US family physicians to indicate their likely management for a case vignette, typical of many seen in primary care: a 30-year-old woman, complaining of urgency, dysuria and blood in the urine for one day, with a history of two previous UTIs but not known to have any urinary tract abnormalities. The 137 doctors recommended 82 different treatment regimens, representing nearly every possible permutation of antibiotic choice, duration, dosage, follow-up, urinalysis and culture. It is likely that when presented only with the biomedical information in this case vignette, these doctors made different assumptions concerning the personal characteristics of the patient and the context in which they were presenting.

This situation is not unique to management of UTI and has been documented for other clinical conditions (Howie, 1976). Variation in management of UTI has also been documented in other countries and between different specialities interested in the clinical problem, such as general practitioners, microbiologists and urologists (Olesen and Oestergaard, 1995). It is likely that the contextual variation for patients seen within and between different speciality settings accounts for much of the variety in management approaches. Nevertheless, there is probably also substantial uncertainty among clinicians regarding which management strategies are supported by evidence.

The medical literature exhaustively covers many aspects of genitourinary symptoms but there are few studies providing the relevant evidence about the commonest symptoms with unselected patients in primary care (Berg et al., 1984; Jacobson et al., 1997). There has been an increased focus in primary care towards addressing not only the biomedical but also the personal and contextual (psychological and social) elements of diagnosis and management (McWhinney, 1996) but this has largely failed to permeate into family practice research on UTI. The most cited research has not addressed the relevant personal, psychological, family and cultural factors which influence management (Berg, 1991; Berg et al., 1984).

When looking at the available evidence about UTI in adult women, however, it is apparent that the clinical 'problem' for the practitioner is not the fact that urinary tract symptoms are so common in primary care but that such presentations are complex, reflecting individual health behaviours, social phenomena and the dynamics between doctors, patients and their families. As with most symptom presentation in primary care, there is an 'iceberg phenomenon' (Hannay, 1979)(*Figure 12.1*). Up to a half of adult women report symptoms of dysuria and frequency at some time, though only one in 10 consults a doctor with these symptoms (Brooks, 1990). There are then two further filtration processes as some of these patients may then require outpatient assessment in secondary care while in others UTI necessitates or complicates admission to hospital (Stamm and Hooton, 1993). Each filtration process is influenced by various factors, one of which is the relatively straightforward biomedical aspect of the presentation. Other features such as the personal characteristics of the patient (including her concern, ideas on causation and expectations for management) and contextual aspects of the presentation (social pressures, family experience of symptoms or treatment) will also contribute to this process and the profile of patients changes at each stage.

As the profile changes, the predictive value of symptoms, the natural history, potential complications and most appropriate management (diagnostic and therapeutic) of UTI vary for each group of patients (Edwards and Stott, 1996; Hannay, 1979). The different denominations of population in these groups make investigations which are mandatory in some settings at the very least difficult to interpret in others such as primary care (Jacobson et al., 1997). Within each of these groups of patients, whether self-managing or in primary or secondary care, there is also a wide range of clinical patterns, each demanding a different approach (Stamm and Hooton, 1993). Research which has not accounted for these contextual variations may be difficult to generalize and apply to primary care but with this caveat, a certain amount of evidence has accrued to guide management of UTI in adult women.

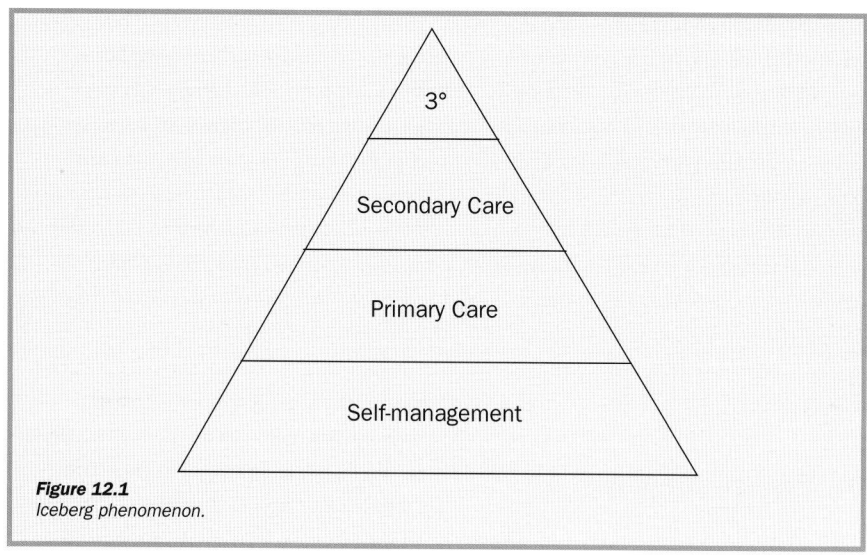

Figure 12.1
Iceberg phenomenon.

Stamm and Hooton (1993) describe five such clinical patterns: young women with acute uncomplicated cystitis, young women with recurrent cystitis, young women with acute uncomplicated pyelonephritis, all adults with complicated urinary infection, and all adults with asymptomatic bacteriuria. The first group of young women with acute uncomplicated cystitis are perhaps the most frequently encountered in primary care and these authors advocated an abbreviated laboratory workup followed by empirical therapy with a three-day regimen of antibiotics for these patients (Stamm and Hooton, 1993).

However, there are several possible strategies even for initial assessment, which include:

- empirical therapy alone;
- therapy based on urinalysis results;
- therapy based on a combination or urinalysis and urine sediment results;
- therapy based on results of culture, with initial therapy while awaiting culture results;
- therapy based on results of culture, without initial antibiotic treatment.

The latter two strategies can also be divided into office-based culture or reference laboratory culture.

From existing evidence, it appears that the

most cost-effective strategy is to treat empirically and only perform further investigation, including urinalysis, if initial treatment fails, though individual patient utilities and the prior probability of UTI will affect this decision (Barry et al., 1977). It is, however, recognized that the clinical presentations differ according to the setting (Berg, 1991; Berg et al., 1984) and the context of the consultation should be taken into account in debates about 'appropriate' management.

II   Clinical diagnosis

Clinical acumen in establishing the diagnosis of UTI has been found to be good in some studies (O'Dowd et al., 1984) but poor in others (Berg et al., 1984). There are certain key characteristics which are relevant to the assessment of all women presenting with frequency, dysuria or other symptoms suggestive of UTI, such as their age, whether they are pre- or postmenopausal, whether they are sexually active and recurrence of chronicity of symptoms, and each individual case must be assessed in order to exclude UTI (Jolleys, 1991). Specific risk factors include the use of the diaphragm as the chosen form of contraception (Strom et al., 1987) and delaying urination during the normal course of the day (Adatto et al., 1979). Urination shortly after sexual intercourse is protective against future attacks of urinary tract symptoms

(Adatto et al., 1979; Strom et al., 1987). No significant associations have been shown between food, drink, clothing, menstrual protection, perineal hygiene, direction of wiping and use of bath preparations and subsequent urinary tract symptoms (Strom et al., 1987). Frequently, however, doctors do not explore these risk factors and the beliefs of patients about causation in routine consultations (Rink, 1998).

There is debate about the value of taking psychological make-up into account in assessing symptoms, some viewing it as helpful in initially distinguishing UTI from the urethral syndrome (O'Dowd et al., 1984) whilst others have not found psychiatric morbidity to be associated with the urethral syndrome (Sumners et al., 1992). Doctors may often note symptoms of frequency and dysuria and balance this with a history of anxiety. When no evidence of infection is found, doctors are more likely then to view patients' emotions as the cause rather than the effect of the conditions (Sumners et al., 1992). Distress and anxiety require tolerance rather than implication in the cause of symptoms. However, the psychiatric co-morbidity should and will influence management decisions about investigation and treatment, though this psychosomatic approach to dealing with these women has perhaps been more evident in specialist than primary care management in the past (Pill and O'Dowd, 1988).

III   Assessment

The advent of urinalysis dipsticks (especially those for leucocyte esterase (LE) or nitrite) since the earlier studies of clinical acumen (Berg et al., 1984; O'Dowd et al., 1984) represents another possible step in initial assessment, with implications for the accuracy of diagnosis and the cost-effectiveness of different management strategies (Barry et al., 1997). Urinalysis is most accurate when using the 'dysjunctive pairing' approach (if either LE or nitrite or both are detected, then UTI is suspected) (Hurlbut and Littenburg, 1991) and if the prior probability of UTI is high (Hashmi et al., 1995). This has been replicated in primary care settings (Jellheden et al., 1996). However, urinalysis studies have usually been undertaken in carefully controlled conditions (Edwards et al., 1997) which are not replicated in real life where intentions and competence are not necessarily matched by performance of investigations (Olesen and Oestergaard, 1995; Winkens et al., 1995). Under these circumstances, the validity of urinalysis is considerably lower than under optimal conditions (Winkens et al., 1995) and negative results cannot reliably exclude UTI (Hurlbut and Littenburg, 1991; Shaw and McGowan, 1997). There is a need for improved 'near patient' investigation, both in terms of accuracy of diagnostic tests and tests which perform well in clinical practice.

There is evidence that home-voided urine specimens are similar in the distribution of pyuria or bacteriuria to clean-catch midstream urines collected under 'ideal' conditions after instruction (Baerheim and Laerum, 1990). These home-voided specimens (which are regularly provided) therefore offer simple opportunities for microbiological diagnosis, including perhaps screening for chlamydial infection (Osterberg et al., 1996). The Kass criterion for UTI (more than 10^5 organisms per millilitre of a recognized pathogen, preferably on two occasions) should, however, be applied with caution as bacteria may be involved in a urethral lesion and not get an opportunity to multiply in the bladder or multiply at different rates. It may be that 10^4 or even 10^2 organisms per millilitre is a more sensitive threshold in women with acute dysuria to diagnose infection (Baerheim and Laerum, 1990) or that we are left with clinical criteria in deciding whether or not to prescribe antibiotics or refer for further investigation (Brooks, 1990).

IV   Treatment

Antibiotic choice should be guided by local pathogen prevalence and sensitivities, but the duration of antibiotic treatment has been reasonably established from current research evidence. Some uncertainty persists about the applicability of this evidence to general practice, arising from the different settings in the primary trials. Some were based in general practice (Brooks et al., 1972; Trienkens et al., 1989) whilst others used student health centres (Hooton et al., 1995), emergency rooms (Greenberg et al., 1986) or elsewhere, so that some authors still advocate single-dose therapy for uncomplicated UTIs in general practice (Bailey, 1990), a view that is supported by decision analysis modelling of alternative strategies if the goal is to reduce not just morbidity but also cost (Carlson and Mulley, 1985). However, two systematic reviews of up to 28 trials support the use of 3–5 days of treatment, shorter durations showing lower cure rates and longer durations being associated with more side-effects (Leibovici and Wysenbeek, 1991; Norrby, 1990).

Recurrent cystitis should be documented by culture at least once and then managed by one of three strategies: continuous prophylaxis, postcoital prophylaxis or therapy initiated by the patient (Stamm and Hooton, 1993). An alternative to antibiotic prophylaxis comes in the form of regular cranberry juice consumption which is popular with patients and has anecdotal supporting evidence in general and trial evidence from an elderly patient group taking 300 ml/day (Avorn et al., 1994). Recurrent UTI in postmenopausal women is often attributed to residual urine after voiding, itself associated with bladder or uterine prolapse and therefore in such cases topically applied oestrogen may be an alternative preventive measure, or referral

for more definitive surgical intervention may be appropriate (Stamm and Hooton, 1993).

Acute uncomplicated pyelonephritis in young women may require antibiotic treatment for up to two weeks though 5–7 days may suffice. Urine culture before and two weeks after completion of therapy is likely to be useful, as with 'complicated' UTI, i.e. infections in an abnormal urinary tract or with resistant pathogens (Stamm and Hooton, 1993).

Primary care patients with asymptomatic bacteriuria are unlikely to encounter problems, except in pregnancy where screening in the first trimester is usually performed. Treatment has been shown to reduce the risks of acute pyelonephritis and associated risks of prematurity or low birthweight infants (Andriole and Patterson, 1991).

Some guidance is available from the literature about the diagnosis, assessment and management of women presenting in primary care with urinary tract symptoms but the issue of management appropriate to the context has not been completely resolved. There is a lack of clear and context-specific evidence about effective management which generates some uncertainty amongst clinicians. With the contextual variations in presentation of symptoms, this contributes to the substantial variation in management strategies found within primary care (Berg, 1991; Olesen and

Oestergaard, 1995) and between specialities (Olesen and Oestergaard, 1995).

There is still a need for more relevant evidence from well-conducted trials with representative patients to confirm 'best management' strategies. Such trials will also require reliable outcome indicators which are relevant to the primary care setting but which are not currently available (Berg, 1991). Patients should be involved in the development of such outcome indicators, a viewpoint which has only rarely featured in the medical literature to date. Given the medical uncertainties, the range of lay views about causation (Rink, 1998) and the fact that the medical approach of 'excluding infection' is inadequate, patient involvement may make an important contribution to research and discussion about effective management (Pill and O'Dowd, 1988).

Evidence from the relevant setting and using relevant outcome measures is a realistic target and important for such a common condition (Barry et al., 1997; Berg, 1991). Full analysis of the costs and benefits is a necessary part of such research (Barry et al., 1997; Carlson and Mulley, 1985). Given the difference in perspectives and patient groups, continuing medical education of general practitioners using hospital specialists as a resource is unlikely to be productive (Olesen and Oestergaard, 1995); however, guidelines on management could be developed and are likely to be popular (van der Voort et al.,

1997). To effect change, the guidelines must be evidence based (Olesen and Oestergaard, 1995) and the development process should closely involve those who will be implementing them (Grimshaw and Russell, 1993). The evidence should also demonstrate benefits which are clear enough to demand change from the current wide variation in practice (Carlson and Mulley, 1985).

V   Childhood urinary tract infection in primary care

Many of the issues of management of childhood UTI are similar to those of managing UTI in adult women. It is relatively common, affecting 3% of girls and 1% of boys before the age of 10 years (Brooks, 1990) but more frequent in fact amongst boys than girls under the age of one year (Winberg et al., 1997). Urine culture is the only way to diagnose UTI accurately (Brooks, 1990) but primary care management of children suspected of having or who could be suffering from UTI shows wide variation (Dighe and Grace, 1984; Fargason et al., 1995; South Bedfordshire Practitioners' Group, 1990a; van der Voort et al., 1997; Vernon et al., 1997a).

The inconsistencies and underdiagnosis of UTI in childhood can, however, have more serious and long-term sequelae, as UTI is implicated in the development of renal scarring and thereby associated with hypertension, problems in pregnancy and renal failure (Jacobson et al., 1989; Jakobsson et al., 1994; Martinell et al., 1990; Smellie et al., 1994). This association with renal scarring thus means that childhood UTI is more than the 'nuisance' that it may be to many adult women and the importance of prompt and effective management is increased. In this context, there appear to be missed opportunities in diagnosis and management (Jadresic et al., 1993; South Bedfordshire Practitioners' Group, 1990b) and the Royal College of Physicians has produced guidelines for the acute management of UTI in childhood (Working Group, 1991).

Indications for examining the urine are as follows.

- unexplained (rectal) temperature above 38.5°C,
- unexplained vomiting or abdominal pain,
- frequency of micturition, dysuria or enuresis,
- failure to thrive,
- prolonged jaundice in the newborn,
- non-specific illness,
- suspected sexual abuse,
- haematuria or hypertension.

After diagnosis further investigations are required to identify the children with renal scars who warrant antibiotic prophylaxis. Opinions vary about the age of child up to which this is required. Consensus suggests children younger than seven require investigation (Working Group, 1991) though recent evidence suggests that the risk of scarring developing after the fourth birthday is virtually zero (Vernon et al., 1997a). Investigations may include ultrasound, plain radiography, intravenous urogram, DMSA scan and cystourethrogram, depending on the child's age. Before investigations are completed all children under the age of seven should receive prophylaxis following immediately on from the therapeutic course of antibiotics for the presenting illness (Working Group, 1991).

However, the guidelines have not been effectively disseminated and most general practitioners are not aware of them (Grimshaw and Russell, 1993; van der Voort et al., 1997). Difficulties are likely to persist even if the guidelines were more readily available, due to some persistent uncertainties amongst general practitioners about the link between UTI and renal scarring and also practical difficulties in establishing the diagnosis.

1. Practical difficulties in diagnosis

Urinary tract infection is most likely to be associated with complications such as renal scarring in the youngest children (aged less than two) (Smellie et al., 1985). These children will usually have non-specific symptoms requiring a high level of awareness of the potential for UTI in children with fever, vomiting, diarrhoea, poor feeding or weight gain and jaundice in neonates (Vernon et al., 1997b). There are practical difficulties in collecting urine in this age group and problems in the availability of laboratory services 'out of hours' are also significant hindrances to establishing the diagnosis (*Drug Therapeutics Bulletin*, 1997; van der Voort et al., 1997).

Various suggestions have been made to facilitate the diagnosis of UTI. Bags attached to the perineum have been used frequently but the specimens collected by this method are often contaminated (Edwards et al., 1997). The use of dipsticks as an initial screening test appears accurate (Hiraoka et al., 1994; Wiggelinkhuizen et al., 1988) but the same concerns as in adults about their validity in the real-life situation persist (Edwards et al., 1997; Winkens et al., 1995). Other approaches include collection of urine from nappies either directly (Vickers et al., 1991) or by syringe from a nappy liner (Vernon, 1995) or using the urinalysis sticks directly onto a panty-liner placed inside a nappy (Edwards et al., 1997). The wide range of options suggests that there are no simple solutions to this difficulty and that perhaps efforts should be directed towards gaining clean-catch specimens for routine microbiological analysis. This does take time and in view of the time pressures in general practice, kits for parents

to undertake collection and the initial urinalysis may be an effective way forward (Edwards et al., 1996; Jones et al., 1993).

The other main obstacle which must also be addressed is the uncertainty among many general practitioners concerning the evidence about whether all children with UTIs are necessarily at risk of scarring or whether treatment will benefit the child (Gordon, 1995; Jones et al., 1993). Although there is evidence suggesting that continuous antibiotic prophylaxis prevents renal scarring, there is no controlled evidence proving that it is effective (Jones et al., 1993). It is possible that the incidence of complications has been overestimated (Gordon, 1990), probably because most studies have used highly selected groups of patients often with the most severe abnormalities of the urinary tract (Houston, 1984; Smellie et al., 1994).

As with adult patients, the filtration process which operates quite effectively from community to primary care and from primary to secondary or tertiary care produces groups of patients with different characteristics and for whom the benefits and costs of investigation and treatment may differ. The natural history of childhood UTI in primary care is still not fully understood (Edwards et al., 1997) and the question about whether children in primary care are the same population of 'at-risk' children as in the hospital series persists (Houston, 1984).

We need a prospective longitudinal study

from general practice of childhood UTI to identify the children at risk and to determine the optimum general practice management for the majority who, in the view of some, may be at greater risk from the 'best current management' than from the disorder itself (Houston, 1984). Over a decade after this view was expressed, we are still no further forward (Edwards et al., 1997).

If this evidence was available to general practitioners to convince them of the association of UTI with renal scarring among the larger number of children with whom they deal, and the value of investigation and active management, then this would stimulate further efforts to increase awareness and improve management as suggested by the Royal College of Physicians (Working Group, 1991). A necessary part of improving management in practice would also be to address the practical difficulties that general practitioners encounter in trying to establish the diagnosis, especially in the acute or 'out of hours' situation (van der Voort et al., 1997).

VI   Conclusion

UTI is common in both children and adult women and is associated with many adverse sequelae. Current management strategies applied in primary care, including each step in diagnosis, therapy and accessing secondary care, are highly varied. This reflects some uncertainty amongst primary care physicians about the best management and a lack of clear, available and evidence-based guidelines. One contribution to this problem arises from the difficulties in interpreting the evidence in the literature and applying it to primary care. There may be great variations in the characteristics of patients encountered in different settings and a further contribution to the range of primary care management comes from the wide contextual variation of patients and their consultations.

Research indicates, for example, that 3–5 days of antibiotic therapy is likely to be the best balance between achieving cure rates for adult women with UTI and minimizing treatment side-effects; however, there is a clear need for further research to address the biomedical condition in the primary care setting and use outcome indicators of benefit relevant to the patient, the doctor and the context of the consultation. If such evidence were available it would be easier to interpret and apply evidence about appropriate management to an individual patient's situation and efforts to improve and standardize management would be justifiable and more likely to be productive.

References

Adatto K, Doebele K, Galland L, Granowetter L (1979) Behavioural factors and urinary tract infection. *JAMA* **241**: 2525–6.

Andriole VT, Patterson TF (1991) Epidemiology, natural history and management of urinary tract infections in pregnancy. *Med Clin North Am* **75**: 359–73.

Avorn J, Monane M, Gurwitz JH, Glynn RJ, Choodnovskiy I, Lipsitz LA (1994) Reduction of bacteriuria and pyuria after ingestion of cranberry juice. *JAMA* **271**: 751–4.

Baerheim A, Laerum E (1990) Home voided urine specimens in women: diagnostic agreement with clean catch midstream specimens. *Scand J Primary Health Care* **8**: 207–11.

Bailey RR (1990) Brief over view of single dose therapy for uncomplicated urinary tract infections. *Chemotherapy* **36** (suppl): 27–30.

Barry HC, Ebell MH, Hickner J (1997) Evaluation of suspected urinary tract infection in ambulatory women: a cost–utility analysis of office based strategies. *J Fam Pract* **44**: 49–60.

Berg AO (1991) Variations among family physicians' management strategies for lower urinary tract infection in women: a report from the Washington Family Physicians Collaborative Research Network. *J Am Board Fam Pract* **4**: 327–30.

Berg AO, Heidrich FE, Fihn SD et al. (1984) Establishing the cause of genitourinary symptoms in women in a family practice. *JAMA* **251**: 620–5.

Brooks D (1990) The management of suspected urinary tract infection in general practice. *Br J Gen Pract* **40**: 399–402.

Brooks D, Garret G, Hollihead R (1972) Sulphadimidine, co-trimoxazole, and a placebo in the management of symptomatic urinary tract infection in general practice. *J Roy Coll Gen Pract* **22**: 695–703.

Brucker PC (1990) Urinary tract infections. *Infect Dis* **17**: 825–32.

Carlson KJ, Mulley AG (1985) Management of acute dysuria. *Ann Intern Med* **102**: 244–9.

Dighe AM, Grace JF (1984) General practice management of childhood urinary tract infection. *J Roy Coll Gen Pract* **34**: 324–7.

Drug & Therapeutics Bulletin (1997) The management of urinary tract infection in children. *Drug Therapeu Bull* **35**: 65–9.

Edwards A, Stott NCH (1996) The incidence and causes of rectal bleeding. *Br J Gen Pract* **46**: 625.

Edwards A, Granier S, van der Voort J (1996) Usefulness of urine dipstick tests: packaging may lead to false positive results. *BMJ* **31**: 1010.

Edwards A, van der Voort J, Newcombe RG, Thayer H, Verrier Jones K (1997) A urine analysis method suitable for children's nappies. *J Clin Pathol* **50**: 569–72.

Fargason CA, Bronstein JM, Johnson VA (1995) Patterns of care received by medicaid recipients with urinary tract infections. *Pediatrics* **96**: 638–42.

Gordon I (1990) Urinary tract infection in paediatrics: the role of diagnostic imaging. *Br J Radiol* **63** (507): 511.

Gordon I (1995) Vesico-ureteric reflux, urinary tract infection and renal damage in children. *Lancet* **346**: 489–90.

Greenberg RN, Reilly PM, Luppen KL, Weinandt WJ, Ellington LL, Bollinger MR (1986) Randomized study of single-dose, three-day, and seven-day treatment of cystitis in women. *J Infect Dis* **153**: 277–82.

Grimshaw JM, Russell IT (1993) Effect of clinical guidelines on medical practice: a systematic review of rigorous evaluation. *Lancet* **342**: 1317–22.

Hannay DR (1997) *The Symptom Iceberg*. Routledge and Kegan Paul, London.

Hashmi P, Ho C, Morgan S, Stephenson JR (1995) Routine analysis in renal transplant patients. *J Clin Pathol* **48**: 383–4.

Hiraoka M, Hida Y, Tuchida S, Kuroda M, Sudo M (1994) Rapid dipstick test for diagnosis of urinary tract infection. *Acta Paediatr Japon* **36**: 379–82.

Hooton TM, Winter C, Tiu F, Stamm WE (1995) Randomized comparative trial and coast analysis of 3-day antimicrobial regimens for treatment of acute cystitis in women. *JAMA* **273**: 41–5.

Houston HLA (1984) Childhood urinary tract infection. *J Roy Coll Gen Pract* **34**: 494.

Howie JRG (1976) Clinical judgement and antibiotic use in general practice. *BMJ* **2**: 1061–64.

Hurlbut TA, Littenburg B (1991) The diagnostic accuracy of rapid dipstick tests to predict urinary tract infection. *Am J Clin Pathol* **96**: 582–8.

Jacobson LD, Edwards A, Granier SK, Butler CC (1997) Evidence based medicine and general practice. *Br J Gen Pract* **47**: 449–52.

Jacobson SH, Eklof O, Eriksson CG, Lins LE, Tidgren B, Winberg J (1989) Development of hypertension and uraemia after pyelonephritis in childhood: 27 years follow-up. *BMJ* **299**: 703–6.

Jadresic L, Cartwright K, Cowie N, Witcombe B, Stephens D (1993) Investigation of urinary tract infection in childhood. *BMJ* **307**: 761–4.

Jakobsson B, Berg U, Svensson L (1994) Renal scarring after acute pyelonephritis. *Arch Dis Child* **70**: 111–15.

Jellheden B, Norrby RS, Sandberg G (1996) Symptomatic urinary tract infection in women in primary health care. *Scand J Primary Hlth Care* **14**: 122–8.

Jolleys JV (1991) Factors associated with regular episodes of dysuria among women in one rural general practice. *Br J Gen Pract* **41**: 241–3.

Jones CL, Walker RG, Powell HR (1993) Recent advances in the management of vesico-ureteric reflux. *J Paediatr Child Hlth* **29**: 325–7.

Leibovici L, Wysenbeek AJ (1991) Single dose antibiotic treatment for symptomatic urinary tract infection in women: a meta-analysis of randomized trials. *Quart J Med* **78**: 43–57.

Martinell J, Jodal U, Lidin-Janson G (1990) Pregnancies in women with and without renal scarring after urinary infections in childhood. *BMJ* **300**: 840–4.

McWhinney I (1996) *A Textbook of Family Medicine.* Oxford University Press, Oxford.

Norrby SR (1990) Short term treatment of uncomplicated lower urinary tract infections in women. *Rev Infect Dis* **12**: 458–67.

O'Dowd TC, Smail JE, West RR (1984) Clinical judgement in the diagnosis and management of frequency and dysuria in general practice. *BMJ* **288**: 1347–9.

Olesen F, Oestergaard I (1995) Patients with urinary tract infection: proposed management strategies of general practitioners, microbiologists and urologists. *Br J Gen Pract* **45**: 611–13.

Osterberg E, Aspevall O, Grillner L, Persson E (1996) Young women with symptoms of urinary tract infection: prevalence and diagnosis of chlamydial infection and evaluation of rapid screening bacteriuria. *Scand J Primary Hlth Care* 14: 43–9.

Pill RM, O'Dowd TC (1988) Management of cystitis: the patient's viewpoint. *Fam Pract* 5: 24–8.

Rink E (1998) Risk factors for urinary tract symptoms in women: beliefs among general practitioners and women and the effect on patient management. *Br J Gen Pract* 48: 1155–8.

Shaw KN, McGowan KL (1997) Evaluation of a rapid screening filter test for urinary tract infection in children. *Pediatr Infect Dis J* 16: 283–7.

Smellie JM, Ransley PG, Normand ICS, Prescod N, Edwards D (1985) Development of new renal scars: a collaborative study. *BMJ* 290: 1957–60.

Smellie JM, Poulton A, Prescod NP (1994) Retrospective study of children with renal scarring associated with reflux and urinary infection. *BMJ* 308: 1193–6.

South Bedfordshire Practitioners' Group (1990a) How well do general practitioners manage urinary problems in children? *Br J Gen Pract* 40: 146–9.

South Bedfordshire Practitioners' Group (1990b) Development of renal scars in children: missed opportunities in management. *BMJ* 301: 1082–4.

Stamm WE, Hooton TM (1993) Management of urinary tract infection in adults. *N Engl J Med* 329: 1328–34.

Strom BL, Collins M, West S, Kreisberg J, Weller S (1987) Sexual activity, contraceptive use, and other risk factors for symptomatic and asymptomatic bacteriuria. *Ann Intern Med* 107: 816–23.

Sumners D, Kelsey M, Chait I (1992) Psychological aspects of lower urinary tract infections in women. *BMJ* 304: 17–19.

Trienekens TAM, Stobberingh EE, Winkens RAG, Houben AW (1989) Different lengths of treatment with co-trimoxazole for acute uncomplicated urinary tract infections in women. *BMJ* 299: 1319–22.

van der Voort J, Edwards A, Roberts R, Verrier Jones K (1997) The struggle to diagnose urinary tract infection in children under two in primary care. *Fam Pract* 14(1): 44–8.

Vernon S (1995) Urine collection from infants: a reliable method. *Paediatr Nurs* 7: 26–7.

Vernon S, Coulthard MG, Lambert H, Keir MJ, Matthews JNS (1997a) New renal scarring in children who at age 3 and 4 years had had normal scans with dimercaptosuccinic acid: follow up study. *BMJ* 315: 905–8.

Vernon S, Foo CK, Couthard MG (1997b) How general practitioners manage children with urinary tract infection: an audit in the former Northern Region. *Br J Gen Pract* 47(5): 297–300.

Vickers D, Ahmad T, Coulthard MG (1991) Diagnosis of urinary tract infection in children: fresh urine microscopy or culture? *Lancet* 338: 767–70.

Wiggelinkhuizen J, Maytham D, Hanslo DH (1988) Dipstick screening for urinary tract infection. *South African Med J* 74: 224–8.

Winberg J, Bergstrom T, Jacobsson B (1997) Morbidity, age and sex distribution, recurrences and renal scarring in symptomatic urinary tract infection in childhood. *Kidney Int* 8S: 101–6.

Winkens RAG, Leffers P, Trienekens TAM, Stobberingh EE (1995) The validity of urine examination for urinary tract infections in daily practice. *Fam Pract* 11: 290–3.

Working Group of the Research Unit (1991) Guidelines for the management of acute urinary tract infection in childhood. *J Roy Coll Phys Lond* 25: 36–42.

Recurrent urinary tract infection

Mary O'Reilly

13

Contents

I   Introduction

Recurrent urinary tract infection (UTI) is a common problem with significant associated morbidity. It is estimated that 40% of women will have a UTI at some time during their adult life (Kunin, 1994) and of those women 27% will experience a recurrence in 6–12 months (Foxman, 1990). In those who are catheterized the recurrence rate is higher, with bacteriuria being universal. The mean time to recurrence of UTI is 60 days (Foxman, 1990). Of these recurrences, 75% are symptomatic, with a majority of the recurrences occurring in a small subgroup of women in whom there is no obvious cause (Mabeck, 1972).

II   Definition

It is necessary to distinguish persistent infection from relapsed infection or reinfection. Persistent UTI is unresolved infection despite treatment, and may be due to a resistant organism or structural abnormality of the genitourinary tract. Abnormalities may include duplex ureters, urinary tract calculus, renal cystic disease, renal abscess and vesicorectal fistula. Relapsed UTI is infection with the same organism, usually within 2 weeks of completing therapy. This may be due to an anatomical abnormality of the renal tract or to unrecognized upper tract infection, such as pyelonephritis or renal abscess, inadequately

treated with short-course therapy. Reinfection implies a new infection. Recurrent UTI is generally considered to be three or more symptomatic episodes over a 12-month period. Most recurrent lower UTI in women is due to reinfection rather than relapse or persistent infection (McGeachie, 1966).

III   Aetiology

Less than 5% of women with recurrent lower tract infections have an anatomical or functional abnormality (Fowler and Pulawski, 1981; Johnson et al., 1992; Hooton and Stamm, 1997). Anatomical abnormalities have been mentioned above, and any cause of incomplete bladder emptying, including neurogenic bladder dysfunction, anticholinergic medications or chronic constipation, which is particularly seen in the elderly and institutionalized group, may be associated with increased incidence of UTI (Nicolle, 1994). In the absence of structural and functional abnormalities several factors have been associated with the pathogenesis of recurrent UTI. These include a maternal history of UTI (Strom et al., 1987) and blood-group secretor status. Diabetes mellitus is associated with a two- to three-fold increase in the frequency of UTI (Kass, 1956). Asymptomatic bacteriuria is increased in women aged over 70 years and women also have an increased risk of upper tract infections (Vejlsgaard, 1966). There are many postulated associations with recurrent UTI in women which have been refuted. These include the use of hot tubs, bubble baths, tight clothing, type of clothing, bicycle riding, volume of fluid consumed and the direction of wiping after defecation (Remis et al., 1987; Strom et al., 1987; Foxman and Chi, 1990). In most cases the reasons for recurrence in women are unclear.

In women, periurethral colonization with bacteria particularly *Escherichia coli*, and the shortened urethra, encourage urethral and bladder colonization and infection (Sobel, 1997). Those women with recurrent UTI have increased periurethral and vaginal bacterial colonization compared with controls (Stamey et al., 1971; Stamey and Sexton, 1975). Two-thirds of recurrent UTI in young women have the same *E. coli* strain in subsequent infections despite successful clearance of bacteria with treatment, and the same isolate is also found in vaginal and faecal flora, suggesting reinfection with the patient's own enteric flora (Russo et al., 1995). Sexual activity is associated with recurrent UTI (Strom et al., 1987). Risk factors include the frequency of sexual activity and the use of spermicidal creams and the diaphragm (Hooton et al., 1996; Strom et al., 1987). Increased sexual activity may be associated with a new partner, which can occur at any age, including the older age group, and a sexual and social history should not be neglected simply on the basis of age.

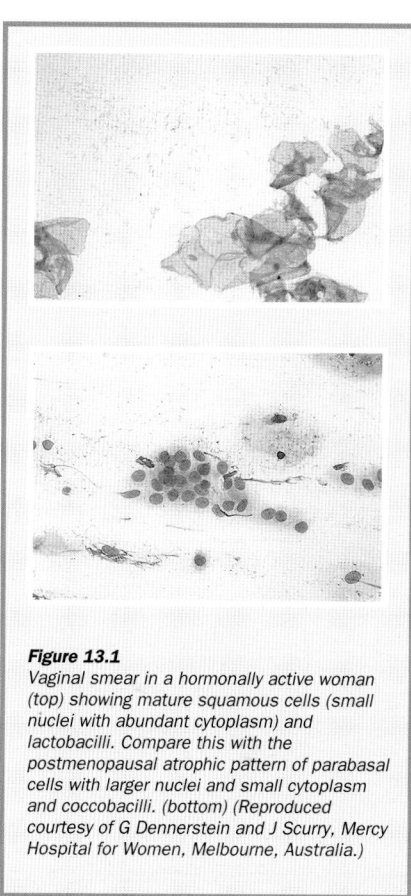

Figure 13.1
Vaginal smear in a hormonally active woman (top) showing mature squamous cells (small nuclei with abundant cytoplasm) and lactobacilli. Compare this with the postmenopausal atrophic pattern of parabasal cells with larger nuclei and small cytoplasm and coccobacilli. (bottom) (Reproduced courtesy of G Dennerstein and J Scurry, Mercy Hospital for Women, Melbourne, Australia.)

Due to changes in hormonal status, postmenopausal women have altered vaginal flora, with increased enteric bacteria (Nicolle, 1994) (*Figure 13.1*). This change in flora is associated with increased incidence of UTI and recurrent UTI (Nicolle, 1994). Raz and Stamm (1993) noted that hormone replacement or topical vaginal oestrogen therapy may be of benefit as it restored the normal vaginal pH and bacterial flora and reduced vaginal colonization with *E. coli* (Raz and Stamm, 1993). They found that topical oestrogen therapy in this group reduced the rate of UTI from 6 infections per year to 0.5 per year.

Recurrent UTI in the elderly may be overdiagnosed given the prevalence of asymptomatic bacteriuria in this group. Bacteriuria occurs in around 2–4% of young women, but is 6–8% in females aged over 60 years and 20% in women aged over 80 years (Schaeffer, 1991). The prevalence is even higher in women who are institutionalized, occurring in 30–50% (Baldassarre and Kaye, 1991). In the elderly the presence of bacteriuria is often incorrectly linked to non-specific symptoms such as behavioural change, confusion or falls. Treatment of asymptomatic bacteriuria of the elderly does not change these symptoms or the mortality associated with UTI (Boscia et al., 1986). Many patients are treated empirically on the basis of abnormal urine analysis or a positive culture, and in this group recurrent UTI is likely to be overdiagnosed and overtreated. This may have adverse consequences, as the elderly experience more adverse drug reactions from antimicrobial therapy (Gleckman, 1995). Other causes of these symptoms need to be considered, particularly if the symptoms do not improve within 48 hours of appropriate therapy.

In the elderly, faecal incontinence with perineal soiling results in increased vaginal and perineal gram-negative colonization, with an increased risk of UTI (Brocklehurst et al., 1977). Other factors that are also implicated in the elderly include renal impairment, with higher urine pH and less bacterial inhibition. Diuretic therapy may also be a factor, as there is a lower urinary osmolality due to dilution and therefore less inhibition of bacteria. Also, with age there is reduced Tamm Horsfall glycoprotein, which coats the pili and reduces adherence of bacteria, and this may result in an increased rate of UTI (Sobel, 1997).

Bacterial factors are also important in the pathogenesis of recurrent UTI. A small number of serogroups of *E. coli* cause a higher proportion of recurrent infections (Measley and Levison, 1991). Several factors are involved, including the P fimbriae, haemolysin, serum resistance and encapsulation, and also the phase variation of the type 1 fimbriae (Svanborg-Eden, 1986; Johnson, 1991; Kunin, 1994). Bacterial virulence factors are found more often in patients with uncomplicated UTI than in healthy patients, and particularly in those with recurrent UTI. Women with some ABO blood groups, non-secretor status, specific human leucocyte antigen (HLA) types and P blood groups seem to be more susceptible to UTI because of enhanced vaginal and urethral colonization with *E. coli* (Kinane et al., 1982). This may relate to specific cell

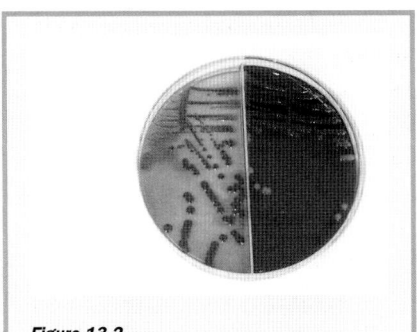

Figure 13.2
Urine culture of E. coli *on split plate containing*
horse blood agar and Maconkey agar
(Reproduced courtesy of H Sheeory, St
Vincent's Hospital, Melbourne, Australia.)

receptor susceptibility promoting adherence to *E. coli* which has been identified in some vaginal and buccal epithelial cells (Schaeffer et al., 1981).

Complicated UTI may be associated with anatomical or functional problems, as outlined previously. *E. coli* (***Figure 13.2***) causes 80% of uncomplicated lower-tract infections in women; however, it is associated with less than one-third of complicated UTI (Stamm et al., 1991; Kunin, 1994). There is an increased rate of other Gram-negative organisms, including *Klebsiella, Enterobacter* and *Proteus*, with increased antibiotic resistance to first-line agents (Stamm et al., 1991). Enterococci are also increased and, depending on the community, vancomycin resistant enterococci (VRE) may be of

concern. *Staphylococcus saprophyticus* is a common cause of uncomplicated cystitis in young women, but is less common in recurrent UTI and is a rarely the cause of complicated UTI.

Methicillin resistance *Staphylococcus aureus* (MRSA) is a rare community pathogen, but is increasing as a nosocomial pathogen. Worthy of note is that the bacterial virulence factors mentioned previously are often absent in women with complicated UTI.

IV   Assessment

A detailed history is important for assessment and further management of patients with recurrent UTI. The number of previous UTI, previous treatment (including antibiotic usage, duration and effectiveness) and any complications of UTI or therapy should be documented. It is important to ascertain, if possible, whether the infection was of the upper or lower tract. The age at the time of first infection, family history of any UTI, urinary tract calculi or structural problems should also be elicited. The patient's voiding pattern, urine continence, bowel pattern and any previous surgery, including urogenital surgery, urinary instrumentation and medication (e.g. antibiotics, antihypertensives, antidepressant therapy, diabetic therapy and hormonal therapy in postmenopausal women) should be recorded. Sexual history and any relationship to UTI is also important, as is a history of other problems such as diabetes or neurological disease. History of any previous investigations performed and management strategies (e.g. antibiotics, urinary antiseptics and cranberry juice) that have been tried previously, and any allergy to or intolerance of any medication should also be documented. Pregnancy, either current or planned, and contraceptive methods should be elicited.

A thorough general and neurological examination is essential. With specific reference to the renal tract, assessment of the renal size and presence of tenderness, whether the bladder is palpable, vaginal examination with assessment for atrophic vaginitis or prolapse and a urine analysis for glycosuria and assessment of the postvoided residual urine volume by bladder scan, should be performed.

Initial investigations required include a midstream urine for microscopy culture and sensitivity on one occasion. For frequently occurring UTI, in general repeated urine cultures are not required except in pregnancy, suspected complicated infections or recent instrumentation or hospitalization. Testing is not cost-effective (O'Connor et al., 1996), and delays therapy. Empirical therapy of cystitis in women without urine culture is not associated with adverse outcomes and is cost-effective (O'Connor et al., 1996). Episodic office urine testing with leucoesterase strips of a urine sample collected prior to self-treatment

can provide verification of the patient's diagnosis. In recurrent lower UTI in women, further imaging is not required; however, in persistent and relapsing infections and upper tract infections, further investigation with renal ultrasound and intravenous urogram to exclude any abnormalities should be performed (see Chapter 3).

V   Management

After thorough clinical assessment, as outlined in *Figure 13.3*, explanation and reassurance is important. Common myths should be dispelled. Underlying conditions should be treated if possible, and women using diaphragms and spermicidal cream should consider alternative contraception. For the elderly, continence and bowel management, perineal hygiene and hydration should be reinforced. In women with catheter-associated infection, catheter management should be reviewed. In postmenopausal women, topical vaginal oestrogens should be considered. Oral hormone replacement has not been trialled; however, small studies suggest that there is a benefit (Parsons and Schmidt, 1982). For women with frequent recurrent UTI three approaches to antibiotic therapy are available: patient-initiated therapy, postcoital therapy or long-term prophylaxis.

For many women with recurrent UTI, frequent or infrequent, episodic therapy prescribed after clinician consultation at the

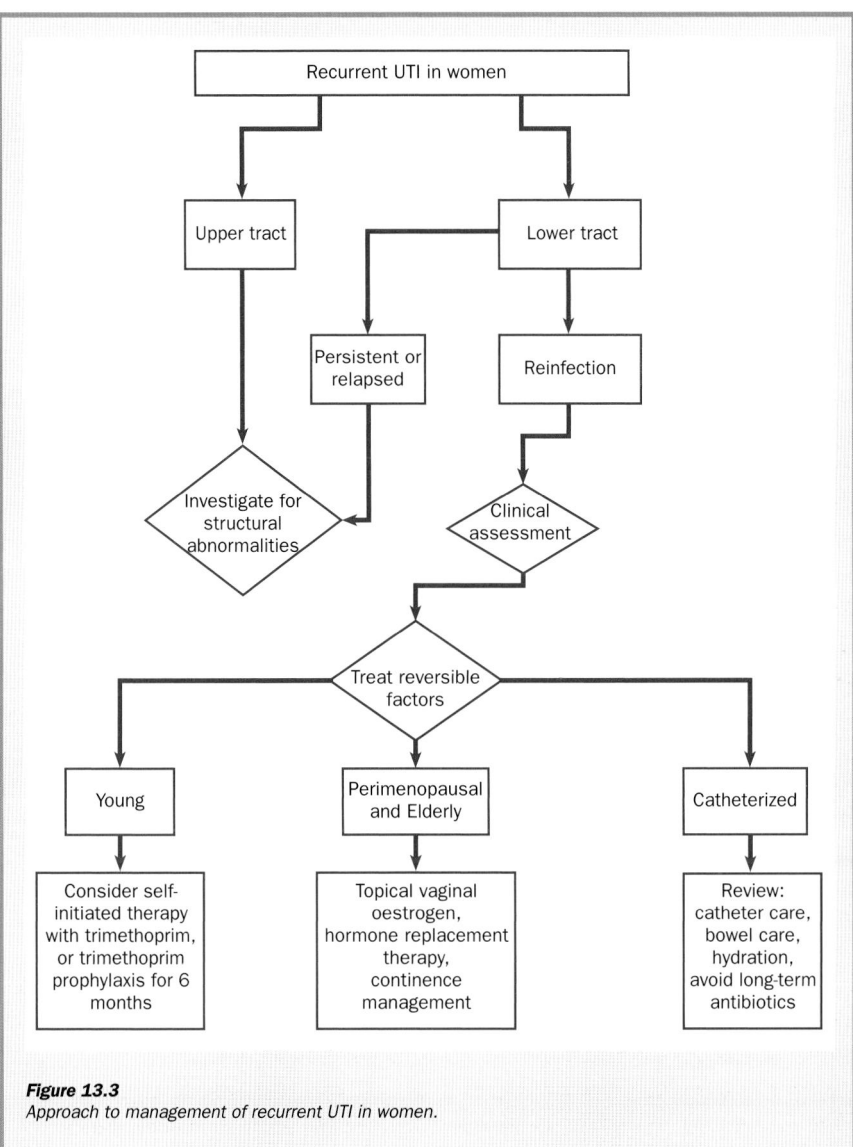

Figure 13.3
Approach to management of recurrent UTI in women.

time of infection is commonly used. This has the disadvantage of delaying therapy, with subsequent prolongation of symptoms, and is uneconomic (O'Connor et al., 1996). An alternative strategy is to provide an empirical antibiotic for the woman to commence at the onset of urinary symptoms. For those women in whom infections are closely associated with coital activity, postcoital antibiotic therapy can be used. Long-term prophylaxis can be used for women with very frequent infections, but this requires significant patient motivation. Antibiotic prophylaxis does not alter the natural history of recurrence, as 40–60% of women develop recurrent infections within 6 months of ceasing prophylaxis (Stapleton and Stamm, 1997).

The choice of antibiotic for the treatment of recurrent UTI, either clinician initiated or self-initiated, should be based on local antibiotic recommendations considering local bacterial flora and sensitivity pattern, patient allergies or intolerances and pregnancy status, cost-effectiveness and simplicity of dose. Treatment needs to be modified to consider previous bacteriology, antibiotic sensitivities and response to therapy. Antibiotic options for women with recurrent UTI include cotrimoxazole, trimethoprim, nitrofurantoin, amoxicillin clavulanate, cephalexin, quinolones and amoxicillin, which is now limited by increasing resistance. β-Lactam antibiotics, including amoxicillin clavulanate, are less effective than cotrimoxazole or

trimethoprim despite a sensitive urinary isolate (Johnson and Stamm, 1989; Norrby, 1990). Cotrimoxazole is used less frequently in some countries due to the availability of trimethoprim, which is effective without the sulphur related toxicity (Kunin, 1994). Due to cost constraints and the possible development of resistance, quinolone antibiotics are only recommended for women with resistant organisms (e.g. *Pseudomonas*) (Harvey et al., 1998).

The duration of therapy is debatable. Single-dose therapy is highly effective in women with acute cystitis (Stamm and Hooton, 1993) but has a higher rate of recurrence and it is less effective in recurrent infections and older women (Nicolle, 1994). Recent reviews of urinary-tract therapy concluded that 3-day regimens of cotrimoxazole, β-lactams or fluoroquinolones were more effective than single-dose therapy (Norrby, 1990; Andriole, 1991). Three-day therapy is also associated with a reduction in rectal flora, the source of infection in most women. More prolonged courses of cotrimoxazole are associated with increased adverse reactions, with no benefit over 3-day therapy (Norrby, 1990). β-Lactams are more effective if given for 5 days. Comparing the various regimens, cotrimoxazole (160/800 mg twice daily) had a significantly higher cure rate than did cefadroxil (500 mg twice daily), amoxicillin (500 mg three times daily) or nitrofurantoin (100 mg four times daily)

(Hooton et al., 1995). There are few data on short-course therapy in postmenopausal women; however, ofloxacin 200 mg/day was more effective than cephalexin 500 mg four times daily for 7 days (Raz and Rozengeld, 1996).

In general, for recurrent UTI at least a 3-day course of trimethoprim or cotrimoxazole or a 5-day course of β-lactams or nitrofurantoin should be prescribed. In the elderly a 7-day course has been suggested (Nicolle and Ronald 1987). Nosocomial pathogens are, in general, more antibiotic-resistant with increased prevalence of enterococci, resistant Gram-negative organisms and *Staphylococcus*. A urine culture should be performed if the patient has recently been hospitalized. Given the rate of nosocomial infections with MRSA, including catheter-associated infections, MRSA may now be a cause of recurrent UTI in the community. Oral therapy for MRSA requires two drugs, as resistance rapidly develops if only one agent is used. Depending on sensitivities and licensing, two out of three antibiotics – rifampicin, fusidic acid and ciprofloxacin (or another quinolone) – should be used.

In pregnant women or those planning pregnancy, safe drugs should be used, namely those that have been taken by a large number of pregnant women and women of childbearing age without any proven increase in the frequency of malformations or other direct or indirect harmful effects on the fetus (Category A drugs). These drugs include amoxicillin, cephalexin and nitrofurantoin. In the elderly there is increased toxicity of some antibiotics: nitrofurantoin is associated with pulmonary and neural toxicity and cotrimoxazole with blood dyscrasias (Gleckman, 1995). Drug interactions also need to be considered – interactions with the oral contraceptive pill in young women, in the elderly interactions of cotrimoxazole with warfarin and methotrexate, and interactions of fluoroquinolones with iron, antacids and theophylline.

Morbidities such as vaginal candidiasis (with amoxicillin or amoxicillin clavulanate), particularly in younger women, and tendonitis (with quinolones) need consideration. Long-term prophylaxis should be considered for those women with three or more UTIs per year. The antibiotics of choice for the prevention of UTIs by long-term prophylaxis include trimethoprim (100–150 mg nocte), cotrimoxazole (40/200 mg nocte), nitrofurantoin (50–100 mg nocte), cephalexin (125–250 mg nocte) and norfloxacin (200 mg nocte) (Stapleton and Stamm, 1997). Nitrofurantoin intermittently sterilizes the urine, and norfloxacin and cotrimoxazole reduce uropathogens in fecal flora (Stamm et al., 1980; Nicolle, 1992). Trimethoprim 100–150 mg nocte for 6–12 months can reduce the rate of UTIs from 2–3 per year to 0.2 per year (Nicolle and Ronald, 1987). Long-term cotrimoxazole appears to be safe and effective (Nicolle, 1992). For women with a UTI related to sexual activity, postcoital prophylaxis can be implemented. Regimens include cotrimoxazole 40/200 mg, nitrofurantoin 50 mg, cephalexin 125–250 mg or cinoxacin 250 mg. For catheterized patients, long-term antibiotic therapy results in selection of resistant organisms and should be avoided. Cranberry juice for prevention of UTIs has received anecdotal support for many years, particularly in long-term care facilities. It acidifies the urine, reduces bacterial adherence and reduces bacteriuria. However, more recently a placebo showed that controlled trial 300 ml/day of cranberry juice is of benefit, reducing bacteuria and pyuria by 42% and persistent bacteriuria and pyuria by 27% (Avorn et al., 1994). There have been no studies on the prevention of symptomatic infection.

VI   Conclusion

Recurrent UTIs pose a significant problem for women of all ages, the problem increasing with increasing age and being particularly a problem in the institutionalized elderly. A thorough understanding and assessment enables a targeted approach and appropriate management of the patient. Preventive strategies are effective, although more research is required.

References

Andriole VT (1991) Use of quinolones in treatment of prostatitis and lower urinary tract infections. *Eur J Clin Microbiol Infect Dis* 10: 342–50.

Avorn J, Monane M, Gurwitz J et al. (1994) Reduction of bacteriuria and pyuria after ingestion of cranberry juice. *JAMA* 271: 751–4.

Baldassarre ZS, Kaye D (1991) Special problems of urinary tract infection in the elderly. *Med Clin North Am* 75: 375–90.

Boscia JA, Kobasa WD, Abrutyn E et al. (1986). Lack of association between bacteriuria and symptoms in the elderly. *Am J Med* 81: 979–82.

Brocklehurst ZC, Bee P, Jones D, Palmer MIC (1977) Bacteriuria in geriatric hospital rates: its correlates and management. *Age Ageing* 6: 240–5.

Fowler JE Jr, Pulawski ET (1981) Excretory urography, cystography, and cystoscopy in the evaluation of women with urinary tract infection: a prospective study. *N Engl J Med* 304: 462–5.

Foxman B (1990) Recurrent urinary tract infection: incidence and risk factors. *Am J Public Health* 80: 331–3.

Foxman B, Chi JW (1990) Health behaviour and urinary tract infections in college-aged women. *J Clin Epidemiol* 43: 329–37.

Gleckman RA (1995) Antibiotic concerns in the elderly. A clinician's perspective. *Infect Dis North Am* 9: 575–89.

Harvey K, Beavis M, Christiansen K et al. (1998) *Therapeutic Guidelines – Antibiotic (1998–1999)*, 10th edn. Therapeutic Guidelines Limited, Melbourne.

Hooton TM, Stamm WE (1997) Diagnosis and treatment of uncomplicated urinary tract infection. *Infect Dis Clin North Am* 11: 551–81.

Hooton TM, Winter C, Tiu F, Stamm W (1995) Randomized comparative trial and cost analysis of 3 day antimicrobial regimens for treatment of acute cystitis in women *JAMA* **273**; 41–5.

Hooton TM, Scholes D, Hughes JP et al. (1996) A prospective study of risk factors for symptomatic urinary tract infection in young women. *N Engl J Med* **335**: 468–74.

Johnson J (1991) Virulence factors in *Escherichia coli* urinary tract infection. *Clin Micro Rev* **4**: 80–128.

Johnson JR, Stamm WE (1989) Urinary tract infections in women: diagnosis and treatment. *Ann Intern Med* **111**: 906–7.

Johnson JR, Vincent LM, Wang K, Roberts PL, Stamm WE (1992) Renal ultrasonographic correlates of acute pyelonephritis. *Clin Infect Dis* **14**: 15–22.

Kass EH (1956) Asymptomatic infections of the urinary tract. *Trans Assoc Am Phys* **69**: 56–63.

Kinane DF, Blackwall CC, Brettle RP et al. (1982) ABO blood group secretor state and susceptibility to recurrent urinary tract infections in women. *Br Med J* **285**: 7–9.

Kunin CM (1994) Urinary tract infections in females. *Clin Infect Dis* **18**: 1–12.

Mabeck CE (1972) treatment of uncomplicated urinary tract infection in non-pregnant women. *Postgrad Med J* **48**: 69–75.

McGeachie J (1996) Recurrent infections of the urinary tract: reinfection or recrudescence. *Br Med J* **1**: 952–4.

Measley RD, Levison ME (1991) Host defense mechanisms in the pathogenesis of urinary tract infections. *Med Clin North Am* **2**: 275–86.

Nicolle LE (1992) Prophylaxis: recurrent urinary tract infection on women. *Infection* **20**(suppl 3): S203–5.

Nicolle LE (1994) Urinary tract infection in the elderly. *J Antimicrob Chemother* **33**(suppl A): 99–109.

Nicolle LE, Ronald AR (1987) Recurrent urinary tract infections in adult women: diagnosis and treatment. *Infect Dis Clin North Am* **1**: 793–806.

Norrby SR (1990) Short-term treatment of uncomplicated lower urinary tract infections in women. *Rev Infect Dis* **12**: 458–67.

O'Connor PJ, Solberg LI, Christianson J, Amundson G, Mosser G (1996) Mechanism of action and impact of a cystitis clinical practice guideline on outcomes and costs of care in an HMO. *J Qual Improvement* **22**: 673–82.

Parsons CL, Schmidt JD (1982) Control of recurrent lower urinary tract infections in the post menopausal woman. *J Urol* **128**: 1224–5.

Raz R, Stamm WE (1993) A controlled trial of intravaginal estriol in post menopausal women with recurrent urinary tract infections. *N Engl J Med* **329**: 753–6.

Raz R, Rozengeld S (1996) Three day course of ofloxacin versus cefalexin in the treatment of urinary tract infections in post menopausal women. *Antimicrob Agents Chemother* **40**: 2200–1.

Remis RS, Gurwith MJ, Gurwith D, Hargrett-Bean NT, Layde PM (1987) Risk factors for urinary tract infection. *Am J Epidemiol* **126**: 685–94.

Russo TA, Stapleton A, Wendercth S, Hooton TM, Stamm WE (1995) Chromosomal restriction fragment length polymorphism analysis of *Escherichia coli* strains causing recurrent urinary tract infections in young women. *Infect Dis J* **172**: 440–5.

Schaefer AT (1991) Urinary tract infections in the elderly. *Eur Urol* **19**(suppl 1): 2–6.

Schaeffer AJ, Jones JM, Dunn JC (1981) Association of in vitro *Escherichia coli* adherence to vaginal and buccal epithelial cells with susceptibility of women to recurrent urinary tract infections. *N Engl J Med* **304**: 1062–6.

Sobel JD (1997) Pathogenesis of urinary tract infection. Role of host defenses. *Infect Dis Clin North Am* **1**: 531–49.

Stamey TA, Sexton CC (1975) The role of vaginal colonisation with enterobacteriaceae in recurrent urinary tract infection. *J Urol* **113**: 214–17.

Stamey TA, Timothy M, Millar M, Mihara G (1971) Recurrent urinary tract infections in adult women. The role of introital enterobacteriaceae. *Calf Med* **115**: 1–19.

Stamm WE, Hooton TM (1993) Management of urinary tract infections in adults. *N Engl J Med* **329**: 1328–34.

Stamm WE, Counts GW, Wagner KF et al. (1980) Antimicrobial prophylaxis of recurrent urinary tract infections: a double-blind, placebo-controlled trial. *Ann Intern Med* **92**: 770–5.

Stamm WE, McKevitt M, Roberts PL, White NZ (1991) Natural history of recurrent urinary tract infections in women. *Rev Infect Dis* **13**: 77–84.

Stapleton A, Stamm WE (1997) Prevention of urinary tract infection. *Infect Dis Clin North Am* **11**: 719–33.

Strom BL, Collins M, West SL, Kreisberg J, Weller S (1987) Sexual activity, contraceptive use, and other risk factors for symptomatic and asymptomatic bacteriuria. *Ann Intern Med* **107**: 816–23.

Svanborg-Eden C (1986) Bacterial adherence in urinary tract infections caused by *Escherichia coli*. *Scand J Urol Nephrol* **20**: 81–8.

Vejlsgaard R (1966) Studies on urinary infection in diabetics. 1. Bacteriuria in patients with diabetes mellitus and in control subjects. *Acta Med Scand* **179:** 173–89.

Acute and chronic nephritis

Kelvin Lynn

14

Contents

X   Renal failure
XI   Renal cystic disease
XII   Xanthogranulomatous pyelonephritis
XIII Malakoplakia
XIV Tuberculosis
    1. Diagnosis
    2. Radiology
    3. Treatment

I Introduction

This chapter discusses infections of the kidney affecting adult women. Urinary infections may affect the lower or upper urinary tract. The localization of any urinary tract infection is usually based on clinical assessment. In addition, urinary tract infections may be single or isolated, or recurrent due to reinfection or relapse.

Urinary tract infection can be classified as complicated or uncomplicated (Bailey, 1994a). Uncomplicated infections occur in a patient with an anatomically and functionally normal urinary tract without complicating associated disease. These urinary tract infections have an excellent long-term kidney outcome. Complicated infections occur in a patient with a structurally or functionally abnormal urinary tract or in a patient with a normal urinary tract but an associated disease, such as diabetes. The most important of these abnormalities are urinary stones, urinary tract obstruction, vesicoureteric reflux (VUR) and papillary necrosis. Patients with complicated urinary tract infection may be at risk of progressive renal damage.

II Prevalence

Urinary tract infections are the commonest bacterial infections treated in primary care and are responsible for considerable morbidity, particularly for women in the sexually-active age group. Apart from the first year of life and over the age of 60 years, urinary tract infections predominantly affect females. The prevalence of acute pyelonephritis in non-pregnant women is not known.

III Pathogenesis

In women, most urinary tract infections are acute and localized to the bladder. Only a minority of women develop upper tract infection (Fünfstück et al., 1997). With the exception of *Staphylococcus saprophyticus*, the organisms responsible for urinary infection come from the patient's large bowel. *Escherichia coli* are responsible for 80–90% of uncomplicated infections (Stamm and Hooton, 1993; Cattell, 1998). *Enterococcus, Proteus, Enterobacter* spp. and *Staph. aureus* are more likely to be associated with a complicated urinary tract infection. Most organisms causing bladder infections, with the possible exception of *Staph. saprophyticus*, can cause upper tract infection. Infections caused by *Proteus* spp. are thought to involve the kidney very frequently. Transfer of organisms into the urinary tract is usually by the transurethral route. Infection of the kidney is almost always secondary to bladder infection. Less commonly, haematogenous spread of organisms, usually *Staph. aureus*, may be responsible for renal or perirenal abscesses.

Both impairment of the local defence mechanisms of the host (e.g. by urinary obstruction or VUR) and bacterial virulence factors, such as the presence of P-fimbriated bacteria, uro-epithelial adhesion and colonization of the periurethral area by uropathogenic microorganisms, are important in determining the clinical symptoms, localization and persistence of infection (Cattell, 1985; Svanborg Edén et al., 1988). Ascent of infection to the kidney is facilitated by VUR, atonic or dilated ureters, medullary susceptibility, urinary obstruction and bacterial virulence factors.

IV   Acute pyelonephritis

In this discussion the term 'acute pyelonephritis' is used to describe infection affecting the renal pelvis and renal tissue resulting from infection originating in the urinary tract (Medical Research Council Bacteriuria Committee, 1979; Talner et al., 1994). Acute pyelonephritis may be complicated or uncomplicated. Pregnancy, associated illness, immunosuppression and possibly VUR increase the likelihood of acute pyelonephritis in the adult female.

1.   Clinical presentation

The clinical diagnosis is made in a woman with fever and rigors, loin pain and flank tenderness. One or both kidneys may be involved. There may be exquisite tenderness over the renal angle and hypochondrium and the pain may radiate to the epigastrium or lower abdomen. Nausea, vomiting and dehydration may be prominent features. Patients with diabetes or those on immunosuppressive therapy, including renal transplant recipients may have few localizing symptoms or signs (Cattell, 1985). The clinical presentation ranges from a young woman with Gram-negative septicaemia and oliguric acute renal failure to one with a cystitis-like illness and mild flank pain. Patients with persisting bacteriuria in association with urinary stones, ileal conduits or neurogenic bladders are often asymptomatic for prolonged periods and then develop fever with or without pain and tenderness. It is presumed that these patients have developed an upper urinary tract infection.

The differential diagnoses of acute pyelonephritis are shown in **Table 14.1**.

2.   Pathology

The kidneys are enlarged and hyperaemic with wedge-shaped areas of intense suppurative inflammation extending from the medulla into the cortex, without significant abnormalities of the intervening renal tissue. Microabscesses, variable in number and size, are present and bacteria may be demonstrated within areas of suppuration (**Figure 14.1**). The tubular lumina are filled with leukocytes and cellular debris resulting in further

Table 14.1
Differential diagnosis of acute pyelonephritis

Acute urinary tract obstruction
Renal colic
Renal and perinephric abscesses
Acute cholecystitis
Lower lobe pneumonia
Appendicitis
Lung abscess
Renal vein thrombosis
Acute glomerulonephritis
Renal infarction
Acute pancreatitis
Pelvic inflammatory disease

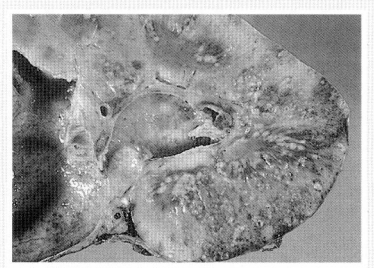

Figure 14.1
Acute pyelonephritis. The cut surface of the kidney reveals multiple abscesses.

extension of the inflammatory process along the nephrons and collecting tubules. The mucosa of the pelvis and calyces may have patchy areas of hyperaemia and inflammation, and sometimes they may be covered by a purulent exudate. The glomeruli are involved in only the most severe cases. Healing takes place when the neutrophilic infiltrate subsides and is replaced by mononuclear cells consisting of macrophages, plasma cells and lymphocytes. Later, fibrotic scars are formed by the proliferation of fibroblasts with deposition of collagen (Blomjous and Meijer, 1998).

3. Natural history and complications

In uncomplicated acute pyelonephritis there is usually an excellent response to appropriate antimicrobial therapy and complete recovery. A few women with severe renal infections may develop cortical scars (Meyrier et al., 1989; Meyrier, 1990). These changes are probably rare and their long-term functional relevance is unknown. If the woman has a complicated infection, such as with stones or obstruction, a different course may result. Obstruction and infection is potentially life-threatening and may cause papillary necrosis, renal or perinephric abscess, or xanthogranulomatous pyelonephritis (Cattell, 1998). Papillary necrosis and acute renal failure are usually seen in women with diabetes, sickle-cell disease or trait, alcoholism or analgesic or non-steroidal anti-inflammatory drug (NSAID) abuse (Meyrier et al., 1989; Jones et al., 1991) (*Figure 14.2*). Acute renal failure may complicate acute pyelonephritis in otherwise healthy young women when

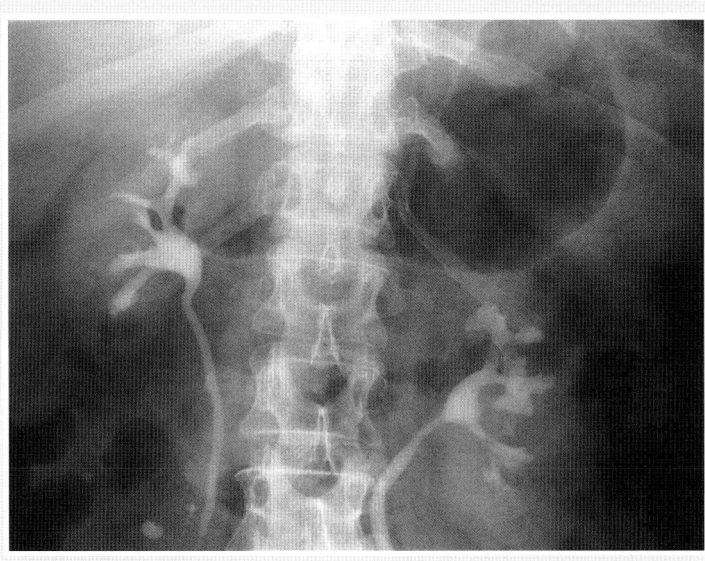

Figure 14.2
Renal papillary necrosis. Intravenous urogram in a 62-year-old woman showing small irregular kidneys and renal papillary necrosis after acute pyelonephritis complicated by a perinephric abscess.

NSAIDs have been given for loin pain thought to be due to renal colic or musculoskeletal disease (Atkinson et al., 1986; Jones, 1992). In all of these complicated kidney infections, eradication of the infecting organism is difficult and relapse is common. It may be impossible to sterilize the urine in patients with renal stones.

Although some authorities have identified focal or multifocal acute bacterial interstitial nephritis as a more severe form of kidney infection, Talner et al. (1994) have argued persuasively that these changes are part of the continuum of acute pyelonephritis. Patients with abnormalities on computed tomography (CT) scanning are usually sicker and have marked clinical signs of renal inflammation. Very severe renal infection may occasionally result in severe focal or multifocal inflammation which, if untreated, may lead to abscess formation. Renal scars may occur on healing (Meyrier et al., 1989).

Recurrent uncomplicated symptomatic or asymptomatic urinary tract infections do not lead to significant renal impairment or hypertension in the long term. Reports of the development or progression of renal scarring in adults with uncomplicated acute pyelonephritis have probably resulted from incorrect radiological diagnoses – either reflux nephropathy unrecognized at initial presentation or incorrect diagnosis in women with papillary necrosis or post obstructive atrophy (Cattell, 1998).

4. Renal imaging

In most women with apparently uncomplicated acute pyelonephritis, renal imaging is not necessary. Investigations of renal morphology should be reserved for those women who do not respond to antibiotic therapy within 48 hours, or for those where there is a strong clinical suspicion of urinary tract obstruction or other underlying abnormality (*Figure 14.3*). The intravenous urogram is normal in about 75% of women with uncomplicated acute pyelonephritis (Fraser et al., 1995). In the remainder, kidney enlargement, decreased opacification or effacement of the collecting system, or delayed calyceal appearance time may be observed. Occasionally a mass lesion is apparent.

Renal ultrasonography is usually normal in women with acute pyelonephritis but is an excellent technique for detecting urinary tract

dilatation. In women with clinically mild kidney infections CT scans, both unenhanced and enhanced, are normal (Talner et al., 1994). With more severe infections, renal enlargement or focal swelling may be seen and, occasionally, there is evidence of parenchymal attenuation with unenhanced scans suggesting haemorrhage. CT scanning with radiocontrast may show one or more wedge-shaped or streaky zones of low attenuation, which may be patchy or homogeneous, extending from the papilla to the kidney capsule (*Figure 14.4*). These changes are thought to be due to focal ischaemia, obstructed tubules and interstitial inflammation. Small areas of fluid attenuation are owing to microabscesses. Perinephric inflammation, evidenced by thickening of Gerota's fascia and stranding in the perinephric fat, may be seen in severe infections. The appearances on CT are time dependent and are modified by antibiotic therapy (Talner et al., 1994). All CT changes may persist for months, even when there is no longer any clinical evidence of inflammation. Focal scars have been demonstrated on CT scanning after acute pyelonephritis in some adults (Meyrier et al., 1989; Meyrier, 1990; Tsugaya et al., 1992; Fraser et al., 1995). Dimercaptosuccinic acid (DMSA) renal scintigraphy is more sensitive than CT in detecting areas of focal ischaemia (Fraser et al., 1995) (*Figure 14.5*). DMSA renal scanning does not distinguish between inflammation and abscess. Gallium

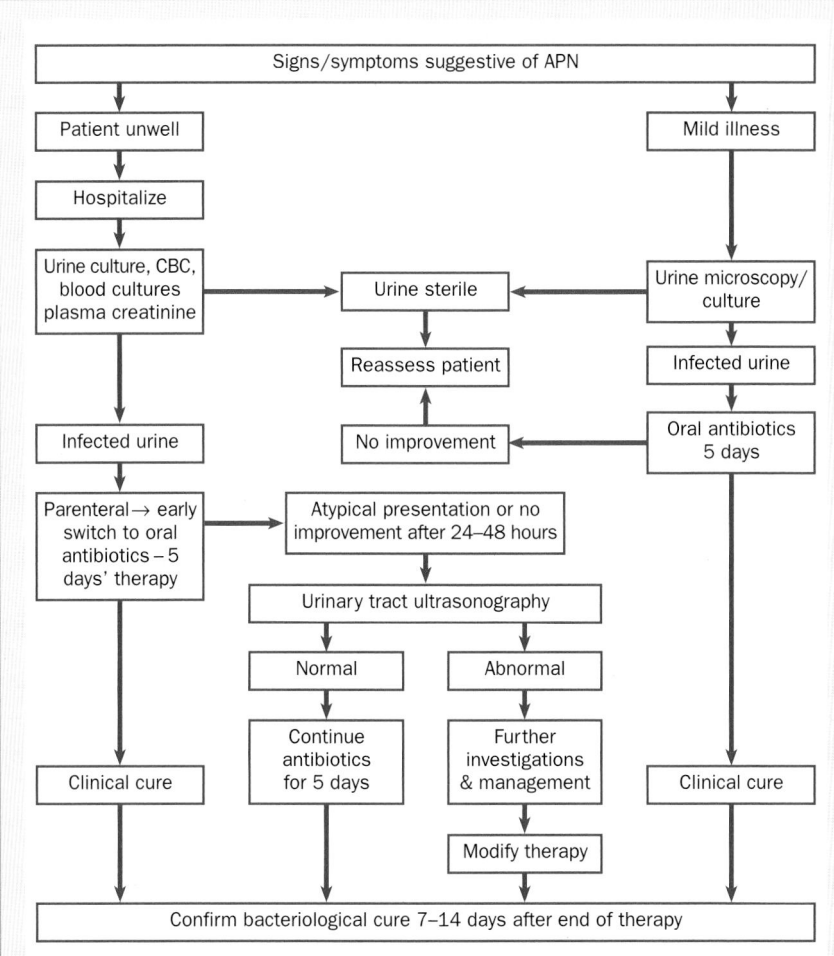

Figure 14.3
Algorithm for management of acute pyelonephritis in the adult female. CBC, complete blood count.

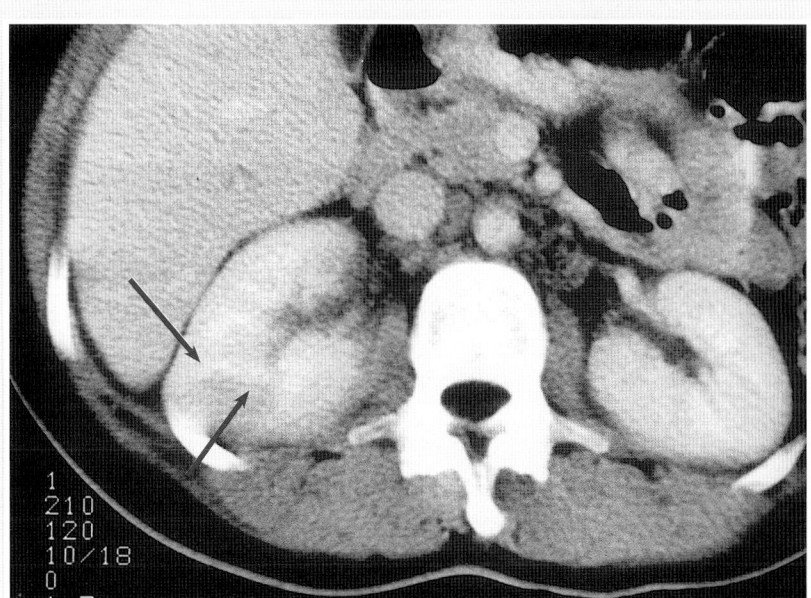

Figure 14.4
CT in acute pyelonephritis. Swollen right kidney with focal areas of reduced enhancement (arrowed) after injection of contrast medium. Left kidney appears normal.

scintigraphy, which is less specific than CT scanning, may show areas of focal or diminished uptake of tracer (Cattell, 1998).

Two prospective studies (Fraser et al., 1995; Bailey et al., 1996) involving hospitalized patients, mainly young women, with acute pyelonephritis provide some information on the likelihood of renal morphological changes after kidney infection (*Table 14.2*). These studies suggest that about

15% of hospitalized patients with acute pyelonephritis may develop permanent morphological changes but provide no information on the long-term potential for deterioration of renal function.

5. Treatment

The management principles of acute pyelonephritis are shown in *Table 14.3* and a

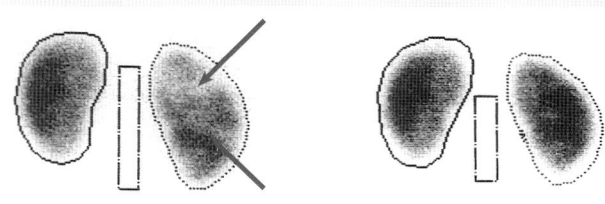

Lt= 53.4%   Rt= 46.5% Lt= 49.8%   Rt= 50.1%

POSTERIOR VIEW   POSTERIOR VIEW

Figure 14.5
DMSA renal scan in acute pyelonephritis. Perfusion defects (arrowed) associated with acute pyelonephritis in the right kidney of a 20-year-old woman shown in scan on the left. Scan on the right obtained three months later when perfusion defects, renal swelling and reduced function had resolved. (Reproduced with permission from Bailey et al. (1996).)

Table 14.2
Renal morphological changes after acute pyelonephritis

Author	Patients (women) (n)	Abnormal IVU on presentation (%)	Abnormal DMSA renal scan on presentation (%)	Abnormal DMSA renal scan > 3 months (%)
Bailey et al (1996)	81 (73)	Not done	37 (46%)	6 of 24 (25%)
Fraser et al. (1995)	164 (142)	59 (36%)	47 of 106* (44%)	27 of 35 (77%)
* 106 patients with normal IVU.				

suggested algorithm for management is shown in *Figure 14.3*. Women with severe symptoms require hospitalization for intravenous fluid therapy and analgesia. The most common reason for admission is vomiting. Tests of renal function, a complete blood count, blood

Table 14.3
Principles of management of women with acute pyelonephritis

> *Establish the diagnosis – complicated or uncomplicated?*
> *Culture the causative organism*
> *Consider whether renal imaging necessary*
> *Uncomplicated infection – appropriate course of antibacterial therapy for 5 days*
> *Complicated infection – individualize therapy, longer course of therapy may be needed*
> *Culture urine 7–10 days after completion of antibacterial therapy*

Table 14.4
Drug regimens for a parenteral treatment of uncomplicated acute pyelonephritis

Aminoglycosides, e.g.		
Gentamicin	*4–7 mg/kg body weight*	*once daily*
Fluoroquinolones, e.g.		
Ciprofloxacin	*250–500 mg*	*12 hourly*
Penicillins, e.g.		
Amoxycillin/clavulanic acid	*1 g/200 mg*	*8 hourly*
Amoxycillin	*1 g*	*8 hourly*
Cephalosporins, e.g.		
Cephazolin	*1 g*	*8 hourly*
Ceftriaxone	*2 g*	*24 hourly*
Other β-lactam antibiotics, e.g.		
Aztreonam	*1 g*	*12 hourly*
Imipenem–cilastin	*550 mg/500 mg*	*8 hourly*

cultures and a pregnancy test (to guide the choice of a suitable antimicrobial agent) should be done as part of the initial assessment. Immediate renal imaging is not usually necessary. Women with uncomplicated acute pyelonephritis should be treated for five days (Bailey, 1994b). The first few doses should be given parenterally if the patient is vomiting.

Antibiotics suitable for initial parenteral therapy include gentamicin, ciprofloxacin or ceftriaxone (*Table 14.4*). There is no place for combined antibiotic therapy in uncomplicated acute pyelonephritis. If a single dose of

Table 14.5
Drug regimens for oral treatment of uncomplicated acute pyelonephritis

Trimethoprim	300 mg	24 hourly
Co-trimoxazole	960 mg	12 hourly
Nitrofurantoin	50 mg	8 hourly
Fluoroquinolones, e.g.		
Ciprofloxacin	250 mg	12 hourly
Norfloxacin	400 mg	12 hourly
Penicillins, e.g.		
Amoxycillin	500 mg	8 hourly
Amoxycillin/clavulanic acid	500 mg/125 mg	12 hourly
Pivampicillin	500 mg	12 hourly
Cephalosporins, e.g.		
Cephalexin	500 mg	8 hourly
Cephradine	500 mg	8 hourly
Cefaclor	250 mg	8 hourly
Cefuroxime axetil	250 mg	12 hourly

gentamicin is used, monitoring blood drug concentrations is unnecessary. A switch to oral therapy after 24 hours is usually possible and most women are well enough for discharge after two days' hospitalization. If it is necessary to continue parenteral treatment, gentamicin dosing should be once daily (Barclay et al., 1994) as this means of administration is safer and more effective than more frequent dosing. The choices of oral antibiotics are shown in *Table 14.5*. Fluoroquinolones may be the antibiotics of choice because of the high blood and urine concentrations achieved after oral use (Karabalut and Drusano, 1993; Moreau et al., 1996). These drugs are not universally available and should not be used in pregnancy or in women with a history of seizures. Although co-trimoxazole has been used extensively for the treatment of urinary tract infections, trimethoprim is as efficacious and avoids the adverse reactions associated with sulphamethoxazole. Nitrofurantoin remains a valuable drug active against most common uropathogens, except *Proteus mirabilis*, and is safe for use in pregnancy. When the patient has renal impairment, trimethoprim or a β-lactam antibiotic is the preferred oral agent.

The duration of antibiotic therapy has received little attention with most reviewers recommending treatment for 10–14 days (Meyrier and Guibert, 1992; Cattell, 1998; Bailey, 1998). Bailey and colleagues reported their extensive experience of the treatment of hospitalized patients with uncomplicated acute pyelonephritis treated for five days. In studies of hospitalized women, 96% were cured with an aminoglycoside and 88% with a fluoroquinolone or a β-lactam antibiotic (Bailey, 1998).

Some women may experience recurrent acute pyelonephritis. Low-dose antimicrobial therapy with nitrofurantoin 50 mg at night, trimethoprim 100 mg at night or co-trimoxazole 0.24 g at night is effective in preventing recurrent urinary tract infections. In patients with renal impairment cephalexin 125 mg at night may be useful. At first, prophylactic therapy should be administered on a nightly basis, but subsequently the frequency may be reduced. Treatment should be for three to six months initially and then according to patient and physician choice.

Treatment of any infection complicating urinary tract obstruction requires relief of the obstruction and often drainage of the urinary tract.

Occasionally, prolonged prophylactic therapy is warranted in women with complicated urinary infections such as those complicating urinary stone disease or urinary obstruction managed with a nephrostomy tube.

V Renal and perinephric abscess

1. Intrarenal abscess

Renal cortical abscess (renal carbuncle) was traditionally considered to result from haematogenous spread of *Staph. aureus* from a primary skin infection to the urinary tract and to predominantly affect young men. Now more than 75% of abscesses are caused by *E. coli*, *Proteus* or *Pseudomonas* spp. and result from ascending urinary infection in diabetics and immunocompromised subjects (Morgan and Nyberg, 1985). Renal and perinephric abscesses are now more commonly seen in women aged between 40 and 60 years (Morgan and Nyberg, 1985). There is usually a long interval between the primary infection and the recognition of the renal abscess. The usual presentation is with fever, weight loss, malaise, loin or hypochondrial pain and tenderness to palpation in the renal angle. Localizing symptoms, however, may be absent and bladder symptoms are uncommon.

Blood and urine cultures are often negative. A modest neutrophil leukocytosis is usual. Infection begins with cortical microabscesses that coalesce to form a large, thick-walled abscess, usually single and unilateral. Rarely the cortical abscess may rupture into the perinephric space but not usually into the collecting system (***Figure 14.6***). Spread of infection is usually confined by Gerota's fascia but rarely infection may

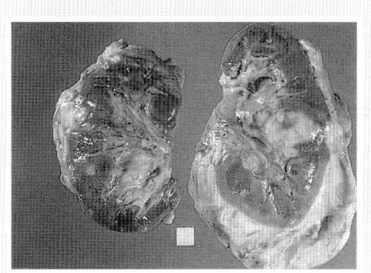

Figure 14.6
*Perinephric abscess. Sectioned kidney
shows perinephric abscess complicating
acute pyelonephritis.*

spread further to cause a subphrenic abscess, empyema, groin or pelvic abscess or psoas abscess.

The differential diagnoses of a renal abscess include severe acute pyelonephritis, an obstructed pyonephrosis, infected renal cysts, a perinephric abscess or a renal tumour.

2.   Perinephric abscess

Perinephric abscesses may arise from either haematogenous spread or from an intrarenal infection (Saiki et al., 1982; Morgan and Nyberg, 1985). Risk factors for the development of perinephric abscesses are, most importantly, renal stones and urinary obstruction, a history of urinary tract surgery or trauma and diabetes. The organisms responsible are the same as for intrarenal

abscesses. As with renal abscesses the diagnosis of a perinephric abscess is usually delayed. Pain, often non-specific, is the most common symptom. Pain may be localized to the renal angle, inguinal region or thigh, or to the abdomen. There may be signs of psoas and lumbar muscle involvement. Up to 25% of patients will have a normal urinalysis. There is usually a mild leukocytosis and anaemia. The differential diagnoses are the same as for an intrarenal abscess. In comparison to those with acute pyelonephritis, patients with a perinephric abscess have a longer duration of symptoms before hospitalization and longer duration of fever after commencement of antibiotic therapy.

3.   Radiological diagnosis

Renal ultrasonography is the investigation of choice for diagnosis and monitoring therapy. When a cortical abscess is fully formed, ultrasonography of the kidney will show a fluid collection which may have a thick wall, contain echoes or a fluid level (*Figure 14.7*). Aspiration is necessary to allow culture of the infecting organism. Before liquefaction occurs, the appearances are those of a solid or semi-solid mass. CT scanning is a more sensitive detector of renal abscess but the changes may be similar to those of a necrotic renal cell carcinoma. CT scanning will demonstrate the extent of any perinephric collection and is very useful when planning drainage (*Figure 14.8*).

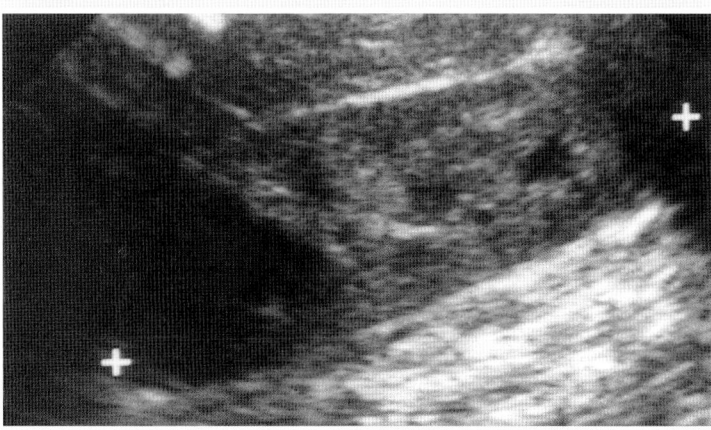

Figure 14.7
Ultrasound of renal abscess. Transverse view of the kidney in a 61-year-old woman presenting with debility and weight loss showing a mass lesion at the upper pole of right kidney. CT showed a thick-walled fluid collection and 45 ml of pus was aspirated.

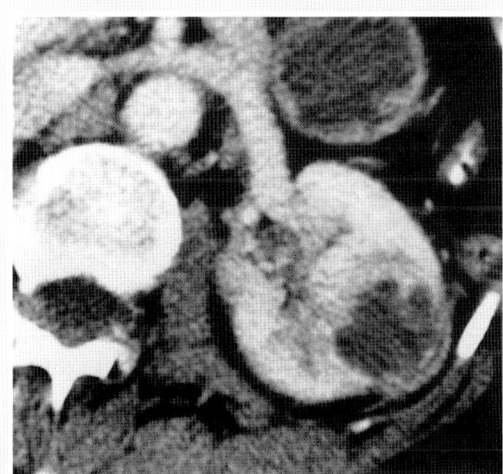

Figure 14.8
CT of renal abscess. CT of the left kidney in a 53-year-old woman with abdominal pain and fever. A focal 2 × 3 cm mass at the mid to upper pole of left kidney is shown after injection of contrast medium. There is abnormal stranding in the adjacent perinephric fat.

Renal imaging cannot distinguish between the classical cortical abscess and that resulting from ascending infection within the urinary tract.

4. Treatment

At the same time that aspiration of the intrarenal abscess is carried out for diagnostic purposes, attempts should be made to remove as much pus as possible followed by insertion of a large bore drain. However, operative drainage of renal and perinephric abscesses with breakdown of loculations of pus is often still necessary (Morgan and Nyberg, 1985). Parenteral antibiotic therapy should be given for at least seven days followed by oral therapy for four weeks. For *Staph. aureus* flucloxacillin (1 g 6-hourly) or vancomycin (1 g 12-hourly adjusted for renal function) intravenously should be followed by oral flucloxacillin (Cattell, 1998). Antibiotic therapy for Gram-negative renal abscess is the same as for acute pyelonephritis (*Tables 14.4 and 14.5*).

VI Urolithiasis

Management of urinary infection complicating urinary stones involves early identification of the infecting organism, assessment of renal function, exclusion of urinary tract obstruction and measurement of the size and position of the stones (Morgan, 1998) (*Figure 14.9*). Urinary infection with stones requires antibiotic treatment before,

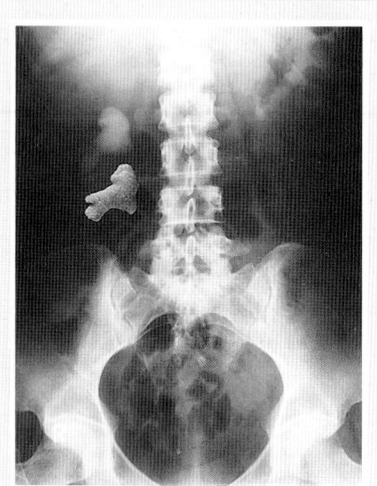

Figure 14.9
Staghorn calculus. Intravenous urogram showing staghorn calculus in right kidney with the surgically removed calculus superimposed.

during and after stone removal. Cure of any infection usually depends on the removal of the stones.

When pyonephrosis or a perirenal abscess complicate urinary obstruction and infection immediate drainage is necessary, usually by percutaneous nephrostomy under local anaesthesia. Definitive removal of urinary stones may not be possible until after drainage of the urinary tract and treatment of infection. Xanthogranulomatous pyelonephritis is a rare complication of urinary infection in the presence of stones.

VII Vesicoureteric reflux (VUR) and reflux nephropathy

The reasons why patients with VUR are prone to urinary infections are not clear. With severe VUR, stasis owing to the large volumes of refluxing urine probably plays a role. Whatever the relative roles of urinary tract infection and VUR in the pathogenesis of reflux nephropathy, new or progressive renal scarring is very uncommon in women (Bailey, 1988). Further progression of reflux nephropathy in adult women is independent of VUR or urinary tract infection.

Young women with acute pyelonephritis associated with onset of sexual activity may be shown to have reflux nephropathy not detected in infancy or early childhood. Correction of any continuing VUR in these patients is usually not warranted as surgery does not reduce the incidence of urinary infections. Antireflux surgery may be indicated in a few women with VUR and recurrent acute pyelonephritis. Urinary infections are usually easily controlled by good microbiological diagnosis, appropriate treatment and follow-up.

VIII Neurogenic bladder and urinary diversion

Women with bladder dysfunction owing to neurogenic disorders or a urinary diversion are prone to frequent urinary infections.

Intermittent self-catheterization, rather than continuous bladder drainage with a urethral catheter, has markedly reduced the incidence of urinary infection in women with a neurogenic bladder (Joiner and Lindan, 1982). Prophylactic antibiotic therapy appears to be ineffective in preventing symptomatic infections in these women. In patients with spinal injuries, clinical localization of urinary infection may be difficult. Asymptomatic bacteriuria should not be treated unless the woman is to undergo instrumentation of the urinary tract or prosthetic surgery, such as total hip replacement. Antibiotic therapy should be reserved for patients with fever, systemic upset and loin pain. Acute pyelonephritis in women with a neurogenic bladder or urinary diversion should be treated as a complicated infection.

IX Renal transplantation

1. Clinical features

Urinary tract infections are the most common bacterial and fungal infections affecting renal transplant recipients. In spite of improvements in assessment and management, urinary tract infection occurs in 35–45% of renal transplant patients and is a common cause of Gram-negative bacteraemia (Tolkoff-Rubin and Rubin, 1997). Acute pyelonephritis in a renal transplant recipient should always be considered a complicated infection.

In the early post-transplant period, infections are usually overt acute pyelonephritis with bacteraemia and a high rate of relapse. Acute pyelonephritis may be painless in renal transplant recipients, probably because of impairment of sympathetic nerve function (Meyrier and Guibert, 1992). In women with severe infection, reversible disturbances of transplant function are common. Later infections are usually limited to the lower urinary tract unless there is a persisting underlying anatomical or functional abnormality.

There are a number of reasons why renal transplantation is associated with a high incidence of urinary tract infection. The recipient may have infected urine at the time of surgery or, rarely, the donor kidney may be infected. Postoperatively, the presence of a urethral catheter and, if there is a ureteric problem, ureteric stents or nephrostomy tubes, increase the likelihood of infection. Early removal of the urethral catheter reduces the incidence of urinary tract infection. Most transplant units remove the urethral catheter 3–7 days after surgery. Ongoing immunosuppression and poor bladder function are further reasons for urinary infection in these patients. The presence of vesicoureteric reflux is probably not important as in experienced hands the type of ureteric implantation does not appear to be related to the incidence of urinary tract infections.

From about three months after transplantation, the pattern of urinary tract infection is not different from that of the general population.

2. Treatment

The management of acute pyelonephritis in the female renal transplant recipient is the same as for other forms of complicated acute pyelonephritis (*see Tables 14.2, 14.4 and 14.5*). Patients with recurrent infections will benefit from long-term antibiotic prophylaxis with nightly trimethoprim 100 mg, co-trimoxazole 480 mg or a fluoroquinolone, e.g. ciprofloxacin 250 mg (Rubin, 1993).

The management of asymptomatic fungal urinary infection involves the removal of any urethral catheter, if possible, and the exclusion of urinary obstruction by fungal balls. Renal transplant patients with candiduria are at risk of candidal pyelonephritis and septicaemia. Pre-emptive treatment of such patients with fluconazole or low-dose amphotericin plus flucytosine is warranted (Tolkoff-Rubin and Rubin, 1997). Fluconazole is active against most *Candida* spp. and achieves high urine concentrations after oral dosing.

X   Renal failure

Urinary tract infections are probably more common in women with chronic renal failure although the reasons for this are unclear. Treatment of acute pyelonephritis in women with renal failure poses significant problems. The dose reduction necessary to avoid toxicity and the reduced urinary excretion of drugs may result in ineffective concentrations in the urine and renal tissue of some antibiotics, such as aminoglycosides. Cephalosporins and β-lactam antibiotics are usually the most effective in the treatment of acute pyelonephritis in women with severe renal failure. In lesser degrees of renal failure, fluoroquinolones, trimethoprim and aminoglycosides are effective.

XI   Renal cystic disease

Acute pyelonephritis is common in patients with polycystic kidney disease and may be recurrent and difficult to eradicate when the infection becomes localized within a cyst (Muther and Bennett, 1981; Bennett et al., 1985). Bleeding into a cyst may cause symptoms similar to those associated with infection.

Infections in simple cysts are uncommon. It may be impossible to distinguish clinically between infection in a simple cyst and a renal abscess. Renal ultrasonography may show a fluid collection containing echoes. Fine-needle aspiration may be necessary to confirm the diagnosis.

XII   Xanthogranulomatous pyelonephritis

Xanthogranulomatous pyelonephritis is an uncommon condition of unknown cause that primarily affects older women and is commonly associated with stones or ureteric obstruction. Bilateral renal involvement is rare. The causative organism is usually *Proteus mirabilis* and less commonly *E. coli, Klebsiella* spp. or *Staph. aureus* or a combination of these organisms. The usual clinical presentation is with loin pain, intermittent fever, weight loss, general malaise and symptomatic anaemia. There is often a history of recurrent urinary tract infection and renal stones, and delays in diagnosis are common. A palpable renal mass is present in about half of those affected. The urine culture is usually positive and anaemia, leukocytosis and abnormal liver function tests may be present.

Intravenous urography usually shows focal or diffuse enlargement of the kidney with focal or multiple space-occupying lesions. There is no or little excretion of contrast in the affected areas. Calyces, when demonstrated, are often distorted or displaced. Urinary stones are present in about 75% of patients. Ultrasonography shows dilated calyces with low-level echoes surrounded by thickened hypoechoic parenchyma. CT scanning shows multiple low attenuation areas of soft-tissue density within the kidney, surrounded by thickened parenchyma and may demonstrate associated perinephric abscesses. The differential diagnoses are renal tuberculosis and renal cell carcinoma. In doubtful cases, modern imaging techniques and positive culture of a fine-needle aspirate usually make the diagnosis (Solomon et al., 1983). The diagnosis is still usually made after nephrectomy. Examination of nephrectomy specimens shows an enlarged kidney with either local or diffuse involvement. The cut surface is yellow with multiple abscesses and the perinephric fat is usually inflamed and adherent. The inflammation may extend into the retroperitoneal space. Histologically, there is diffuse replacement of the renal parenchyma with large foamy lipid-containing macrophages (xanthoma cells), neutrophils, plasma cells and necrotic debris. Foreign-body giant cells are frequently present. Antibiotics rarely eradicate the infection. Usually there is such extensive kidney damage that nephrectomy is necessary. Fortunately, the condition is usually unilateral and recurrence after nephrectomy has not been reported (Claes et al., 1987).

XIII   Malakoplakia

This rare condition usually involves the bladder but also may extend up the ureters to the pelvis and kidney (Long and Althausen, 1989). Malakoplakia occurs more commonly in women and the elderly and is usually secondary to urinary tract infection with *E. coli* or, more rarely, *Proteus mirabilis* or *Klebsiella pneumoniae*. Patients usually present with a history of recurrent or persistent frequency, dysuria and haematuria. Renal parenchymal involvement, which is more common in immunocompromised patients, may present with systemic upset, fever, loin pain and a palpable mass. Ureteral stenosis may occur with resultant obstructive uropathy or pyonephrosis.

The diagnosis is based on the cystoscopic finding of round yellow or red intravesical plaques which, on biopsy, show the diagnostic features of submucosal aggregates of macrophages containing inclusion bodies – the Michaelis–Gutmann body. The lesion is thought to result from a defect in the bactericidal function of monocytes and macrophages (Stevens and McClure, 1982). Intravenous urography may show small filling defects which may be indistinguishable from ureteropyelitis cystica or multiple epithelial tumours. Aggressive and prolonged antibacterial therapy is necessary. A course of six weeks followed by low-dose prophylaxis for twelve months has been recommended (Matthews et al., 1986).

XIV   Tuberculosis

Genitourinary tuberculosis may involve any part of the female genitourinary tract. Renal tuberculosis is an important form of non-lung tuberculosis which usually, but not exclusively, affects young adults. Renal

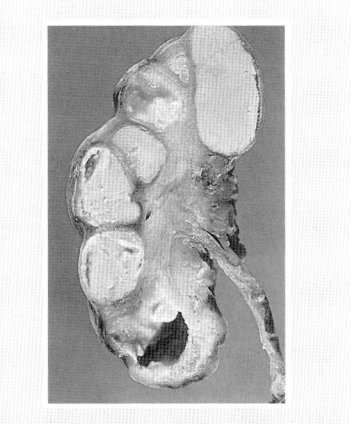

Figure 14.10
Renal tuberculosis. Kidney showing caseous necrosis and cavitation that has destroyed virtually all of the normal renal tissue.

reach the kidney by haematogenous spread, usually from the lungs, but occasionally from other sites such as the gut. Renal tuberculosis may occur at the same time as pulmonary presentation or many years after the apparent cure of the lung disease. The infection is frequently accompanied by involvement of the lower urinary tract, particularly the bladder.

There are two types of renal tuberculosis: miliary tuberculosis, as part of a general systemic involvement; and nodular or cavitating tuberculosis, with only the kidney affected (***Figure 14.10***).

The clinical presentations are summarized in *Table 14.6*. Up to 30% of patients do not have any genitourinary symptoms.

tuberculosis is usually caused by *Mycobacterium tuberculosis* or, more rarely, *M. bovis* or *M. africanum*. The organisms

1. Diagnosis

Examination of the urine reveals pyuria and haematuria with routine culture being sterile.

Table 14.6
Presentation of renal tuberculosis

Incidental finding as part of assessment of patient with pulmonary tuberculosis
Incidental finding of sterile pyuria
Symptoms of bladder inflammation
Haematuria
Renal colic from blood clot or sloughed renal papilla
Constitutional symptoms
Back pain and lumbar mass
Chronic renal failure
Acute renal failure due to tubulointerstitial nephritis
Genital tuberculosis

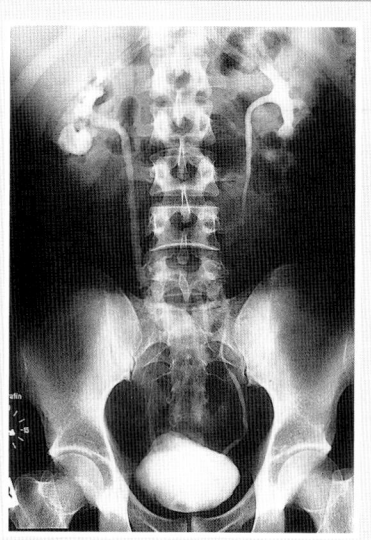

Figure 14.11
Renal tuberculosis. Intravenous urogram showing dilated and irregular right lower pole calyces with a filling defect suggestive of a sloughed renal papilla. The right upper pole calyces are irregular and slightly clubbed. The right ureter is irregular and slightly dilated to the level of the iliac vessels. The mucosa of the bladder appears thickened. The left kidney and upper urinary tract are normal.

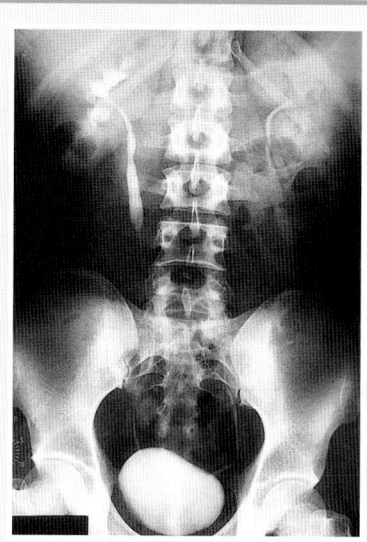

Figure 14.12
Renal tuberculosis. Intravenous urogram in same patient as shown in Figure 13.11 after antituberculous chemotherapy showing a stricture in the mid-lumbar right ureter with fullness and irregularity proximally but reduced dilatation of the calyces.

Bacteriological diagnosis requires the collection of three early-morning urine specimens and culture for acid-fast bacilli on Lowenstein–Jensen slopes. Newer techniques such as Bactec radiometric culture (Middlebrook et al., 1977) or the polymerase chain reaction (van Vollenhoven et al., 1996)

allow more rapid diagnosis. Renal function is usually normal but may be impaired if there is widespread parenchymal damage and patients may reach end-stage renal failure.

2. Radiology

Typically, urinary tract tuberculosis involves multiple sites (***Figure 14.11***). All patients

Table 14.7
Radiological features of renal tuberculosis

Dilatation of all or part of the pelvicalyceal system
Irregularity of minor calyces
Irregular cavities which may communicate with a calyx via an irregular track
Renal calcification
Ureteric stricture, frequently multiple, with proximal dilatation
Autonephrectomy as evidenced by a grossly distorted, calcified kidney on plane radiograph
Thick-walled, low-capacity bladder
Secondary VUR

should have a chest radiograph. Intravenous urography is the method of choice for renal imaging when tuberculosis is suspected. An intravenous urogram will document the extent of disease and the response to therapy (*Figure 14.12*). Both ultrasonography and CT scanning may show many of the renal abnormalities. The cardinal radiological features of renal tuberculosis are shown in *Table 14.7*.

3.   Treatment

Management of renal tuberculosis involves accurate assessment of the extent of disease, the nature and extent of ureteric obstruction, adequate bacteriological diagnosis, and assessment of renal function. Antituberculous chemotherapy is the mainstay of treatment. Routine radical surgery is not indicated in most patients. Surgery, if undertaken, does not obviate the need for chemotherapy. Cure should be possible in all patients. The renal functional outcome is related to the degree of renal parenchymal damage.

References

Atkinson LK, Goodship THJ, Ward MK (1986) Acute renal failure associated with acute pyelonephritis and consumption of non-steroidal anti-inflammatory drugs. *Br Med J* **292**: 97–8.

Bailey RR Vesicoureteric reflux and reflux nephropathy. In: Schrier RW, Gottschalk GW, eds. *Diseases of the Kidney*, 4th edn. Boston: Little, Brown, 1988: 747–83.

Bailey RR (1994a) Management of uncomplicated urinary tract infections. *Int J Microb Agents* **4**: 95–100.

Bailey RR (1994b) Duration of antimicrobial treatment and the use of drug combinations for the treatment of uncomplicated acute pyelonephritis. *Infection* **22**: S50–S52.

Bailey RR Cost-effectiveness and the management of uncomplicated urinary tract infections. In: Brumfitt W, Hamilton-Miller JMT, Bailey RR, eds. *Urinary Tract Infections*. London: Chapman & Hall Medical, 1998: 265–79.

Bailey RR, Lynn KL, Robson RA, Smith AH, Maling TMJ et al. (1996) DMSA renal scans in adults with acute pyelonephritis. *Clin Nephrol* **46**: 99–104.

Barclay ML, Begg EJ, Hickling KG (1994) What is the evidence for once-daily aminoglycoside therapy? *Clin Pharmacokinet* **27**: 32–48.

Bennett WM, Elzinga L, Pulliam JP, Rashad AL, Barry JM (1985) Cyst fluid antibiotic concentrations in autosomal-dominant polycystic kidney disease. *Am J Kidney Dis* **6**: 400–4.

Blomjous CEM, Meijer CJLM Pathology of urinary tract infections. In: Brumfitt, W, Hamilton-Miller JMT, Bailey RR, eds. *Urinary Tract Infections*. London: Chapman & Hall Medical, 1998: 17–35.

Cattell WR (1985) Urinary tract infections in adults – 1985. *Postgrad Med J* 61: 907–13.

Cattell WR The patient with urinary tract infections. In: Davison AM, Cameron JS, Grunfeld J, Kerr DNS, Ritz E, Winearls CG, eds. *Oxford Textbook of Clinical Nephrology*, 2nd edn. New York: Oxford University Press, 1998: 1252–9.

Claes H, Vereecken R, Oyen R, van Damme B (1987) Xanthogranulomatous pyelonephritis with emphasis on computerized tomography scan: retrospective study of 20 cases and literature review. *Urology* 29: 389–93.

Fraser IR, Birch D, Fairley KF, John S, Lichtenstein M et al. (1995) A prospective study of cortical scarring in acute febrile pyelonephritis in adults: clinical and bacteriological characteristics. *Clin Nephrol* 43: 159–64.

Fünfstück R, Smith JW, Tschäpe H, Stein G (1997) Pathogenetic aspects of uncomplicated urinary tract infection: recent advances. *Clin Nephrol* 47: 13–18.

Joiner E, Lindan R (1982) Experience with self intermittent catheterisation for women with neurological dysfunctions of the bladder. *Paraplegia* 20: 147–53.

Jones BF, Nanra RS, White KH (1991) Acute renal failure due to acute pyelonephritis. *Am J Nephrol* 11: 257–9.

Jones SR (1992) Acute renal failure in adults with uncomplicated acute pyelonephritis: case reports and review. *Clin Inf Dis* 14: 243–6.

Karabalut N, Drusano GL Pharmacokinetics of the quinolone antimicrobial agents. In: Hooper DC, Wolfson JS, eds. *Quinolone Antimicrobial Agents*, 2nd edn. Washington, DC: American Society of Microbiology, 1993: 195–223.

Long JP, Althausen AF (1989) Malacoplakia: a 25-year experience with a review of the literature. *J Urol* 141: 1328–31.

Matthews PN, Greenwood RN, Hendry WF, Cattell WR (1986) Extensive pelvic malacoplakia: observations on management. *J Urol* 135: 132–4.

Medical Research Council Bacteriuria Committee (1979) Recommended terminology of urinary-tract infection. *BMJ* ii: 717–19.

Meyrier A, Condamin M, Fernet M, Labigne-Roussel A, Simon P et al. (1989) Frequency of development of early cortical scarring in acute primary pyelonephritis. *Kidney Int* 35: 696–703.

Meyrier A. (1990) Long-term risks of acute pyelonephritis. *Nephron* 54: 197–201.

Meyrier A, Guibert J (1992) Diagnosis and drug treatment of acute pyelonephritis. *Drugs* 44: 356–67.

Middlebrook G, Reggiardo Z, Tigertt WD (1977) Automatable radiometric detection of growth of *Mycobacterium tuberculosis* in selective media. *Am Rev Resp Dis* 115: 1066–9.

Moreau JL, Royer-Morrot MJ, Lozniewski A, Trackoen G, Delavault P et al. (1996) Penetration of pefloxacin and its desmethyl metabolite into the uroepithelium after a 800 mg single oral dose in human patients. *Eur J Clin Pharm* 49: 401–5.

Morgan RJ Surgical management of urinary tract infections. In: Brumfitt W, Hamilton-Miller JMT, Bailey RR, eds. *Urinary Tract Infections*. London: Chapman & Hall Medical, 1998: 317–31.

Morgan WR, Nyberg LM (1985) Perinephric and intrarenal abscesses. *Urology* 26: 529–36.

Muther RS, Bennett WM (1981) Cyst fluid antibiotic concentrations in polycystic kidney disease: differences between proximal and distal cysts. *Kidney Int* 20: 519–22.

Rubin RH (1993) Infectious disease complications of renal transplantation. *Kidney Int* 44: 221–36.

Saiki J, Vaziri ND, Barton C (1982) Perinephric and intranephric abscesses: a review of the literature. *West J Med* 136: 95–102.

Solomon A, Braf Z, Papo J, Merimsky E (1983) Computerized tomography in xanthogranulomatous pyelonephritis. *J Urol* 130: 323–5.

Stamm WE, Hooton TM (1993) Management of urinary tract infections in adults. *N Engl J Med* 329: 1328–34.

Stevens S, McClure J (1982) The histochemical features of the Michaelis–Gutmann body and a consideration of the pathophysiological mechanisms of its formation. *J Pathol* 137: 119–27.

Svanborg Edén C, Hausson S, Jodal U, Lidin-Janson G, Lincoln K et al. (1988) Host–parasite interaction in the urinary tract. *J Infect Dis* 157: 421–6.

Talner LB, Davidson AJ, Lebowitz RL, Palma L, Goldman SM (1994) Acute pyelonephritis: Can we agree on terminology? *Radiology* 192: 297–305.

Tolkoff-Rubin NE, Rubin RH Urinary tract infection in the renal transplant recipient. In: Bergan T, ed. *Urinary Tract Infections. Infectiology*. Basel: Karger, 1997: 27–33.

Tsugaya M, Hirao N, Sakagami H, Ohtaguro K, Washida H (1992) Renal cortical scarring in acute pyelonephritis. *Brit J Urol* 69: 245–9.

van Vollenhoven P, Heyns CF, de Beer PM, Whitaker P, van Helden PD et al. (1996) Polymerase chain reaction in the diagnosis of urinary tract tuberculosis. *Urol Res* 24: 107–11.

Instrumentation and catheterization: risks and remedies

Peter L Dwyer and Suzanne M Garland

15

Contents

I Introduction

Instrumentation of the lower urinary tract by urethral catheterization is the commonest procedure performed in hospitals, occurring in one in five of all admissions (Stevens et al., 1981). Urinary tract infection (UTI) occurs in approximately one in three of all patients catheterized in hospital and is the cause of 40% of all hospital-associated infections (Haley et al., 1985). Urinary tract instrumentation and catheterization is implicated in 80% of all nosocomially acquired genitourinary tract infections (Meares, 1991). Women with catheter-associated bacteriuria may be asymptomatic or be unwell with pyrexia and urinary tract symptoms. Urinary infections usually respond quickly to catheter removal and/or antibiotic treatment but can occasionally lead to acute and chronic pyelonephritis, bacteremia and death and have significant financial implications for both hospital and community health services. Platt et al. (1982) found that patients with hospital-associated UTIs had three times the mortality rate of matched non-bacteriuric patients. Moreover, women with bacteremic UTI who had an indwelling urethral catheter have a higher mortality rate than non-catheterized bacteremic patients (Kreger et al., 1980). Women with urinary tract infection have a 1–4% risk of bacteremia, which has a one in 10 mortality rate (Bryan and Reynold, 1984).

Bladder catheterization is generally used for temporary or long-term bladder drainage by either the urethral or percutaneous suprapubic route. Pathogenic micro-organisms may enter the bladder from the periurethral or perineal areas at the time of catheter insertion. Nevertheless, the technique of catheterization in the normal healthy bladder may not be of such relevance, as randomized studies of sterile to non-sterile urethral catheterization technique have shown no statistical difference in outcome of development of UTI (Carapeti et al., 1996). With indwelling catheters uropathogenic micro-organisms can also gain access into the bladder along the catheter–mucosal interface or intraluminally along the inner surface of the catheter from colonized drainage systems or catheter junction sites. In women, most catheter-associated urinary tract infections occur secondary to intraluminal catheter spread of organisms of anorectal origin, which subsequently colonize the periurethral area and the urinary tract (Daifuku and Stamm, 1984). In males the majority of catheter-related infections occur via the intraluminal route, are not of anorectal origin and often result from cross-infection. Cross-infection from patient to patient can also occur through the use of inadequately sterilized equipment such as cystoscopes or urodynamic equipment (Climo et al., 1997). Instrumentation of the lower urinary tract is also performed for a variety of diagnostic and therapeutic indications. Diagnostic procedures used in the evaluation of lower urinary tract function and structure which require instrumentation include cystourethroscopy, and urodynamic and radiological investigations. Increasingly, lower urinary tract instrumentation may also be used for placement of semipermanent devices such as urethral or ureteric stents, and urethral occlusive valves or plugs which are used to normalize urinary tract function (*Figure 15.1*). One of the major problems of all these implants is urinary tract colonization by bacteria growing in biofilms and encrustations, with or without calculi formation, which protect these organisms from antimicrobial agents.

More recently the bloodborne virus epidemics of HIV/AIDS and hepatitis B and C have refocused medical attention on the importance of good infection control practices such as appropriate aseptic techniques, instrument sterilization and standard (previously known as 'universal') blood and body fluid precautions. All contact with blood and body substances should be seen as a potential source of infection. The risks of cross-infection associated with medical procedures have become highly emotive public health issues in various countries since reports of patients becoming HIV positive following simple surgical procedures (Centers for Disease Control, 1992; Chant et al., 1993;

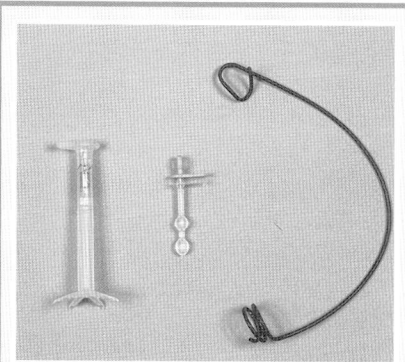

Figure 15.1
Devices implanted into the urinary tract to normalize urinary function. From the right: a ureteric stent (Bard) for ureteric obstruction; the Viva intraurethral plug (Pharma-plast International) for stress incontinence; and the urethral valve prosthesis (Influence Inc.) for urinary retention secondary to an acontractile bladder.

Incident Investigation Team, 1997). This does highlight the importance of an appropriate level of eradication of micro-organisms, firstly by mechanical cleaning, and secondly by disinfection or sterilization of instruments used in the lower urinary tract.

II Single urethral catheterization

Single in/out urethral catheterization may be performed:

- to overcome a temporary impairment of bladder emptying such as may occur postoperatively or following epidural anesthesia;
- to collect urine for microscopy and culture when other approaches to obtain a clean voided midstream specimen have failed;
- to estimate the postvoid residual volume when ultrasonic estimation is not possible;
- prior to surgery to ensure the bladder is empty, so that it will neither be damaged nor be an obstruction for surgical access.

The risk of UTI following in/out urethral catheterization has been estimated to be between 1% and 2% (Turck et al., 1962) but may be higher in women with incomplete bladder emptying (Dwyer and Welstab, 1993), in pregnancy and postpartum (Brumfitt et al., 1961) and when immunological competence has been compromised by drugs, age or disease, e.g. diabetes.

In healthy women urethral catheterization using an aseptic technique introduces only a small quantity of micro-organisms into the bladder which are readily cleared by the normal urinary tract defenses. In high-risk patients or when significant bacteriuria is already present, single-dose antibiotic prophylaxis with nitrofurantoin, trimethoprim or trimethoprim sulfamethoxazole would be appropriate. For short term indwelling urinary catheterization, strict adherence to a closed catheter drainage system assists in preventing development of a UTI.

III   Urodynamic and radiological evaluation of the lower urinary tract

Urodynamic studies are common investigative procedures used in both sexes for the assessment of urinary incontinence, voiding difficulties and other lower urinary tract symptoms. The storage and emptying functions of the lower urinary tract are evaluated by measuring the pressure–volume relationship during bladder filling and pressure–urinary flow relationship during bladder emptying. Small-diameter (8 Fr) urethral catheters are inserted to measure bladder and urethral pressure during bladder filling and emptying. A further catheter is placed in either the vagina or rectum to measure abdominal pressure. Intravesical pressure is calculated by subtracting intra-abdominal pressure from total bladder pressure. Radiological visualization of the lower urinary tract can be performed synchronously with urodynamic pressure measurements by filling the bladder with radiolucent material or as a separate procedure (micturating cystourethrography). In both procedures the duration of catheterization is approximately 30 minutes.

Significant bacteriuria has been reported to occur in 15% (Payne et al., 1988) to 18% (Baker et al., 1991) of women following urodynamic investigations. The incidence of bacteriuria is considerably higher following urodynamic studies than in/out or short-term indwelling urethral catheterization. Urodynamic investigations take longer to perform and may involve multiple catheterizations. Urodynamic equipment and catheters can also be a source of infection (Climo et al., 1997) when tubing lines and transducers are inadequately sterilized and reused. Although significant bacteriuria may be detected on a clean-catch urine specimen a few days following urodynamic studies, most patients do not develop symptomatic infections, as bacteria clear spontaneously with the physiological flushing of bladder emptying. Prospective studies (Baker et al., 1991; Cundiff et al., 1999) have shown that routine antibiotic prophylaxis is not effective in preventing UTIs following multichannel urodynamic investigations.

In our urogynecology department the prevalence of unsuspected bacteriuria (>10^5 organisms per ml) in women presenting for urodynamic evaluation was reported as 7.3% (Dwyer and Welstab, 1993). Bacteriuria was significantly more prevalent in women with impaired bladder emptying (19%) than in women with normal micturition (5.4%). *Escherichia coli* (63%) and *Klebsiella pneumoniae* (15%) were the commonest

organisms isolated. There was no difference between the type of organisms isolated in women with normal and those with impaired micturition. In view of this high incidence of unsuspected UTI, we recommend routine testing of urine prior to urodynamic evaluation so that therapy can be initiated and guided by susceptibility results. Alternatively, dip reagent strips can be used at the time of assessment to detect pyuria (wbc esterase), protein and nitrates which can indicate an underlying Gram-negative bacteriuria but will not detect (the less frequent) Gram-positive infection. Antibiotic prophylaxis should be used in women with significant bacteriuria or high-risk patients who have diabetes, voiding dysfunction or a history of recurrent UTIs.

IV Endoscopic instrumentation of the urinary tract

Cystourethroscopy may be performed in the diagnostic assessment of lower urinary tract structure, to exclude anatomical abnormality or urological disorders as a cause of patient symptoms. Endoscopy is also a valuable therapeutic tool in the female, with procedures such as bladder biopsy for diagnostic purposes to exclude malignancy (*Figure 15.2*), injections of bulking agents into the urethra for stress incontinence (Gax-collagen or particulate silicone), transvesical injections of phenol in the treatment of

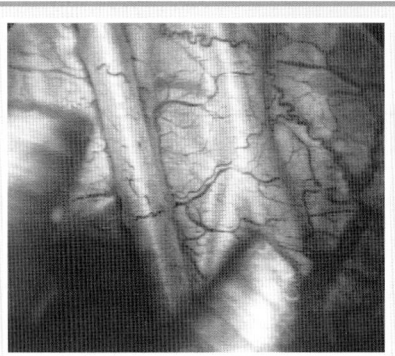

Figure 15.2
Cystoscopic photography of a biopsy forceps and trabeculated bladder wall.

unstable bladder, resection of bladder tumors, removal of foreign bodies or calculi and ureteric catheterization.

Women with sterile urine undergoing diagnostic cystoscopy have a low risk of developing bacteriuria although there are potential added risks from the irrigating fluid and urinary tract trauma. Appell et al. (1980), in a male population, found a 38.7% incidence of urinary infection after transurethral resection of bladder tumor, compared with 11.2% after transurethral prostate resection and 4.7% after routine cystoscopy. In one review of transurethral surgery, Christensen and Madsen, 1990) found that patients with preoperative bacteremia have a 60% change of developing

bacteremia with a 10% risk of septicemia. Women undergoing endoscopic urinary tract surgery should be screened preoperatively for bacteriuria and, if present, should be treated according to the sensitivity profile for the pathogen identified. If immediate surgery is required for women with bacteriuria, gentamicin 5–7 mg/kg intravenously should be given daily (Victorian Drug Usage Advisory Committee, 1998).

Antibacterial chemoprophylaxis for women with sterile urine having transurethral surgery is more controversial, although most authorities believe it is useful in reducing infection rates following surgery. Antibiotics should be used that cover the spectrum and resistance of organisms causing urinary tract infection locally. Suitable prophylactic antibiotics for endoscopic transurethral surgery, vaginal and abdominal gynecological surgery are cephalothin 2 g or cephazolin 1 g intravenously, at the time of induction plus either tinidazole 2 g 6–12 hours prior to induction or metronidazole 500 mg as an intravenous infusion at the time of induction. Alternatively, cefotetan 2 g or cefoxitin 2 g intravenously can be used as a single agent at the time of induction (Victorian Drug Usage Advisory Committee, 1998).

V   Long-term bladder catheterization

Indwelling bladder catheters are estimated to be used in one in 10 patients in nursing homes (Warren et al., 1989) and hospitals (Kunin and M'Cormach, 1966). Bacteriuria is an inevitable consequence of long-term catheterization; following urethral catheterization there is a 5–10% daily increment in the prevalence of bacteriuria increasing to virtually 100% in women with long-term urethal catheterization (Kunin and M'Cormach, 1966). Following catheter removal, the bacteriuria will resolve spontaneously in a third of cases (Harding et al., 1991). The remainder continue to have asymptomatic bacteriuria with many eventually developing symptomatic UTIs.

Over the last 25 years the prevalence of catheter-associated UTIs has decreased considerably (Stamm, 1991). Various reasons for this include less frequent catheterization of shorter duration, increasing use of chemoprophylaxis and better catheter care by more informed nursing and medical staff. In the 1960s, the change from open to closed urinary drainage systems halved infection rates (Kunin and M'Cormach, 1966). Although the introduction of disposable closed drainage systems has prevented infection, breaking of closed urinary systems still occurs. A recent survey of 1153 nursing staff in Danish hospitals (Zimakoff et al., 1995) found that 25% of respondents opened the drainage system to collect urine for analysis, 58% to perform bladder washouts and 76% to change the catheter bags. These violations of catheter care occur despite national guidelines stressing

the importance of maintaining a closed system. These indiscretions in catheter care have led to the development of sealed drainage systems, which are more expensive but may still be cost-effective overall with the resultant lower incidence of UTI.

Other strategies such as daily application of antiseptics or antimicrobials to the periurethral area, use of antibiotic urethral lubricants, and prophylactic antiseptics or antibiotics for bladder irrigation and in drainage bags have not been shown to be effective in reducing infection rates and are not recommended.

Changes to catheter design have been made to reduce the risk of urinary infection and other catheter-related problems. Latex catheters, which may be responsible for inflammatory urethral strictures with long-term usage, have been replaced by smoother and more biocompatible catheters made from teflon, silicone, silicone elastimar coated latex and hydrogel coated latex (*Figure 15.3*). These newer catheters are easier to insert, are less irritant to urethral and bladder mucosa and cause less catheter encrustation, but have not been shown to reduce the incidence of catheter-associated infections. Although catheters impregnated with antibiotics were not found to reduce the incidence of catheter-related UTI (Butler and Kunin, 1968), more recently silver alloy-coated catheters had a lower infection rate compared to conventional catheters. In a study by Lindberg and

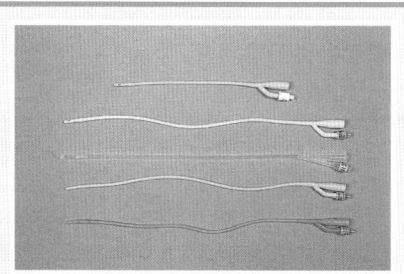

Figure 15.3
Various types of indwelling male and female Foley catheters: latex, teflon, silicone and silver oxide coated.

Lundeberg (1990) where 221 patients were catheterized for up to six days, the incidence of bacteriuria was 10% in patients catheterized with silver-coated latex catheters compared to 37% in patients catheterized with teflon-coated latex catheters. Silver has a broad-spectrum antimicrobial activity although the exact mode of its action is unknown. Gabriel et al. (1995), in an in vitro study using a radiolabeled leucine cell assay, found reduced adherence of bacteria to silver-treated silicone or latex catheters compared with the standard latex or silicone catheters. In contrast, a further study by Johnson et al. (1990) failed to show any improvement in

infection rates in patients using the silver alloy-coated catheters.

Collection leg bags and catheter valves have made the use of long-term catheterization less intrusive on normal living. A one-way catheter valve inserted into the end of the catheter replacing the closed collection system has been shown to improve patient satisfaction (92% vs 35%), without increasing the risk of infection (Wilson et al., 1997).

Permanent indwelling catheters should be the treatment of last resort because catheter-related problems such as infection, catheter blockage with bypass and stone formation are common and have a serious deleterious effect on lifestyle and general health. Therefore, proper evaluation by experienced medical personnel is essential before the decision is made for long-term catheterization, with all other therapeutic options having been considered or tried. Newer treatments for genuine stress incontinence and detrusor instability make the need for a permanent indwelling catheter uncommon. Intractable urinary incontinence or urinary retention, usually in the elderly or the mentally or neurologically impaired, are the major indications for long-term bladder catheterization. In women with urinary retention from neurogenic or non-neurogenic causes, intermittent urethral or suprapubic catheterization may be better options for short-term and long-term needs (Dwyer and Desmedt, 1994). Other methods to facilitate impaired bladder emptying are simple advice, e.g. double voiding, abdominal tapping, vibrating devices (the Queen's Square stimulator; Dasgupta et al., 1997) and the use of drugs which improve bladder emptying. The goals of bladder management strategies are social continence, with improvement in quality of life, while preserving normal renal function.

Catheter-associated bacteriuria generally only requires treatment if there are signs of systemic infection. For symptomatic patients, treatment of bacteriuria is with appropriate oral or systemic antibiotics and removal and/or replacement of the urethral catheter. Bacteria grow in biofilms on the inner surface of catheters and promote encrustation and stone formation, particularly by *Proteus* and *Morganella* species. Catheter encrustation can cause catheter blockage and stasis and may protect bacteria from bacterial agents, so a change of catheter is important for bacteria eradication.

VI Intermittent urethral catheterization

Intermittent catheterization was introduced in the mid-1960s to replace indwelling catheters in spinal injury patients with chronic urinary retention. It resulted in a lower incidence of UTI and an improvement in quality of life (Guttman and Frankel, 1964). In 1972 Lapides et al. described the method of clean

intermittent catheterization where patients were taught to pass clean, non-sterile urethral catheters per urethra at regular intervals during the day (*Figure 15.4*). This method of bladder emptying is now the treatment of choice in all patients with chronic urinary retention who have adequate manual dexterity and ability to learn this relatively simple technique.

Clean intermittent catheterization (CIC) is an excellent method to ensure regular bladder emptying, to minimize the risk of UTI and bladder distension from chronic urinary retention which can lead to upper urinary tract dilatation and damage. Bakke et al. (1977), in a prospective study of 170 patients (84 men and 86 women) with a mean duration of CIC use of 8.8 years, found that 65% of patients had had no symptoms of urinary tract infection, 29% had minor symptoms whilst 6% had had major symptoms of infection. Bacteriuria was found in 61% of urine samples, with *Escherichia coli* being the dominant organism in women and Gram-positive cocci in men. The incidence of sterile urine was 31% in patients who did not use antibiotics compared to 54% in patients using antibiotics. Women reported more infection than did men and patients with UTI had the highest mean catheterization volume. These authors conclude that patients using CIC need to catheterize sufficiently often to ensure that the mean volume of each catheterization is less than 400 ml (in adults)

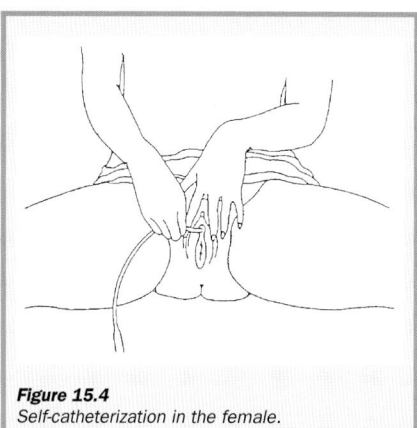

Figure 15.4
Self-catheterization in the female.

VII Transcutaneous suprapubic catheterization

The bladder can be accessed for temporary or long-term bladder drainage by the transcutaneous suprapubic route. Suprapubic catheters have been shown to be associated with a lower incidence of urinary infection and to be more comfortable for postoperative patients (Bonnano et al., 1970). It is not known whether the lower incidence of UTI is secondary to the avoidance of repeated urethral catheterization or to the lower density and diversity of skin flora of abdominal skin compared to periurethral area. As yet, the advantages of short-term bladder drainage by the transabdominal route have not been shown to apply to long-term use.

There are a variety of suprapubic catheters available. Small-diameter suprapubic catheters (Bonnano, Becton-Dickinson Ltd.; Stamey, Cook Inc.; Cystocath, Dow Corning Corp.) are commonly used for postoperative bladder drainage and are passed through small suprapubic stab incisions into the distended bladder under local, regional or general anesthesia (*Figure 15.5*). For more long-term bladder drainage, a wider diameter Foley silastic catheter can be passed into the bladder using a specifically designed trocar (Addi-Cath) in a similar manner. If the bladder cannot be distended beyond 300 ml, due to either severe detrusor instability or bladder fibrosis, the suprapubic catheter should be

and that antibiotics should be used sparingly and only for symptomatic UTI. Antibiotic therapy needs to be based on culture and sensitivity results (with the urine collected with a needle and syringe from the sample arm of the catheter, not from the bag of the collection system) and the catheter needs to be removed as soon as possible. Repeated courses of antibiotics lead to the development of antimicrobial-resistant bacterial strains as well as yeast infections due to *Candida* species without reducing morbidity from UTI.

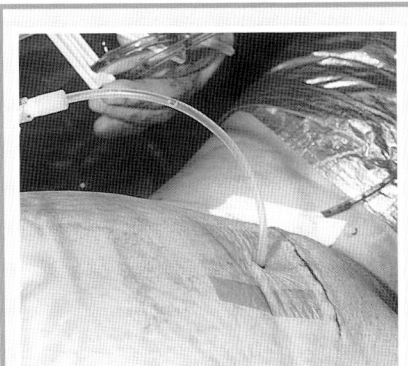

Figure 15.5
Postoperative bladder drainage following a Burch colposuspension using a Stamey suprapubic catheter.

In a survey of practices of bladder drainage amongst gynecologists in the British Isles published in 1988, Hilton found that 51% of gynecologists preferred the urethral route for routine postoperative bladder drainage, 39% the suprapubic route and 10% had no preference. There was also a trend of preference for the suprapubic catheterization in the younger and more recently graduated gynecologists.

VIII   Postoperative bladder drainage

Normal bladder function may be impaired following surgery as a result of surgical trauma, edema, partial bladder dennervation or pain. Bladder impairment may also be secondary to physical or mental impairment, anesthetic drugs or regional anesthesia. If urinary retention occurs postoperatively, early detection and adequate bladder drainage are required to prevent bladder distension which can cause prolonged urinary dysfunction and urinary infection. Sonography is increasingly becoming available on all postoperative wards and avoids the need for repeated urethral catheterization to detect urinary retention. The risk of impaired voiding following abdominal or pelvic surgery needs to be assessed to decide whether bladder drainage is necessary and, if so, by which route and for how long.

inserted by open cystotomy, by cutting down onto a bladder sound passed transurethrally into the bladder (Feneley, 1983). In meta-analysis of studies comparing suprapubic to transurethral catheterization following vaginal surgery, Schiotz (1992) found that the incidence of postoperative bacteriuria (with or without clinical infection) ranged from 12.5% to 44.5% for suprapubic catheterization and 37.2% to 50.7% for urethral catheterization. Patients with a suprapubic catheter can void with the catheter in situ and have residual urine measured without catheter removal, which reduces patient discomfort and saves nursing time.

The urinary tract is the commonest source

of infection following abdominal and gynecological surgery with bacteriuria and/or symptomatic UTI reported in 35–50% of all women postoperatively who do not receive surgical chemoprophylaxis (Ireland et al., 1982; Schiotz, 1994). In many women the bacteriuria is asymptomatic, the bacteriuria clearing without treatment in most cases (Schiotz, 1994). However, postoperative urinary catheterization is not the only reason for this as there is a high incidence of bacteriuria (Ireland et al., 1982) following pelvic surgery in women who do not have the postoperative catheterization. Urinary infection may also be related to trauma to the lower urinary tract during gynecological surgery or impaired bladder emptying which does not result in urinary retention and catheterization.

Intraoperative chemoprophylaxis is in common use and has been shown to reduce postoperative pyrexia and morbidity (van der Wall et al., 1992) although it remains to be proven whether once-only antibiotics are of any value in the prevention of UTI in women with continuous postoperative bladder drainage. Continuation of antibiotic prophylaxis in patients with a urinary catheter is not recommended because this practice leads to colonization of more resistant bacterial strains.

Postoperative UTI can be minimized by the judicious use of postoperative bladder drainage for the shortest duration and only when necessary, the use of suprapubic rather than urethral bladder drainage, and perioperative prophylactic antibiotics.

IX   Infection control and urogenital instrumentation

In any healthcare setting, the primary aims of infection control are to prevent transmission of infection from patient to patient or between healthcare workers and to prevent staff acquiring infections from patients or transmitting infection to patients. Infection control is largely a matter of risk management and involves balancing the costs and consequences of specific infection control procedures against benefits that arise from their application.

There are various levels of micro-organism eradication, which are appropriate to different clinical situations. *Sterilization* means the complete destruction and eradication of micro-organisms, including bacterial spores. Sterilization is generally achieved by autoclaving (steam under pressure), a process which must be monitored and quality controlled according to strict standards. Newer systems for heat-sensitive equipment include low temperature peraretic acid (e.g. Steris) and hydrogen peroxide plasma (e.g. Sterrad) sterilization. *Disinfection*, however, means inactivation of vegetative bacteria, viruses and fungi but not necessarily of bacterial spores. In contrast, *cleaning* (an essential step prior to sterilization or disinfection) is the removal of soil and hence the reduction in numbers of micro-organisms from the surface and is usually achieved by washing in detergent.

1. Appropriate instrument processing

Good infection control is more than just implementation of standard precautions. It requires an understanding of safe work practices and quality assurance, as well as an assessment of the risk of infection for any particular procedure under investigation. Therefore, appropriate processing of instruments and equipment will depend largely on the risk of infection associated with the procedures for which they are to be utilized.

(i) High-risk procedures

For high-risk (critical) procedures – that is, those which involve penetration of skin, membranes or other tissues – prevention of contamination of the site with endogenous microbial flora and avoidance of cross-infection of bloodborne pathogens are essential. In this setting, it is imperative that any instrument used is sterile and is either a single-use sterilized item or a reusable item that has been decontaminated and then sterilized (Royal Australian College of GPs,

1994; Australian Standard, 1998). Hence, for any instrument which is to be utilized in an invasive procedure involving either sterile sites or puncture of skin or mucous membranes, disinfection only is an inappropriate and potentially litigious practice.

Therefore, for any invasive urogynecological procedure (e.g. bladder biopsy or resection, suprapubic urinary catheter installation), any instrument utilized for skin or mucous membrane puncture must be sterilized, preferably by steam autoclave. For instruments which cannot be autoclaved, other alternatives such as ethylene oxide, peracetic acid (Steris system) or hydrogen peroxide (Sterrad system) sterilization should be considered. Those clinicians who opt to purchase their own table-top steam sterilizer must ensure that it is one which complies with the appropriate standards for the country and also that they monitor and quality control the instrument as per accepted guidelines.

The low temperature plasma sterilization (Sterrad) system uses a lower temperature (<45°C) hydrogen peroxide plasma to achieve rapid sterilization for heat- and moisture-sensitive devices. This low humidity system allows for processing of moisture-sensitive devices without damaging sophisticated electronic circuitry and can be used to sterilize metal as well as non-metal instruments. The hydrogen peroxide is vaporized during the procedure and broken down to form oxygen and water vapor; hence no toxic byproducts are released. The turnaround time of sterilization is within a 75 minute cycle.

The peracetic acid sterilization (Steris) system is also a relatively new low-temperature sterilization system, the active ingredient of which is peracetic acid, a liquid chemical sterilant which is an effective biocide with no toxic residue, and is suitable for heat-sensitive endoscopic equipment. This is an automated wet system (items are wet when removed for sterilization) and hence particularly suited for heat sensitive endoscopes which will tolerate <55°C and where a fast turnaround is required.

(ii)   Medium-risk procedures

Medium-risk (or semicritical) instruments include those used in contact with intact mucous membranes; for example, vaginal specula, vaginal ultrasound, cystoscope or pressure transducer. Instruments used where the level of risk is semicritical require, at minimum, high-level disinfection but preferably sterilization. Before disinfection, however, the instruments must be cleaned and dried; instruments must not be stored in disinfectants. Methods of high-level disinfection include *thermal* disinfection (a minimum of 5 minutes uninterrupted boiling) or *chemical* disinfection (20 minutes immersion in 2% activated glutaraldehyde and then thorough rinsing with flowing water

before patient use). Glutaraldehyde, a cold disinfectant, is bactericidal, fungicidal, slowly sporicidal and variably tuberculocidal. However, attempts are being made to phase out the use of glutaraldehyde because of safety issues with respect to toxicity of fumes and sensitivity of healthcare workers to the disinfectant (skin and eye irritation). These risks can be controlled, however, by ensuring proper ventilation, good work practices and personal protective equipment (gloves, goggles, etc.) (Australian Standard, 1998).

Potential sources of infection associated with vaginal transducers include those organisms transmitted by blood and genital secretions such as HIV, HBV, HCV, CMV, *Neisseria gonorrhoeae*, *Chlamydia trachomatis* and *Trichomonas vaginalis*. Whilst, in general, covers for vaginal ultrasound transducers are recommended (Garland and de Crepigny, 1996), it is recognized that 3% of gloves and 7% of condoms used to sheath a transducer show evidence of perforation after removal (Jimenez and Duff, 1993). Therefore, it is imperative that as well as ensuring an appropriate cover, appropriate cleaning of the transducers between patients is carried out (Garland and de Crispigny, 1996)

Non-flexible cystoscopes are readily autoclavable and hence this is the preferred method. For flexible cystoscopes which cannot be autoclaved, high-level disinfection with glutaraldehyde is recommended.

(iii)   Low-risk procedures

Low-risk instrumentation involves contact with intact skin (e.g. abdominal ultrasonography). In these situations it is sufficient to clean either with an alcohol wipe, which kills vegetative bacteria and lipid-containing viruses and is fungicidal and tuberculocidal, or clean with soap and water, and allow to dry (Royal Australian College of GPs, 1994; Australian Standard, 1998).

X   Conclusion

Urinary infection is a potential complication of urinary tract instrumentation with possibly serious sequelae. Instrumentation of the urinary tract is one of the commonest procedures performed and is used for short- and long-term bladder drainage and for the investigation and treatment of urinary disorders. Adequate infection control, chemoprophylaxis and appropriate use of urinary catheters can reduce the incidence of UTI caused by instrumentation.

References

Appell RA, Flynn JT, Paris AM, Blandy JP (1980) Occult bacterial colonization of bladder tumours. *J Urol* 124: 345–6.

Australian Standard (1988) Cleaning, disinfection and sterilization of reusable medical and surgical intruments and equipment, and maintenance of associated environments in health care facilities. AS4187, 1998, second edition, Sydney.

Baker KR, Drutz HP, Barnes MD (1991) Effectiveness of antibiotic prophylaxis in preventing bacteriuria after multichannel urodynamic investigations: a blind randomized study in 124 female patients. *Am J Obstet Gynecol* 165: 679–81.

Bakke A, Digranes A, Hoisaeter PA (1997) Physical predictors of infection in patients treated with clean intermittent catheterization: a prospective 7 year study. *Br J Urol* 79: 85–90.

Bonanno PJ, Landers DE, Rock DE (1970) Bladder drainage with the suprapubic catheter needle. *Obstet Gynecol* 35: 807–12.

Brumfitt W, Davies BI, Rosser E (1961) Urethral catheter as a cause of urinary infection in pregnancy and puerperium. *Lancet* ii: 1059–62.

Bryan CS, Reynold K (1984) Hospital-acquired bacteremic urinary tract infection: epidemiology and outcome. *J Urol* 132: 494–8.

Butler HK, Kunin CM (1968) Evaluation of polymyxin catheter lubricant and impregnated catheters. *J Urol* 100: 560–8.

Carapeti EA, Andrews SM, Bentley PG (1996) Randomised study of sterile versus non sterile urethral catheterization. *Ann Roy Coll Surg Engl* 78: 59–60.

Centers for Disease Control (1992) Update: Investigations of patients who have been treated by HIV-infected health-care workers. *Morbid Mortal Wkly Rep* **41**: 344–6.

Chant K, Lowe D, Rubin G et al. (1993) Patient to patient transmission of HIV in private surgical consulting rooms (letter). *Lancet* **342**: 1548–9.

Christensen MM, Madsen PO (1990) Antimicrobial prophylaxis in transurethral surgery. *Urology* **35** (suppl): 11–14.

Climo MW, Pastor A, Wong ES (1997) An outbreak of *Psuedomonas aeruginosa* related to contaminated urodynamic equipment. *Infect Control Hosp Epidemiol* **18**: 509–10.

Cundiff G, McClennan M, Bent AE (1999) Randomized trial of antibiotic prophylaxis for combined urodynamics and cystourethroscopy. *Obstet Gynecol* **93**: 749–52.

Daifuku R, Stamm WE (1984) Association of rectal and urethral colonization with urinary tract infection in patients with indwelling catheters. *JAMA* **252**: 2028–30.

Dasgupta P, Haslam R, Goodwin R, Fowler CJ (1997) The 'Queen's Square bladder stimulator'. A device for assisting emptying of the neurogenic bladder. *Br J Urol* **80**: 234–7.

Dwyer PL, Desmedt E (1994) Impaired bladder emptying in women. *Aust NZ J Obstet Gynaecol* **34**: 73–8.

Dwyer PL, Welstab J (1993) Urinary tract infection and impaired bladder emptying in the female. *Int Urogynecol J* **4**: 328 (abst).

Feneley RC (1983) The management of female incontinence by suprapubic catheterisation with or without urethral closure. *Br J Urol* **55**: 203–7.

Gabriel MM, Sawant AD, Simmons RB, Ahearn DG (1995) Effects of silver on adherence of bacteria to urinary catheters: in vitro studies. *Curr Microbiol* **30**: 17–22.

Garland SM, de Crespigny L (1996) Prevention of infections in obstetric and gynaecological ultrasound practice. *Ultrasound Obstet Gynaecol* **7**: 1–4.

Guttman I, Frankel H (1964) The value of intermittent catheterization in the early management of traumatic paraplegia and tetraplegia. *Paraplegia* **4**: 63–84.

Haley RW, Culver DH, Waite JW, Morgan WM, Emori TG (1985) The national nosocomial infection rate. A new need for new vital statistics. *Am J Epidermiol* **121**: 159–67.

Harding GKM, Nicolle LE, Ronald AR et al. (1991) How long should catheter acquired urinary infection in women be treated? A randomised controlled trial. *Ann Intern Med* **114**: 713–19.

Hilton P (1988) Bladder drainage: a survey of practices among gynaecologists in the British Isles. *Br J Obstet Gynaecol* **95**: 1178–89.

Incident Investigation Teams and Others (1997) Transmission of hepatitis B to patients from four infected surgeons without hepatitis B e antigen. *N Engl J Med* **336**: 178–84.

Ireland D, Tacchi D, Bint AJ (1982) Effect of single dose prophylactic co-trimoxazole on the incidence of gynaecological postoperative urinary tract infection. *Br J Obstet Gynaecol* **89**: 578–80.

Jimenez R, Duff P (1993) Sheathing of the endovaginal ultrasound probe: is it adequate? *Infect Dis Obstet Gynaecol* **1**: 37–9.

Johnson JR, Roberts PL, Olsen RJ, Moyer KA, Stamm WE (1990) Prevention of catheter associated urinary tract infections with a silver oxide-coated urinary catheter: clinical and microbiological correlators. *J Infect Dis* **162**: 1145–50.

Kreger BE, Craven DE, Carling PC, McCabe WR (1980) Gram negative bacteremia: III. Reassessment of etiology, epidemiology and ecology in 612 patients. *Am J Med* **68**: 332–43.

Kunin CM, M'Cormach RC (1966) Prevention of catheter-induced urinary tract infection by sterile closed drainage. *N Engl J Med* **274**: 1155–61.

Lapides J, Diokno AC, Silber S, Lowe B (1972) Clean intermittent self-catheterization in the treatment of urinary tract disease. *J Urol* **107**: 458–61.

Linberg H, Lundeburg T (1990) Silver alloy coated catheters reduce catheter associated bacteriuria. *Br J Urol* **65**: 379–81.

Meares EM (1991) Current patterns in nosocomial urinary tract infections. *Urology* **37** (3 suppl): 9–12.

Payne SR, McKenning ST, Pead LJ, Timoney AG, Doenhollander D, Maskell RM (1988) Microbiological look at urodynamic studies. *Lancet* **ii**: 1123–6.

Platt R, Polk BF, Murdock B, Rosner B (1982) Mortality associated with nosocomial urinary tract infection. *N Engl J Med* **307**: 637–42.

Royal Australian College of General Practitioners Practice Management Committee (1994) *Sterilisation/Disinfection Guidelines for General Practice*, 2nd edn. RACGP, Melbourne.

Schiotz HA (1992) Urinary tract infection after vaginal repair surgery. *Int Urogynecol J* **3**: 185–90.

Schiotz HA (1994) Urinary tract infection and bacteriuria after gynecological surgery: experience with 24 hour Foley catheterization. *Int Urogynecol J* **5**: 345–8.

Stamm WE (1991) Catheter associated urinary tract infection: epidemiology, pathogenesis and prevention. *Am J Med* **91** (suppl 3B): 65–71.

Stevens GP, Jacobson JA, Burke JP (1981) Changing patterns of hospital infections and antibiotic use. Prevalence surveys in a community hospital. *Arch Intern Med* 141: 587.

Turck M, Goffe B, Petersdorf RG (1962) The urethral catheter and urinary tract infection. *J Urol* 88: 834–7.

van der Wall E, Verkooyen RP, Mintjes-de Groot J et al. (1992) Prophylactic ciprofloxacin for catheter-associated urinary tract infection. *Lancet* 339: 946–51.

Victorian Drug Usage Advisory Committee (1988) *Therapeutic Guidelines: Antibiotic*, 10th edn. Therapeutic Guidelines Limited, Melbourne, p 302.

Warren JW, Steinberg L, Hebel JH, Tenney JH (1989) The prevalence of urethral catheterization in Maryland nursing homes. *Arch Intern Med* 149: 1535–7.

Wilson C, Sandhu SS, Kaisary AV (1997) A prospective randomized study comparing a catheter value with a standard drainage system. *Br J Urol* 80: 915–17.

Zimakoff JD, Pontoppidan B, Larsen SO, Poulsen KB, Stickler DJ (1995) The management of urinary catheters: compliance of practice in Danish hospitals, nursing homes and home care to national guidelines. *Scand J Urol Nephrol* 29: 299–309.

Alternative therapies

Christopher Maher and Donna Gilmour

16

Contents

I Introduction

The doctor of the future will give no medicine, but will interest his patient in the care of the human frame, in diet and in the cause and prevention of disease.

Thomas Edison

Increasingly patients are seeking alternatives to orthodox medicine for the management of common ailments. In 1986, 22% of Australians had used alternative therapies (VSDC, 1986). Almost a decade later up to half of Australia's population used $621 million worth of alternative medicines a year (The Age, 1996). One-fifth of the Australian population spent an additional $309 million a year on alternative medicine practitioners. A large telephone survey in the USA found that 34% of respondents had used unconventional therapy and one-third of these individuals had visited an alternative therapist in the preceding year (Eisenberg et al., 1993). In Australia, the most common users of alternative medicine were well-educated women aged 15–34 years. Eighty-five percent of the individuals who visited alternative medicine practitioners were satisfied with the treatment they received (VSDC, 1986).

The aim of this chapter is to describe and evaluate the more common alternative therapies used for urinary tract infection (UTI). We have strived to achieve a balance in presenting information from orthodox and alternative literature.

II Philosophy

Although recent awareness and popularity of alternative therapies imply that they are relatively new phenomena, ancient cultures have relied on alternative therapies such as acupuncture, herbal medicine and massage for centuries (Shealy, 1996). As early as 400 BC, Hippocrates promoted three fundamental premises to healing:

- an illness is due to bodily dysfunction;
- the environment of the patient must be closely studied to arrive at a satisfactory diagnosis and prognosis;
- our own natures are the physicians of our illness (Millenson, 1995).

Plato believed that the causes of many diseases were unknown to the physicians of the time because they were ignorant of the whole being and that the part or organ involved in the illness could never be well unless the whole person was well (Millenson, 1995). These early teachings form the basis of alternative approaches which stress seeing the mind, body and environment as inseparable and that the individual is essentially able to heal him- or herself given the right set of conditions or opportunity (Shealy, 1996).

A common theme of alternative therapies is the presence of a 'vital energy' or 'life force'. The aim of most alternative therapies is to correct the imbalance in this life force by a variety of means. For example, the acupuncturist liberates blocked energy pathways or meridians within the body by the insertion of needles at specific points (Shreeve, 1986). The naturopath corrects a patient's energy imbalance by stimulating the innate healing power the individual possesses and by helping the individual correct those elements of his or her lifestyle that are most likely to be contributing to the disorder (Shreeve, 1986). Orthodox medicine tries to simplify disease and illness into specific organ or system dysfunction and target treatment to the underlying cause. Alternative medicine tries to see the individual in a holistic manner, focusing on multiple areas in which to correct the individual's energy imbalance and thus restore the whole being.

III   Herbal medicine

Plants have been used for medicinal purposes since the earliest recorded history (Murray and Pizzorno, 1990). Approximately 25% of all pharmaceutical drugs contain elements derived from plants (Murray and Pizzorno, 1990). Similar to the philosophy of other alternative therapists, herbal therapists believe that herbs affect the whole being and are not just organ or disease specific (Hoffmann, 1996). Herbs are felt not only to exert their effects on a physical level but also to enhance the 'life force' or 'vital energy' of the

individual (Hoffmann, 1996). Herbalists believe their remedies work synergistically and that purifying or isolating the individual ingredients would limit the holistic healing properties of herbal medicines (Hoffmann, 1996). The three main types of medicinal herbs used for UTI are urinary antiseptics, diuretics and demulcents (Yarnell, 1997). Demulcents act to soothe or allay irritation of inflamed or abraded surfaces.

1.   Cranberry (Vaccinum macrocarpon)

Although it originated as alternative therapy, cranberry juice now has a widespread reputation as a simple, non-pharmacological means to prevent or treat UTI (*Figure 16.1*). As early as 1914, investigators were studying and reporting on its possible mechanisms of action in UTI (Blatherwick, 1914). Initial clinical reports suggested that cranberry was effective either because it acidified the urine (Fellers et al., 1933) or because of its benzoic acid content, which is converted to hippuric acid in the urine (Bodel et al., 1959). However, to maintain a consistent urinary pH of 5.5 which would be associated with an antibacterial effect, one would have to drink at least 1500 ml of cranberry juice per day (Kahn et al., 1967).

In vitro laboratory studies have demonstrated high molecular weight

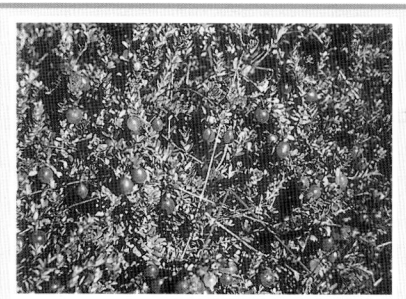

Figure 16.1
Cranberry (Vaccinum macrocarpon).

substances in cranberry juice that inhibit or block bacterial adherence to urinary epithelial cells (Sobota, 1984; Zafriri et al., 1989). The active ingredient is present in cranberry and blueberry juices but absent in most other fruit juices (Ofek et al., 1991). In vitro microbiology studies with electron microscopy have confirmed cranberry's short-term effects on inhibiting the P-fimbrial adhesion of *Escherichia coli* and have demonstrated a long-term effect on reducing the fimbrial expression of *E. coli* (Ahuja et al., 1998). Howell and Vorsa (1998) identified proanthocyanidins (condensed tannins) as the active compounds in cranberries that are responsible for preventing uropathogenic phenotypes of P-fimbriated *E. Coli* from adhering to the urinary tract.

In a large prospective, double-blind, placebo-controlled randomized clinical trial, Avorn et al. (1994) evaluated the effect of cranberry juice cocktail on the presence of bacteriuria and pyuria in elderly women. One hundred and fifty three women were randomly assigned to consume 300 ml/day of cranberry juice cocktail or 300 ml of a placebo drink that was indistinguishable in taste, appearance and vitamin C content. The investigators were able to demonstrate that subjects randomized to cranberry juice cocktail were about half as likely (42%) as controls to have bacteriuria–pyuria. In addition, women with a bacteriuria–pyuric sample who were taking the cranberry juice cocktail were only about a quarter as likely as controls (27%) to continue to have a bacteriuria–pyuric urine sample in the following month. Both findings were statistically significant at $p = 0.004$ and $p = 0.006$, respectively.

In summary, Avorn et al. (1994) demonstrated that in elderly women, regular ingestion of cranberry juice was effective in preventing and treating bacteriuria–pyuria. This study did not evaluate the effects of cranberry on symptomatic UTIs. The investigators themselves noticed that most subjects with bacteriuria were asymptomatic and that many subjects with symptoms referable to the urinary tract did not have bacteriuria or pyuria. The mean age of the women in this study was 78.5 years and these findings may not be generalizable to younger women or to women with recurrent UTI. However, given the facts that a reduction of bacteriuria–pyuria was demonstrated, that bacteriuria–pyuria is a risk factor for UTI and that cranberry juice is a well-tolerated non-toxic substance, recommending it for other women with or at risk of UTI is reasonable until evidence demonstrates otherwise.

2. Bearberry (Arctostaphylos uva-ursi)

Bearberry or Uva-ursi belongs to the same plant family, Ericaceae, as cranberry. Bearberry is a small evergreen shrub indigenous to Asia, the northern USA, Canada and Europe (O'Connel, 1996). The antimicrobial action of bearberry is attributed to arbutin, which is converted to the antiseptic hydroquinone in the urine (Bradley, 1992). Bearberry is also purported to soothe, tone and strengthen the membranes of the urinary system (Bradley, 1992). Most of the studies on the pharmacology of bearberry have not been published in English and are thus not accessible for review.

There is one clinical trial published in English involving 57 women with recurrent UTIs (Larsson et al., 1993). This was a double-blind randomized controlled trial in which women were allocated to a herbal mixture of bearberry and dandelion extract or to placebo. Treatment with the herbal mixture

for one month significantly reduced the recurrence of cystitis during the subsequent one-year follow-up period. There were no cases of cystitis in the herbal group and a 23% incidence of cystitis in the placebo group ($p = 0.05$). No significant adverse effects were reported by participants. Enthusiasm about using this herb as a prophylactic measure must be tempered by a few reports suggesting potentially toxic long-term effects of hydroquinones, including nephrotoxicity and suppression of β-lymphocyte maturation (King et al, 1989; Lau et al., 1996).

3. Buchu (Agathosma betulina)

Buchu is native to the Cape Province of South Africa. The active constituents are present in the dried leaves of the shrub, which are collected while the plant is bearing fruit (O'Connel, 1996). Purported benefits for UTI include urinary antiseptic and diuretic effects, but no studies are available to confirm these effects (Bradley, 1992). Buchu continues to be a popular herb prescribed by many herbal practitioners for UTI. It is contraindicated in pregnancy. On occasion, buchu may cause gastrointestinal side-effects (O'Connel, 1996). We could not find any laboratory or clinical trials to confirm the effects of buchu on the urinary tract.

4.   Goldenseal (Hydrastis canadensis)

Berberine is an alkaloid derived from goldenseal which has been traditionally used as an antimicrobial agent (*Figure 16.2*). Activity has been demonstrated in vitro against *Streptococcus pyogenes*, enterotoxigenic *E. coli* and uropathogenic *E. coli* (Rabbani et al., 1987, Sun et al., 1988a,b). In vitro studies suggest that berberine's mechanism of action against uropathogenic *E. coli* involves suppression of the synthesis and assembly of fimbrial adhesions (Sun et al., 1988a). The loss of fimbriae would result in decreased adhesion to uroepithelial cells and thus decreased risk of infection.

At present, there are no clinical trials on the efficacy of berberine in the treatment of UTI. Berberine's use in pregnancy is discouraged because it may affect uterine muscle tone (O'Connel, 1996).

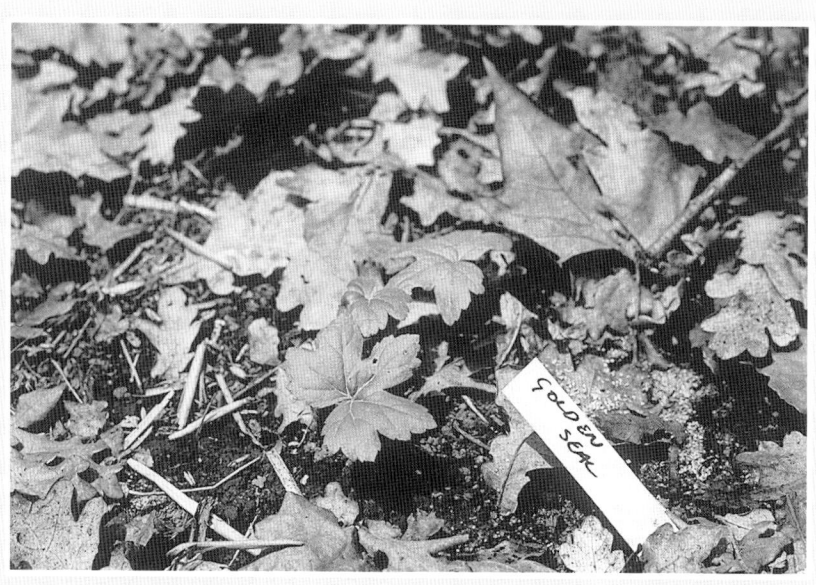

Figure 16.2
Goldenseal (Hydrastis canadensis).

5.   Cornsilk (Zea mays)

Cornsilk is the silken threads from ripe corn or maize, a plant indigenous to Central America and cultivated worldwide (*Figure 16.3*). Purported actions on the urinary system include a mild diuretic effect and a soothing or demulcent effect (Bradley, 1992). There are few studies reported in the English literature on the pharmacology and mechanisms of action of cornsilk. There have been no clinical trials on its use for cystitis.

6.   Juniper, dandelion, parsley and celery seed

Herbalists recommend juniper (*Figure 16.4*), dandelion, parsley and celery seed for UTI because of their diuretic properties. We could not find any clinical studies on the use of these herbs for UTI. According to herbal theory, diuretics are beneficial for the management of UTI because of increased elimination of bacteria and toxins (Shreeve, 1986). Herbalists also believe that the resulting dilute urine is less irritating to the inflamed urinary tract mucosa (Shreeve, 1986). In orthodox medicine, UTIs are not managed with diuretics.

IV   Acupuncture

Acupuncture is an ancient Chinese system of medicine involving the stimulation of specific points on the body to enhance the flow of vital energy or 'chi' along pathways called meridians (Shreeve, 1986). Chi expresses itself in two mutually complementary modalities, called Yin and Yang. The Chinese character of Yin translates as 'the dark side of the mountain' and represents such qualities as darkness, passiveness, cold and stillness. The character for Yang translates literally as 'the bright side of the mountain' and represents qualities such as warmth, activity, light and expression. A dynamic balance between the Yin and Yang aspects of the body is characterized by a healthy state. In acupuncture all disharmonies are reduced to a pattern of imbalance of Yin and Yang (Williams, 1996).

Acupuncture points are situated along the meridians, each of which is primarily Yin or Yang. The bladder meridian is primarily Yang. It starts on the nose, runs upward, over the top of the head, down the back of the chest, torso and leg and ends along the last joint of the large toe. The acupuncturist determines where the imbalance between Yin and Yang lies and decides which quality to tranquilize and which to stimulate. The shape, temperature, speed of insertion and direction of rotation of the needle all vary depending on which element is stimulated (Shreeve, 1986).

While acupuncture has a long tradition in the management of chronic pain and disease, there is a paucity of information about its success for treating UTI.

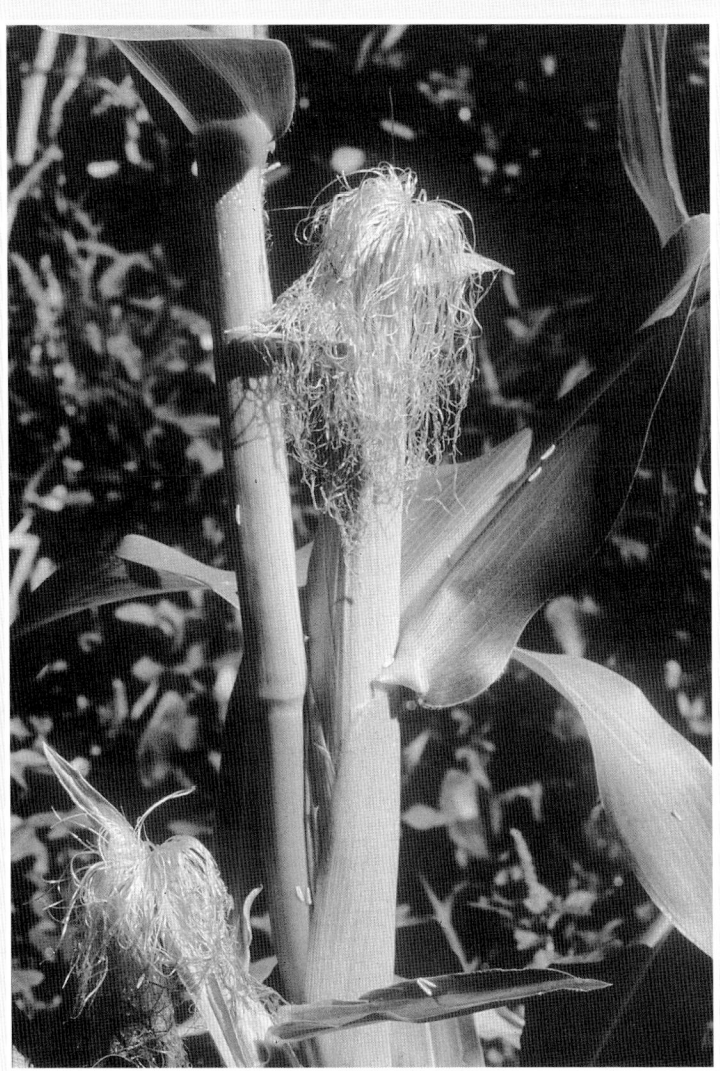

Figure 16.3
Cornsilk (Zea mays).

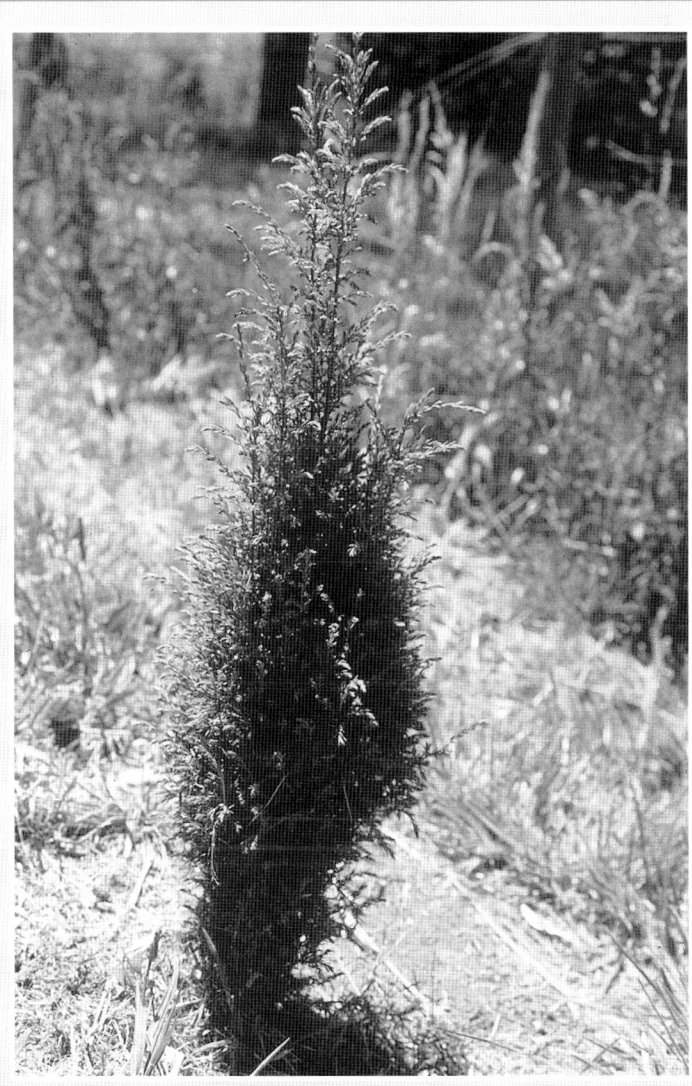

Figure 16.4
Juniper (Juniperis communis).

V Reflexology

Reflexology is the application of gentle manipulation or pressure to certain areas of the hands and feet to help correct illness, soothe pain and calm the mind. Reflexologists believe that there are areas called reflex points on the hands, face and feet, which correspond to each organ and structure of the body (*Figure 16.5*). These reflex areas are thought to be joined by channels of energy through nerve endings just beneath the skin. By gently manipulating the relevant area, reflexologists re-establish balance in the way the body functions (Bradford and Chamberlain, 1995).

One small prospective clinical trial involving 24 patients with UTI, 12 of whom received antibiotics and foot massage and 12 of whom received antibiotics only, demonstrated that the time to disappearance of symptoms after initiation of treatment was significantly longer in the control group (Yu-lian, 1996). Problems with this study include the small sample size, the fact that patients were not blinded to their treatment status and the absence of a placebo control group.

VI Relaxation and hypnotherapy

Studies have shown that there is a statistically significant association of personality traits such as obsessionality, neuroticism and anxiety in women with recurrent UTI (Hunt and Woller, 1992; Rees and Farhounard, 1977). These studies have only determined an association and not a relationship of cause and effect. Although not completely regarded as alternative therapies, relaxation techniques and hypnotherapy have been used to assist individuals with recurrent UTI manage anxiety (Shreeve, 1986). Using hypnotherapy and relaxation therapy for reducing the anxiety associated with recurrent UTI is reasonable because of the established roles these techniques have for the management of anxiety in general (Stanley, 1994; Williams and Chamberless, 1994). Whether these therapies definitely benefit patients with recurrent UTI needs to be determined in a prospective clinical trial.

VII Homeopathy

Homeopathy is a type of alternative medicine that treats a disease with a dilute preparation of an agent or drug that will cause symptoms similar to the disease being treated. The fundamental principle of homeopathy is that 'like cures like' (Hammond, 1995).

Two homeopathic remedies commonly recommended for cystitis are Cantharides and Staphisagria. Cantharides is derived from the Spanish fly, which is a traditional aphrodisiac. The Spanish fly lives on olive trees and honeysuckle all over southern Europe and western Asia. The whole insect, dried and

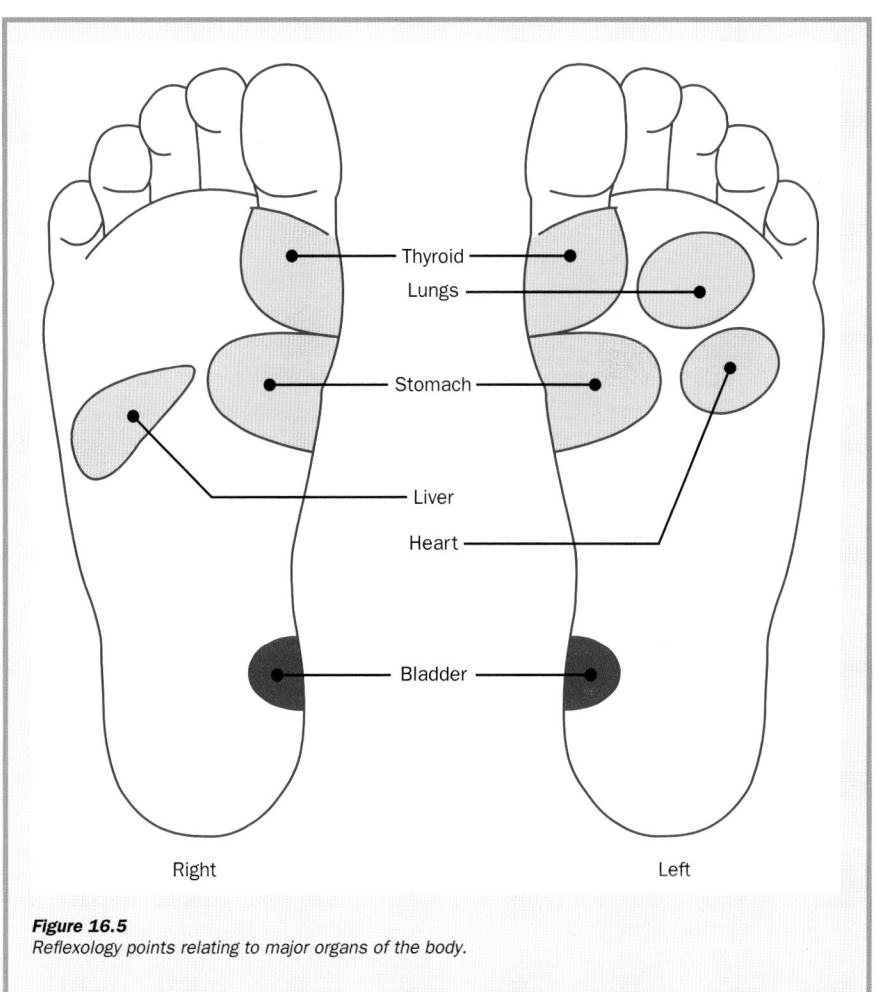

Figure 16.5
Reflexology points relating to major organs of the body.

powdered, is used to make the remedy
(Hammond, 1995). Cantharides is commonly
recommended for cystitis in the presence of

dysuria, haematuria and painful urination
(Jamil, 1997). Staphisagria is derived from the
palmated larkspur and the remedy is made

from the seeds of the fruit (Hammond, 1995). Staphisagria is typically recommended for 'honeymoon cystitis' and cystitis during pregnancy (Jamil, 1997). We found multiple descriptions of these two agents throughout the homeopathic literature but there were no references to any studies on the mechanism of action, efficacy, side-effects or safety.

VIII Naturopathy

Fundamental to the practice of naturopathic medicine is the belief that the body can heal itself given the proper opportunity (Murray and Pizzorno, 1990). Naturopaths believe that the symptoms accompanying UTI are not directly caused by the bacteria, but rather are a result of the body's attempt to defend and heal itself. Symptoms such as dysuria, haematuria, and pain are thus seen in a positive light as a sign of the body marshalling its innate defensive forces against harmful agents (Shreeve, 1986). Orthodox medicine often focuses on eradicating disease and symptoms, whereas naturopathic medicine focuses on assisting the individual's capacity to prevent and overcome illness by establishing the life force or vital energy balance not only in the body but also in the mind and spirit.

The naturopath's approach to UTI would consist of recommending a wholefood diet, eliminating processed foods, caffeine and alcohol. The naturopath would also encourage the elimination of bodily toxins via the skin, lungs, kidneys and bowel. Methods that may be used to encourage toxin elimination include skin brushing with a rough hemp glove or natural bristle brush, deep breathing with yoga exercises, flushing out the urinary tract with increased fluid consumption and consuming a high-fibre diet to empty the large bowel of its toxin-producing stagnant contents. The naturopath would also pay particular attention to the individual's mental and spiritual elements to re-establish emotional harmony (Shreeve, 1986).

We found numerous guides, encyclopaedias and anecdotes describing the approaches of naturopathic medicine but we could not find any reports documenting its compliance, safety or efficacy.

IX Aromatherapy

Aromatherapy consists of the use of aromatic oils and essences from plants and herbs to treat ailments. These oils can be in a number of vehicles and are commonly administered via mist, massage or orally. We found very few articles about the use of aromatherapy specifically for UTI, except in a small number of self-help guides. Sandalwood oil was recommended as a massage or in a warm bath to ease discomfort from UTI (Jamil, 1997). Sandalwood oil was also purported to be an effective diuretic and urinary tract antiseptic when administered orally (Leung, 1980). Lavender essence is reported to have wide-ranging antibacterial effects for UTI (Shreeve, 1986). Coriander blended with other oils is thought to soothe the inflammation associated with UTI (Keville and Green, 1983). Frankincense oil apparently has antiseptic and anti-inflammatory properties for UTIs (Keville and Green, 1983).

Except for an unreferenced comment that large doses of sandalwood can be toxic (Murray and Pizzorno, 1990), we could not find any other references for dosages, efficacy or safety of this therapy.

X Conclusion

The majority of alternative therapies lack significant scientific validation of their efficacy for the treatment of UTI. However, because of increasing consumer interest and demand, rather than discouraging and discarding alternative therapies for UTI as unproven and invalid, we should try to evaluate them formally for their safety and efficacy. We might find some new effective treatments for the management of this common condition.

References

Ahuja S, Kaack B, Roberts J (1998) Loss of fimbrial adhesion with the addition of *Vaccinum macrocarpon* to the growth medium of P-fimbriated *Escherichia coli*. *J Urol* **159**: 559–62.

Avorn J, Monane M, Gurwitz JH et al. (1994) Reduction of bacteriuria and pyuria after ingestion of cranberry juice. *JAMA* **271**: 751–4.

Blatherwick NR (1914) The specific role of foods in relation to the composition of the urine. *Arch Intern Med* **14**: 409–50.

Bodel PT, Cotran R, Kass EH (1959) Cranberry juice and the antibacterial action of hippuric acid. *J Lab Clin Med* **54**: 881–8.

Bradford N, Chamberlain G (1995) *Pain Relief During Childbirth*. Harper Collins, London, pp 199–203.

Bradley PR (1992) *British Herbal Compendium, Volume I*. British Herbal Medicine Association, Bournemouth, pp 211–13.

Eisenberg DM, Kessler RC, Foster C, Norlock FE, Calkins DR, Delbanco TL (1993) Unconventional medicine in the United States. *N Engl J Med* **328**: 246–52.

Fellers CR, Redmon BC, Parrott EM (1933) Effect of cranberries on urinary tract acidity and blood alkali reserve. *J Nutr* **6**: 455–63.

Hammond C (1995) *The Complete Family Guide to Homeopathy*. Element Books, Brisbane, pp 12–60.

Hoffmann D (1996) *The Complete Illustrated Holistic Herbal: A Safe and Practical Guide to Making and Using Herbal Remedies*. Element Books, Brisbane, pp 12–24.

Howell A, Vorsa N, Der Marderosian A, Foo LY (1998) Inhibition of adherence of P-fimbriated *Escherichia coli* to uroepithelial cell surfaces by proanthocyanidins extracts from cranberries. *N Engl J Med* **339**: 1085–6.

Hunt JC, Woller G (1992) Psychological factors in recurrent uncomplicated urinary tract infection. *Br J Urol* **69**: 460–4.

Jamil T (1997) *Complementary Medicine: A Practical Guide.* Butterworth Heinemann, Melbourne, pp 203–5.

Kahn HD, Panariello VA, Saeli J, Sampson JR, Schwartz E (1967) Effect of cranberry juice on urine. *J Am Diet Assoc* **51**: 251–4.

Keville K, Green M (1983) *Aromatherapy: A Complete Guide to the Healing Art.* The Crossing Press, Freedom, USA, pp 52–6.

King AG, Landreth KS, Wierda D (1989) Bone marrow stromal cell regulation of B-lymphopoiesis. II. Mechanisms of hydroquinone inhibition of pre-B cell maturation. *J Pharmacol Exp Ther* **250**: 582–90.

Larsson B, Jonasson A, Fianu S (1993) Prophylactic effect of UVA-E in women with recurrent cystitis: a preliminary report. *Curr Ther Res* **53**: 441–3.

Lau SS, Peters MM, Kleiner HE et al. (1996) Linking the metabolism of hydroquinone to its nephrotoxicity and nephrocarcinogenity. *Adv Exp Med Biol* **387**: 267–73.

Leung A (1980) *Encyclopaedia of Common Natural Ingredients Used in Foods, Drugs and Cosmetics.* Wiley, New York, pp 292–317.

Millenson JR (1995) *Mind Matters: Psychological Medicine in Holistic Practice.* Eastland Press, Seattle, pp 1–27.

Murray MT, Pizzorno JE (1990) *An Encyclopaedia of Natural Medicine.* Macdonald, London, pp 255–9.

O'Connel J (1996) *Traditional herbal compendium.* PhD Thesis, pp 109–18.

Ofek I, Goldhar J, Zafriri D (1991) Anti-*Escherichia coli* adhesin activity of cranberry and blueberry juices. *N Engl J Med* **324**: 1599.

Rabbani GH, Butler T, Knight J, Sanyal SC, Alam K (1987) Randomised controlled trial of berberine sulfate therapy for diarrhea due to enterotoxigenic *Escherichia coli* and *Vibrio cholera. J Infect Dis* **155**: 979–84.

Rees DL, Farhoumand N (1977) Psychiatric aspects of recurrent cystitis in women. *Br J Urol* **49**: 651–8.

Shealy CN (1996) *The Complete Family Guide to Alternative Medicine.* Element Books, Brisbane, pp 7–10.

Shreeve C (1986) *Cystitis: The New Approach.* Thorsons, Wellingborough, pp 50–107.

Sobota AE (1984) Inhibition of bacterial adherence by cranberry juice: potential use for the treatment of urinary tract infections. *J Urol* **131**: 1013–16.

Stanley R (1994) The use of hypnosis in the treatment of anxiety disorders: general considerations and contraindications. In: *Hypnosis in the Management of Anxiety Disorders* (ed. BJ Evans),

Australian Journal of Clinical and Experimental Hypnosis, Heidelberg, Australia, pp 33–40.

Sun D, Abraham SN, Beachey EF (1988a) Influence of berberine sulfate on synthesis and expression of pap fimbrial adhesin in uropathogenic *Escherichia coli. Antimicrob Agents Chemother* **32**: 1274–7.

Sun D, Courtney H, Beachey EH (1988b) Berberine sulfate blocks adherence of *Streptococcus pyogenes* to epithelial cells, fibronectin, and hexadecane. *Antimicrob Agents Chemother* **32**: 1370–4.

The Age (1996) Annual spending nears $1b on alternative health. *The Saturday Age* February 20.

VSDC (1986) *Inquiry into Alternative Medicine and the Health Food Industry.* Victorian Social Development Committee, Victoria, Australia.

Williams KE, Chamberless DL (1994) Behavioural therapies. In: *Anxiety and Related Disorders: A Handbook* (eds BB Wolman and G Stricker), Wiley, Brisbane, pp 363–70.

Williams T (1996) *The Complete Illustrated Guide to Chinese Medicine.* Element Books, Brisbane, pp 21–9.

Yarnell E (1997) Botanical medicine for cystitis. *Altern Complement Ther* **3**: 269–75.

Yu-lian Z (1996) Clinical observation on treatment of infection of urinary tract by foot massage. *1996 Beijing International Reflexology Conference*, p 17 (abst).

Zafriri D, Ofek I, Adar R, Pocino M, Sharon N (1989) Inhibitory activity of cranberry juice on adherence of type 1 and type P fibriated *Escherichia coli* to eukaryotic cells. *Antimicrob Agents Chemother* **33**: 92–8.

Research priorities

Allan Ronald

17

Contents

I   Introduction

Urinary tract infections (UTIs) are common in females with an estimated annual global incidence of at least 150 million, costly with regard to direct and indirect health costs and controversial in respect to optimal strategies for management. During a two-decade span from 1960 to 1980, substantive advances occurred in our understanding of urinary infection epidemiology, pathogenesis and management (Harding and Ronald, 1994). During these decades, at least 100 investigators made significant scientific contributions to the field. Research sources were allocated to urinary infection, groups of investigators were located in at least 30 sites around the world and consensus conferences occurred at regular frequent intervals, creating discussion and excitement in the field.

Since 1980, research interest in urinary infections has waned, the number of scientists active in this field has gradually decreased and fewer important observations are being made (Ronald and Sanche, 1997). I estimate that fewer than 15 research sites currently receive competitive grants to support UTI research. Why has this occurred?

First, numerous clinical trials in patients with acute urinary symptoms, particularly acute bacterial cystitis in females, identified treatment regimens that have largely solved the management of this common recurring illness. Also, excellent epidemiologic and pathogenesis research has identified the risk factors that precipitate these infections. Prevention strategies by modifying risk factors, using antimicrobial prophylaxis and providing women with intermittent treatment have all largely 'contained' this disease burden and it no longer creates the impetus for further research.

Second, it was recognized that urinary infections in functionally normal urinary tracts, at least in adults, rarely progress to endstage renal disease or to serious consequences such as hypertension. The contribution of UTIs to complications of pregnancy was recognized and strategies were devised in the 1970s to screen and treat these infections. As a result, UTIs are now 'passé' with regard to their contributions to morbidity and mortality.

Third, the overall disease burden of acute and recurrent UTIs has never been adequately identified with good population-based studies and almost no health services research has been carried out. As a result, we have limited appreciation of UTI morbidity. Variability in provision of care has not been well documented and current care status strategies have not been assessed. Without this information, we assume that most patients with urinary infections are being managed in an appropriate cost-effective way. However, health services research has not confirmed this and at least one study suggests that treatment is highly variable and often inefficient (Berg, 1984).

Fourth, the substantive advances that could arise from additionally funded basic research on UTI pathogens and the host response to them is not well appreciated. Although the development of a vaccine would be an excellent outcome of basic research, almost certainly further understanding of pathogenesis as it relates to both bacterial virulence and determinants of clinical illness would enable additional strategies to be developed that would lead to improvement in the management of patients with urinary infection. Only a few laboratories are currently investigating the molecular and cellular biology of UTIs. Very few animal model studies are being funded. Basic research continues to be the foundation for innovative ideas and major significant advances in all areas of clinical medicine. If it is not well supported, significant advances in clinical research are much less likely.

Fifth, our leadership in maintaining awareness of urinary infection has not been as effective during the past two decades. As a result, the priorities of funding agencies, the training of new investigators and the overall enthusiasm for urinary infection within organizations and at major infectious disease meetings are markedly less than they were during earlier decades.

What initiatives can alter this trend? This chapter will identify some goals that could be accomplished and lead to enhanced interest and academic excellence in the field.

II   Significant research achievements since 1980

Despite a reduced research investment in UTIs, the past two decades have seen advances in understanding and managing them. Among these I would include the following.

Acute bacterial cystitis in women can be adequately treated with short three-day courses with excellent outcomes, both clinical and bacteriologic cures and few adverse effects, particularly if trimethoprim/sulfamethoxazole or the quinolones are selected for therapy (Hooton and Stamm, 1997). The emergence of resistance during therapy is rare and in uncomplicated acute bacterial cystitis, an optimal response is achieved with these regimens, with cures in about 95% of women.

Closed drainage systems introduced during the 1960s and 1970s are now being used routinely for short-term (<30 days) catheterization with markedly reduced probability that patients will be infected. Although further studies are required, patients who do acquire infection during catheterization should be treated on catheter removal as these infections usually do not resolve spontaneously (Harding et al., 1991).

The *risk factors* for acute bacterial cystitis in women were largely determined by studies by Stamm, Hooton and others in superb sequential studies that have investigated the contribution of sexual intercourse, spermicides, nonoxyl-9 impregnated condoms and bacterial floral changes in the vagina and perineum (Stapleton and Stamm, 1997). Although some of these risk factors may be difficult to modify, the information is valued by women with recurring cystitis. Myths about unproven associations between cystitis and bathing, menstrual hygiene, tight underwear and other factors that were part of a urinary infection folklore but had no basis in fact have also been debunked.

The *laboratory diagnosis* of urinary infection had rested on the premise of bacterial numbers. This was too artificial and studies, particularly from the Seattle group, have identified the range of bacterial numbers that can be associated with acute cystitis and have also drawn attention to the importance of pyuria (Stapleton and Stamm, 1997). Although a number of investigators have attempted to identify 'short cuts' with automation and more sophisticated instrumentation for the diagnosis of UTI, these have largely proved to be not sustainable. In addition, some studies have provided evidence that urine cultures are not necessary or cost-effective for women with recurring episodes of bacterial cystitis and that follow-up cultures do not contribute to care (Stapleton and Stamm, 1997). These latter observations need to be validated in population-based studies.

Strategies for the *management of UTIs in pregnancy* with screening and treatment programs have been widely implemented and are largely successful. As a result, acute pyelonephritis is unusual during the third trimester in patients who have received prenatal care.

The futility of treating *asymptomatic bacteriuria in elderly females* has been demonstrated by at least two investigative groups, and strategies are now needed to convince caregivers that this common finding does not require active management (Abuttyn et al., 1994).

Imaging choices have been well identified. Most patients with UTI do not require imaging. However, in patients where imaging is necessary, a helical computed tomography (CT) scan, usually with contrast, is the definitive technology to diagnose calculi, abscesses and underlying explanations for infection (Kaplan et al., 1997). The old strategy of using ultrasound, intravenous pyelography and nuclear imaging often prior to CT scanning is no longer an appropriate approach. Again, further population-based studies and health sciences research are necessary to ensure the implementation of appropriate imaging processes.

We have increased our knowledge base in a number of areas but remain remarkably ignorant. Among these I would include the following.

Bacterial virulence factors. Despite substantial progress in understanding

Escherichia coli and its virulence, we have largely ignored other urinary pathogens and few studies have identified their pathogenicity determinants.

The studies by Svanberg and her colleagues have characterized *cytokine responses* and their importance in determining local and systemic symptoms (Hedges and Svanberg, 1994). However, almost certainly only a small portion of what we need to know about host response has been learned to date.

The management of *acute uncomplicated pyelonephritis* has become relatively routine, particularly with outpatient oral regimens. The recent study by Talan et al. (1998) identifies optimal duration of treatment and provides some evidence that the fluoroquinolones, specifically ciprofloxacin, are a superior choice for acute pyelonephritis. However, further studies are needed to determine how this common problem should be managed with development and testing of algorithms to establish cost-effective parameters.

Vaginitis and urinary infection are perceived by patients as commonly occurring together. We have still not sorted out the ties between the symptoms, signs and changes in microbial flora. In particular, the importance of H_2O_2-producing lactobacilli and their potential role in preserving normal vaginal flora and preventing UTIs have not been adequately studied prospectively and currently there are no proven therapeutic options.

Despite the existence of large numbers of patients with UTIs who either should not or cannot be treated based on our current knowledge, we still have limited information on the *natural history* of this illness and the role of bacterial virulence determinants and host response. Are there organisms which can asymptomatically colonize the urinary tract, perhaps exclude other pathogens and persist indefinitely to the benefit of the patient?

Diabetes and urinary infections are common co-morbidities. Efforts to understand their linkages and optimal management require far more input than has been provided to date.

Physician practice has largely been ignored but at least one study shows great variability and inadequate understanding of management advances (Berg, 1984). Almost no studies have taken into account patient satisfaction with their treatment. Health services research should be a priority as it will determine and ultimately mold public opinion and facilitate changes in policies, payment systems and practice of physicians.

III Important UTI subject areas where we are largely ignorant

Complicated UTIs occur in the practice of all physicians and are very common consultations for infectious disease physicians, urologists, gynecologists and nephrologists. Despite their common occurrence, we have almost no information on most aspects of complicated urinary infections. Pathogenesis, cost-effective management, natural history and population-based morbidity are all areas in which no information is available. Unfortunately, our lack of information has not prevented us from being opinionated and, in retrospect, frequently 'wrong' about strategies for managing these patients. Both medical and surgical approaches to these patients should be studied by investigators using randomized clinical trials, well-defined outcomes and correlates of bacterial virulence determinants and host response. Instead, we have depended upon anecdotes and personal clinical experiences to manage these patients. Unfortunately, we know from history that these opinions are frequently in error (Ronald and Harding, 1997).

Population-based studies of illness burden have not been carried out to any extent for UTIs (Nicolle et al., 1996). These are a priority for both uncomplicated and complicated UTIs and require expertise in using administrative health databases and also should be carried out prospectively in defined populations at risk of complicated UTIs.

Management of the *chronically catheterized patient* has not been adequately studied. Complications do arise in this population and the cost of care is substantial. When should catheters be changed? Can we prevent complications from chronic catheter care with other strategies? Does cranberry juice change the natural history of infections in catheterized patients? Are there any other useful or necessary interventions? What is the role of the suprapubic catheter? None of these questions has been answered prospectively and we wallow in our ignorance.

IV   Suggestions for addressing the UTI research dearth

Several of these may be redundant suggestions and others may have already failed. However, from my perspective, the following are areas in which a response might encourage more urinary infection research.

Population-based studies and *health services studies* on the disease burden and the response of caregivers and patients. There are still large gains to be made by improving our understanding of UTIs and health care money would be better used to provide support for organizations to address strategies for improved care. Out of this, advocacy groups and activists may arise who would contribute to ongoing discussions about prioritization of research and targeting these priorities within the budgets of funding agencies.

Substantial monies continue to be spent on *'research' by pharmaceutical companies* as they fulfil regulatory agency requirements and explore the potential usefulness of new therapeutic products for UTIs. Unfortunately, most of these studies have not provided worthwhile outcomes and most newer treatment regimens are only 'equivalent' to established ones. No advances in either science or patient care take place as a result. Perhaps a consortium of pharmaceutical companies and investigators could initiate studies that would address more significant issues, with the possibility of improved care and alternative uses for drugs, enabling enhanced pharmaceutical profits.

Managed care organizations in the USA collect large amounts of data on patients. With limited monies, studies could be undertaken that would determine the natural history and enable both medical and surgical controlled trials to be carried out.

Organizations, either existing ones or new ones, need to address *research priorities* and be advocates for additional funding. The Clinical Evaluation of Drug Efficacy in Urinary Tract Infection is a multinational group that addresses some of the opportunities and challenges of urinary infection. However, other study groups and research conferences should be a priority. In 1990, the Infectious Disease Society of America (IDSA) with a contract from the US Food and Drug Authority, established a group to review and establish regulatory guidelines for drugs to be used for the management of UTIs. More recently, the IDSA has established through its Practice Guidelines Committee a subcommittee to establish treatment guidelines for uncomplicated UTI. These committees and structures are important in that they provide a venue for investigators to share information and ideas, set standards and facilitate research planning. However, additional strategies may be necessary to address research gaps and facilitate advocacy for research funding.

The apparent failure of many existing investigators to train the *next generation of scientists* needs to be reviewed. Only a handful of scientists have trained and mentored a new generation of investigators; these few successful sites need to augment their training activities and new ones need to be created. Too few urologists and gynecologists are serious UTI investigators. Additional basic scientists in microbiology and molecular and/or cellular biology need to be trained and, in most instances, be incorporated into UTI research groups. Several additional research groups need to be established around a core of excellent scientists.

V   Conclusion

Urinary infection research is underresourced with inadequate human and fiscal commitment. The challenge to all of us in the field is to become advocates for our patients, with granting agencies and with each other to create more opportunities through training, through conferences, through improved research management and through effective advocacy to double over the next five years the amount of research being carried out globally on UTIs. The burden of disease and the importance of UTIs for individuals and for populations demand no less.

References

Abuttyn E, Mossey J, Berlin JA et al. (1994) Does asymptomatic bacteriuria predict mortality and does antimicrobial treatment reduce mortality in elderly ambulatory women? *Ann Intern Med* **120**: 827.

Berg AO (1984) Variations among family physicians' management strategies for lower urinary tract infections in women: a report from the Washington Family Physicians' Collaborative Research Network. *J Am Board Fam Pract* **4**: 327.

Harding GKM, Ronald AR (1994) The management of urinary infections. What have we learned in the past decade? *Int J Antimicrob Agents* **4**: 83–8.

Harding GKM, Nicolle LE, Ronald AR et al. (1991) How long should catheter-acquired urinary tract infection in women be treated? A randomized controlled study. *Ann Intern Med* **114**: 713–19.

Hedges S, Svanberg C (1994) The mucosal cytokine response to urinary tract infection. *Int J Antimicrob Agents* **4**: 89–93.

Hooton TM, Stamm WE (1997) Diagnosis and treatment of uncomplicated urinary tract infection. *Infect Dis Clin North Am* **11**: 551–81.

Kaplan DM, Rosenfield AT, Smith RC (1997) Advances in the imaging of renal infection: helical CT and modern coordinated imaging. *Infect Dis Clin North Am* **11**: 681–705.

Nicolle LE, Friesen D, Harding GKM, Roos LL (1996) Hospitalization for acute pyelonephritis in Manitoba, Canada during the period from 1989–1992: impact of diabetes, pregnancy and aboriginal origin. *Clin Infect Dis* **22**: 1051–6.

Ronald AR, Harding GKM (1997) Complicated urinary tract infections. *Infect Dis Clin North Am* **11**: 583–92.

Ronald AR, Sanche SE (1997) Urinary tract infections: some research priorities. In: *Urinary Tract Infections* (ed. T Bergan), Karger, New York, pp 132–7.

Stapleton A, Stamm WE (1997) Prevention of urinary tract infection. *Infect Dis Clin North Am* **11**: 719–33.

Talan DA, Stamm WE, Reuning-Scherer J, Faulkener L, Church D and the Pyelonephritis Study Group (1998) Treatment of acute uncomplicated pyelonephritis (AUP): a randomized double-blind trial comparing 7 versus 14 day therapy. Abstract presented at the Interscience Conference on Antimicrobial Agents and Chemotherapy, San Diego, CA.

Index